PRACTICAL
RHINOLOGY

PRACTICAL RHINOLOGY

Editor

Nicholas Jones Nottingham, UK

Assistant editors

Scott M Graham Iowa City, USA

James N Palmer Philadelphia, USA

Dharmbir S Sethi Singapore

Daniel B Simmen Zurich, Switzerland

Aldo C Stamm São Paulo, Brazil

Peter–John Wormald Adelaide, Australia

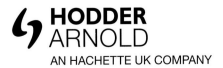

HODDER
ARNOLD

AN HACHETTE UK COMPANY

First published in Great Britain in 2010 by
Hodder Arnold, an imprint of Hodder Education,
an Hachette Livre UK Company,
338 Euston Road, London NW1 3BH

http://www.hodderarnold.com

Hachette Livre UK's policy is to use papers that are natural, renewable
and recyclable products and made from wood grown in sustainable
forests. The logging and manufacturing processes are expected to
conform to the environmental regulations of the country of origin.

Whilst the advice and information in this book are believed to be true
and accurate at the date of going to press, neither the author[s] nor the
publisher can accept any legal responsibility or liability for any errors
or omissions that may be made. In particular, (but without limiting the
generality of the preceding disclaimer) every effort has been made to
check drug dosages; however it is still possible that errors have been
missed. Furthermore, dosage schedules are constantly being revised and
new side-effects recognized. For these reasons the reader is strongly
urged to consult the drug companies' printed instructions before
administering any of the drugs recommended in this book.

British Library Cataloguing in Publication Data
A catalogue record for this book is available from the British Library

Library of Congress Cataloging-in-Publication Data
A catalog record for this book is available from the Library of Congress

ISBN-13   978 1 444 10861 3

1 2 3 4 5 6 7 8 9 10

Commissioning Editor: Gavin Jamieson
Project Editors: Jane Tod and Stephen Clausard
Production Controller: Joanna Walker
Cover Design: Helen Townson
Indexer: Laurence Errington

Typeset in 10 on 12pt Minion by Phoenix Photosetting, Chatham, Kent
Printed and bound in Italy by Printer Trento

What do you think about this book? Or any other Hodder Arnold
title? Please visit our website: www.hodderarnold.com

Contents

Preface

This book is not meant to be an all encompassing encyclopaedia of rhinological conditions. It is meant to be practical and relevant to most doctors treating rhinological conditions.

In all honesty it was my intention to compile a book that addressed the difficulties which are posed by the variety of ways patients present with different nasal symptoms, and give guidance on how to arrive at a correct diagnosis. It is thanks to Scott Graham that this proposal was, in part, jettisoned as he convinced me that few surgeons would be interested in such a text. He suggested that I approached some of the world's leading rhinologists and put together a text that incorporates most of the current relevant problems that rhinologists face and present this in, what we hope is, a digestible format. So please forgive omissions of some of the less common conditions and the absence of a structured evidence based approach, although we have tried to include the evidence base where it exists. We hope you will find this of use in your day to day work.

Nicholas Jones
2010

This new practical book has been keenly anticipated as the list of contributors reads like a "Who's Who" in Rhinology.

Practical applied anatomy, clinical examination, conservative therapy, the latest technology open the book and are very well illustrated.

The following chapters deal with all the surgery in and around the nose and the paranasal sinuses.

Surgery of the orbit, skull base, sella and of skull base tumors is discussed in detail.

The frontal sinus is addressed with a special chapter that looks at good long term results.

Importantly, complications are presented in detail as everybody faces these accidents sooner or later.

Paediatric rhinology, the sense of smell, postoperative management and guidance for patients, which is not always in the center of the surgeon's attention, provide an important finale.

Excellent figures and photographs make this book a wonderful resource for the beginner and the advanced surgeon, and a good practical resource before surgery with answers for many specific questions.

I am sure it will be a very successful publication because of its practical qualities in a time when political influences make it difficult for us to have enough time for our patients.

Professor Wolfgang Draf FRCS
Director of the Department of Ear, Nose and
Throat Diseases
Head and Neck Surgery
International Neuroscience Institute at the
University of Magdeburg (INI)
Hanover, Germany

Contributors

Boaz Forer MD
Department of Otolaryngology, Singapore General Hospital, Singapore

Scott M Graham MD
Professor, Department of Otolaryngology, Head and Neck Surgery, University of Iowa, Iowa City, and Director, Division of Rhinology, University of Iowa Hospitals and Clinics, Iowa, USA

Nicholas Jones BDS MD FRCS FRCS (ORL)
Special Professor, University of Nottingham, Queens Medical Centre, University Hospital, Nottingham, UK

João F Nogueira Jr MD
Resident, Sao Paulo ENT Center, Hospital Professor Edmundo Vasconcelos, Sao Paulo, Brazil

James N Palmer MD
Associate Professor and Director, Division of Rhinology, Department of Otorhinolaryngology, Head and Neck Surgery, University of Pennsylvania, Philadelphia, USA

Vijay R Ramakrishnan MD
Assistant Professor, Department of Otolaryngology, University of Colorado, Denver, Colorado, USA

Dharmbir S Sethi FRCSEd FAMS
Clinical Associate Professor, National University of Singapore, and Senior Consultant, Singapore General Hospital, Singapore

Maria L S Silva MD
ENT resident, São Paulo ENT Center, Hospital Professor Edmundo Vasconcelos, São Paulo, Brazil

Daniel B Simmen
ORL Zentrum, Centre for Rhinology, Skull Base Surgery and Facial Plastic Surgery, Hirslanden Clinic, Zurich, Switzerland

Aldo C Stamm MD
Director of São Paulo ENT Center, Hospital Professor Edmundo Vasconcelos, and Associate Professor, Federal University of São Paulo, São Paulo, Brazil

Jeffrey D Suh MD
Assistant Professor, Department of Surgery, Division of Otolaryngology–Head and Neck Surgery, UCLA School of Medicine, Los Angeles, California, USA

Marc A Tewfik MD, MSc, FRCSC
Assistant Professor, Department of Otolaryngology – Head and Neck Surgery, McGill University, Montreal, Canada

Erik K Weitzel MD MC USAF
San Antonio Military Medical Center, Department of Otolaryngology – Head and Neck Surgery, Ste 1 Lackland AFB, Texas, USA

Peter-John Wormald MD FRCS FRACS FCS(SA)
Professor and Chair, Department of Otolaryngology – Head and Neck Surgery, Adelaide and Flinders Universities, Adelaide, Australia

Applied surgical anatomy of the nasal cavity and paranasal sinuses

DHARMBIR S SETHI

GENERAL CONSIDERATIONS

A thorough understanding of the anatomy of the paranasal sinuses and an awareness of the variations in these complex structures are essential in order to perform safe and effective sinonasal surgery. In recent years, endoscopic sinus surgery has gained worldwide acceptance. Although this modality of treating sinonasal pathology is minimally invasive, it has a steep learning curve and is not necessarily safer than headlight or external approaches. Catastrophic complications may occur in the hands of the inexperienced with an inadequate understanding of the anatomy. It is, therefore, essential to have a good grasp of the endoscopic anatomy of the nasal cavity and the paranasal sinuses. As anatomy viewed through the lens of an endoscope can be distorted, it is also essential to understand the gross anatomy. Excellent textbooks on detailed anatomy of the paranasal sinus are available but they cannot replace the need for training in wet cadaver laboratories. Performing these dissections first hand under supervision before embarking on endoscopic surgery is the key to understanding the anatomy. Surgeons in training are encouraged to attend workshops offering cadaver dissections (Fig. 1.1). This chapter describes the gross and endoscopic sinus anatomy that is relevant to the endoscopic sinus surgeon.

PARANASAL SINUSES

The paranasal sinuses comprise the frontal, maxillary, ethmoid and the sphenoid sinuses. The sinus drainage pathways divide the paranasal sinuses into anterior and

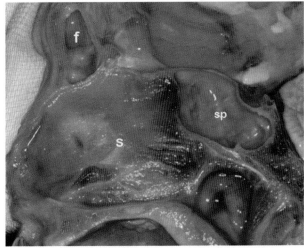

Figure 1.1 Sagittal section of a fresh cadaver head showing the intact nasal septum (s), right frontal sinus (f) and the sphenoid sinus (sp).

posterior systems that are anatomically separated by the basal lamella of the middle turbinate (see page 2). The anterior drainage system drains the frontal, maxillary and anterior ethmoids, and the posterior system drains the posterior ethmoids and the sphenoid. Pathology may involve one or more of these drainage systems.

NASAL TURBINATES

The lateral nasal wall has three prominent projections called turbinates (Fig. 1.2). The inferior turbinate is an

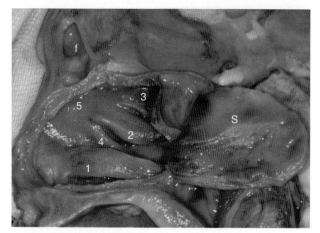

Figure 1.2 The nasal septum (S) has been separated from its attachments and retracted medially and posteriorly to reveal the right lateral nasal wall. Note the turbinates: the inferior turbinate (1), the middle turbinate (2) and the superior turbinate (3). Other anatomical structures of note are the agger nasi (5) and the uncinate process (4). The right frontal sinus (f) is also visible.

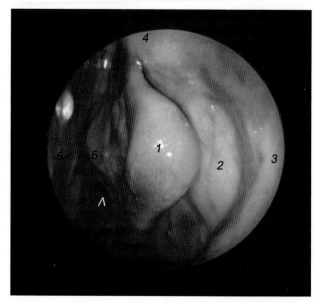

Figure 1.3 Endoscopic view of the left nasal cavity. Note the middle turbinate (1), uncinate process (2), prominence of the nasolacrimal duct (3), agger nasi (4), nasal septum (5), superior turbinate (6) and the olfactory cleft (7). Note the groove between the uncinate process and the nasolacrimal duct. This corresponds to the attachment of the uncinate to the nasolacrimal bone. The arrowhead is pointing to the sphenoid ostium.

independent bone, whereas the middle and the superior turbinates are part of the ethmoid complex. Occasionally, a fourth turbinate termed the supreme nasal turbinate is present. The recesses between these turbinates and the nasal wall are the called the meati, termed the inferior meatus, the middle meatus and the superior meatus, respectively.

Inferior turbinate

This structure is attached to the lateral nasal wall. Only one structure drains into the inferior meatus, the nasolacrimal duct (NLD).

Middle turbinate

The middle turbinate is approximately 4 cm long and it is about 14.5 mm, 12.5 mm and 7 mm high in its anterior, middle and posterior segments, respectively. The attachment of the middle turbinate is divided into three segments: the anterior third is attached sagittally to the skull base (Fig. 1.3) and inside the cranial cavity it continues as the lateral lamella of the cribriform plate (a vertical flange of variable length that is attached to the fovea ethmoidalis – part of the frontal bone – and is often quite thin). As the attachment of the middle turbinate continues posteriorly it turns laterally towards the lamina papyracea (see below) and then goes on to form a coronally oriented middle third of the basal lamella (Fig. 1.4). The posterior third of the middle turbinate attaches to the lamina papyracea as far as the perpendicular plate of the palatine bone; this part of the attachment is almost horizontal. The varying orientation of the attachment of the middle turbinate

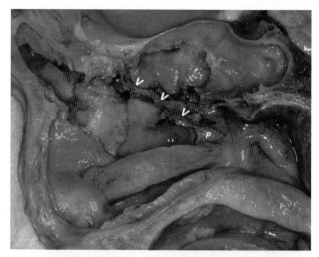

Figure 1.4 The arrowheads are pointing to the basal lamella, which separates the anterior group of the paranasal sinuses from the posterior group. p, palatine bone.

accounts for its stability and an understanding of this structure will help prevent destabilization of the turbinate by excessive resection.

The middle meatus is the final common drainage pathway for the frontal, anterior ethmoid and maxillary sinuses.

Superior turbinate

This structure is sagittally oriented and attached to the skull base. The natural sphenoid ostium is located posterior to the inferior half of the superior turbinate within the sphenoethmoid recess.

AGGER NASI CELL

Derived from the Latin word *agger* for 'nasal mound', this cell, which is pneumatized in 98 per cent of patients, is the most anterior and consistent of all ethmoid cells (Fig. 1.5).

Endoscopically, an eminence on the lateral nasal wall anterosuperior to the origin of the middle turbinate defines the location of the agger nasi. The agger nasi is bounded laterally by the lacrimal bone, anteriorly by the frontal process of the maxilla and medially by the uncinate process (see below); posteriorly it is related to the ethmoid infundibulum. Superiorly it forms the anterior boundary of the frontal recess and serves as an important landmark in the intraoperative identification of the frontal recess.

NASOLACRIMAL DUCT

The lacrimal sac is closely related to the agger nasi cell, being located slightly lateral and anterior to it. The lacrimal sac is usually 15 mm in height and 5–8 mm of this extends superior to the anterior insertion of the middle turbinate on the lateral wall (Figs 1.6–1.9). The NLD courses from the lacrimal sac down to its opening in the inferior meatus. The eminence anterior to the uncinate process is formed by the NLD. The intraosseous portion of the NLD is approximately 12 mm in length. The opening of the NLD in the inferior meatus is located about 15 mm above the nasal floor and approximately 1 cm behind the anterior end of the inferior turbinate. As the NLD descends it curves slightly posteriorly and is closely related to the

anterior fontanelle. Any attempt to extend the middle meatal antrostomy anteriorly into the anterior fontanelle places the NLD at risk.

UNCINATE PROCESS

The uncinate process is a thin, almost sagittally oriented, boomerang-shaped bony leaflet. It forms part of the lateral nasal wall between the middle and the inferior turbinates in an anterosuperior to posteroinferior orientation. It is attached anteriorly to the posterior edge of the lacrimal bone and inferiorly (by several bony pedicles) to the superior edge of the inferior turbinate. It has a free posterosuperior border (Fig. 1.10). Its superior attachment is variable:

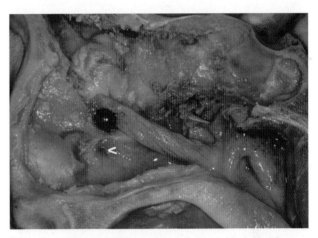

Figure 1.6 The anterior end of the inferior turbinate has been truncated and retracted superiorly to expose the inferior meatus. The arrowhead is pointing to the opening of the nasolacrimal duct in the inferior meatus.

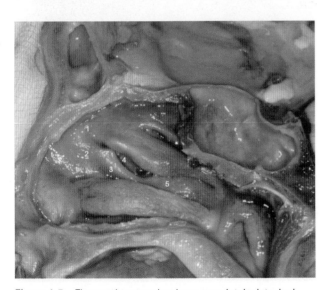

Figure 1.5 The nasal septum has been completely detached to reveal the lateral nasal wall. Note the agger nasi cell (1), nasolacrimal duct (2), uncinate process (3), bulla ethmoidalis (4) and the posterior fontanelle (5).

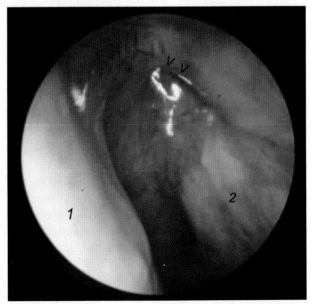

Figure 1.7 Endoscopic view of the opening of the nasolacrimal duct (arrowheads) in the left inferior meatus. Also seen are the inferior turbinate (1) and the lateral nasal wall (2).

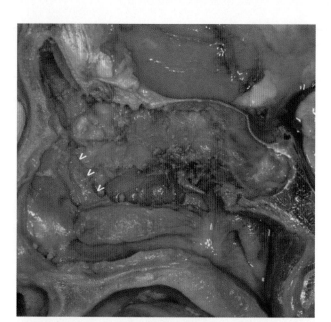

Figure 1.8   The overlying mucosa and the bone have been removed to expose the nasolacrimal duct (arrowheads).

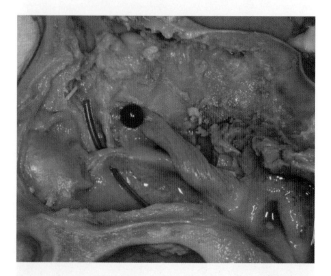

Figure 1.9   The lacrimal sac and nasolacrimal duct have been incised open. The blue probe is showing the nasolacrimal duct and its opening. The white probe is showing the location of the common canaliculus on the lateral wall of the lacrimal sac.

it may be attached to the lamina papyracea, the roof of the ethmoid sinus or the middle turbinate. Often there is more than one attachment. The superior attachment of the uncinate process determines the drainage of the frontal recess. The uncinate process may also present with many anatomical variations, including medial and lateral rotations. Occasionally, it may be rotated anteriorly, mimicking the middle turbinate to give the impression of a double middle turbinate. Together with the agger nasi, the uncinate process forms the first of the four lamellae on the lateral wall.

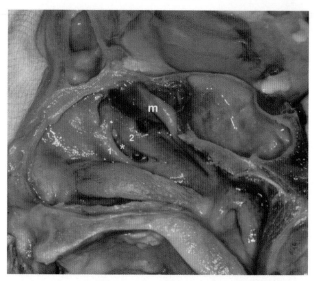

Figure 1.10   The middle turbinate (m) has been reflected medially and superiorly, upon its lateral attachment called the basal lamella, to reveal the middle meatus. Note the uncinate process (1) and the bulla ethmoidalis (2). The cleft between the posterior free border of the uncinate process and the anterior wall of the bulla is called the hiatus semilunaris anterioris (asterisk).

THE ETHMOID COMPLEX

Bulla ethmoidalis

The bulla ethmoidalis is the most prominent of the anterior ethmoid air cells and is readily identified posterior to the uncinate process (Figs 1.11 and 1.12). The bulla is variable in size and is pneumatized in 60–70 per cent of cases (thus

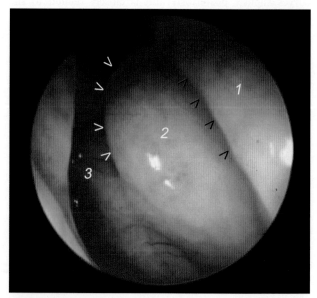

Figure 1.11   Endoscopic view of the left middle meatus showing the hiatus semilunaris superioris (white arrowheads) and the hiatus semilunaris inferioris (black arrowheads). Also seen are the uncinate process (1), bulla ethmoidalis (2) and the basal lamella (3).

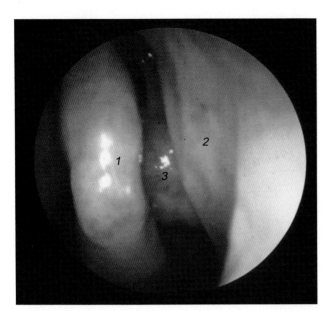

Figure 1.12   Close-up view of the left middle meatus showing the middle turbinate (1), uncinate process (2) and the bulla ethmoidalis (3).

termed bulla). When it is not pneumatized, it is termed the lateral torus. The bulla measures about 18 mm (range 9–23 mm) in length and is 5.4 mm (range 2–13 mm) high. Not infrequently the bulla may be highly pneumatized, extending to the skull base superiorly and the ground lamella posteriorly. The bulla ethmoidalis is closely related

to three recesses: the ethmoid infundibulum, the retrobullar recess and the frontal recess (see below). The anterior wall of the bulla ethmoidalis forms the posterior limit of the ethmoid infundibulum and its posterior wall forms the anterior wall of the retrobullar recess. The anterior and posterior walls of the bulla ethmoidalis merge superiorly to first form the bulla lamella, which can be attached to the skull base immediately anterior to the anterior ethmoid artery, and then continue as the posterior limit of the frontal recess (Fig. 1.13). It is important to remember that the lateral wall of the bulla ethmoidalis is formed by the lamina papyracea (Fig. 1.14). Inferiorly and posteriorly the bulla ethmoidalis may fuse with the basal lamella, in which case the retrobullar recess may be obliterated or is absent.

Lamina papyracea

As stated above, the lateral wall of the ethmoid complex is formed by the lamina papyracea, which is literally paper thin so that the orbital fat imparts a yellowish colour to it. The medial rectus muscle may, occasionally, be located in close contact with the lamina (Figs 1.15 and 1.16). The lamina thickens towards the orbital apex to form the optic tubercle protecting the optic nerve. The optic nerve courses in close proximity to the medial orbital wall in this location.

Hiatus semilunaris inferioris

The two-dimensional cleft between the posterior free border of the uncinate process and the anterior wall of the bulla ethmoidalis is called the hiatus semilunaris

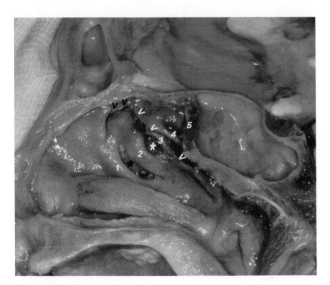

Figure 1.13   The middle turbinate has been trimmed from its attachments. The anterior third of the middle turbinate is attached to the skull base (black arrowheads) and the middle third and the posterior third curve laterally to form the basal lamella, which inserts onto the lamina papyracea (white arrowheads). Note the five lamellae: uncinate process (1), bulla ethmoidalis (2), basal lamella of the middle turbinate (3), lamella of the superior turbinate (4) and the anterior wall of the sphenoid (5). The white asterisk indicates the hiatus semilunaris superioris and the black asterisk the hiatus semilunaris inferioris.

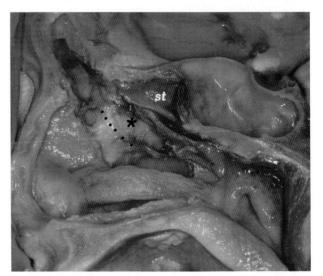

Figure 1.14   The bulla ethmoidalis has been removed, with the dotted line indicating the line of attachment of the anterior wall of the bulla ethmoidalis (asterisk) to the lamina papyracea, which also forms the lateral wall of the bulla ethmoidalis. The superior turbinate (st) is still intact.

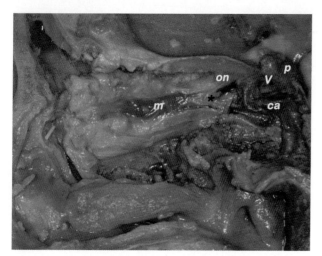

Figure 1.15   The lamina papyracea has been removed and the periorbita incised to expose the orbital contents related to the lateral wall. Note the orbital fat and the medial rectus (m) in close proximity to the lateral wall posteriorly. The asterisk indicates the anatomical location of the orbital apex. The medial wall of the cavernous sinus has been opened to expose the contents of the cavernous sinus. The cavernous portion of the internal carotid artery (ca) is the most medial structure in the cavernous sinus. The pituitary gland (p) has been retracted medially and superiorly to show the third (arrowhead) cranial nerve, which is lateral to the carotid artery. Note the optic nerve (on) anterosuperiorly on the lateral wall of the sphenoid sinus.

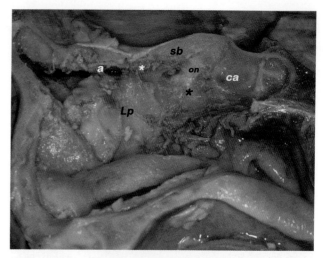

Figure 1.16   A complete sphenoethmoidectomy has been done delineating the lamina papyracea (Lp) laterally and the skull base (sb) superiorly. Note the location of the anterior ethmoid artery (a), the posterior ethmoid artery (white asterisk), the optic nerve (on), the orbital apex (black asterisk) and the carotid artery (ca).

inferioris. Its dimensions are variable and it can measure 14–22 mm in length and 0.5–3 mm mediolaterally. The hiatus semilunaris inferioris is located from 1–10 mm (43 per cent) to 11–20 mm (47 per cent) behind the anterior attachment of the middle turbinate. This two-dimensional cleft leads laterally into a three-dimensional space called the ethmoid infundibulum (see Fig. 1.10).

Hiatus semilunaris superioris

A cleft may be identified between the posterior aspect of the bulla ethmoidalis and the basal lamella, termed hiatus semilunaris superioris (see Fig. 1.13). It leads laterally into a very variable three-dimensional space called the retrobullar recess.

Ethmoid infundibulum

The ethmoid infundibulum, a three-dimensional space, is bounded medially by the uncinate process, posteriorly by the anterior wall of the bulla ethmoidalis and laterally by the lamina papyracea (Fig. 1.17). In about 86 per cent of cases the infundibulum ends superiorly in a blind recess, called the terminal recess (recessus terminalis), formed by the superior attachment of the uncinate process lateral to the lamina papyracea. In cases in which a terminal recess is

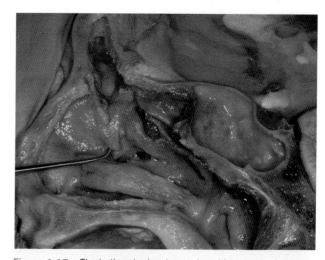

Figure 1.17   The ball probe has been placed in a recess lateral to the uncinate process. This three-dimensional recess bounded laterally by the lamina papyracea and limited superiorly by the terminal recess is called the ethmoid infundibulum.

present, the frontal recess drainage pathway will be medial to the uncinate process. In about 14 per cent of cases, in which the terminal recess is absent, the infundibulum continues anteriorly and superiorly into the frontal recess, which drains directly into the ethmoid infundibulum. Other structures that drain into the ethmoid infundibulum are the anterior ethmoid cells including the agger nasi cell, any frontal cells and the maxillary sinus.

Note that the lateral wall of the ethmoid infundibulum is the lamina papyracea. When the uncinate process is removed and the ethmoid infundibulum is opened, the surgeon will encounter the lamina papyracea, which is an important intraoperative landmark.

Retrobullar recess

A small, variable, space may exist superior and posterior to the bulla ethmoidalis separating it from the skull base and the basal lamella: this is referred to as the retrobullar recess. The boundaries of this recess are: the posterior wall of the bulla ethmoidalis anteriorly, the basal lamella posteriorly, the skull base superiorly and the lamina papyracea laterally (Fig. 1.18). This recess opens medially through the hiatus semilunaris superioris. Removing the bulla ethmoidalis and keeping the basal lamella intact opens the retrobullar recess (Fig. 1.19). Three important landmarks are encountered in this recess: the skull base superiorly, the anterior ethmoid artery traversing the skull base and the lamina papyracea laterally.

Posterior ethmoid cells

Located posterior to the basal lamella the posterior ethmoid cells are larger in size and fewer in number than the anterior ethmoid cells. The boundaries of the posterior ethmoid cells are formed by the basal lamella anteriorly, lamina papyracea laterally, skull base superiorly and superior turbinate medially (Figs 1.20 and 1.21). The posterior ethmoid cells drain under the superior turbinate into the superior meatus. The relationship of the posterior ethmoid cells with the sphenoid sinus depends on the presence or absence of a sphenoethmoid cell, also known

as Onodi cell (Fig. 1.22). The sphenoid sinus is usually located inferiorly and medially, and *not* posteriorly, in relation to the posterior ethmoids. The size of this cell complex depends on the degree of encroachment by the anterior ethmoid cells anteriorly and the sphenoid posteriorly. A posterior ethmoid cell may pneumatize posterolaterally and posterosuperiorly in relation to the anterior wall of the sphenoid. This is a sphenoethmoid cell. In this situation, the sphenoid sinus will be located

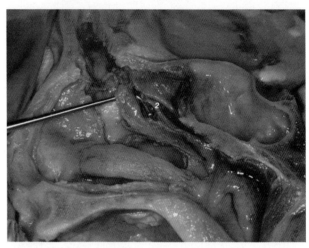

Figure 1.19   The anterior wall of the bulla ethmoidalis has been removed but the posterior wall has been retained. A probe has been passed through an opening in the posterior wall of the bulla, which drains into the retrobullar recess. Note the recess (ball probe) between the posterior wall of the bulla ethmoidalis (1) and the basal lamella (2).

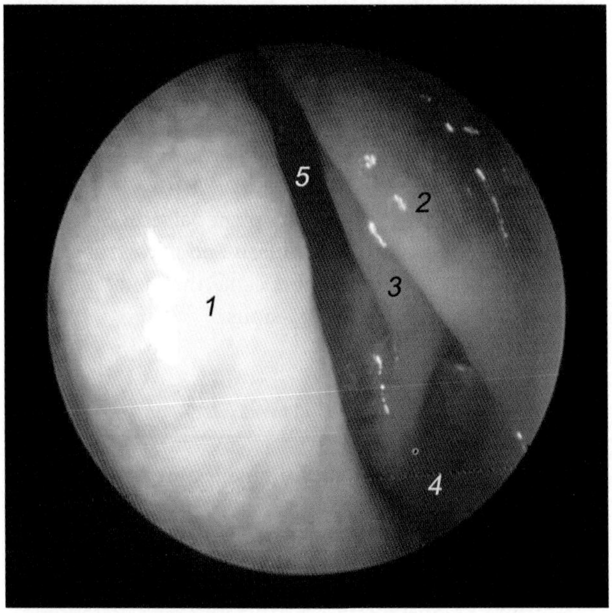

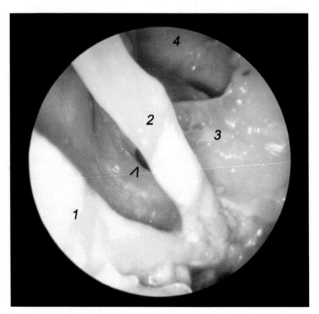

Figure 1.18   Endoscopic view of the left middle meatus. The retrobullar recess is a three-dimensional recess (5) bounded anteriorly by the posterior wall of the bulla ethmoidalism (3) and posteriorly by the basal lamella (4). Also seen are the middle turbinate (1) and uncinate process (2).

Figure 1.20   Endoscopic view of the left posterior ethmoid cells (3) bounded medially by the superior turbinate (2) and superiorly by the skull base (4). Note the sphenoid ostium (arrowhead) medial to the superior turbinate in the sphenoethmoid recess. Also seen is the middle turbinate (1).

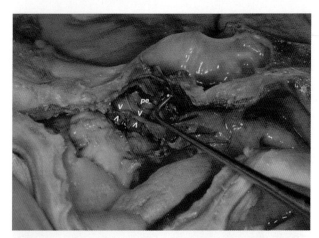

Figure 1.21   The superior turbinate has been lifted revealing the posterior ethmoid cells (pe). The probe has been placed in the sphenoid ostium (asterisk). Note the basal lamella (arrowheads).

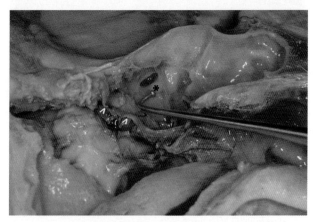

Figure 1.22   The posterior ethmoid cells have been removed. Note the optic nerve (black asterisk) at the posterior superior aspect of the lateral wall of this posterior ethmoid cell. This is likely to be a sphenoethmoid (Onodi) cell.

inferiorly and medially to this cell and *not* posterior to it (Fig. 1.22).

Ethmoid roof

The ethmoid roof is formed mainly by frontal bone. Its average thickness is 5 mm and it slants posteriorly at an angle of 15°. The ethmoid roof has several 'crater-like' impressions on it created by the ethmoid cells. These impressions are called the foveae. The most anterior fovea is often referred to as the fovea ethmoidalis.

The fovea ethmoidalis has important anatomical relationships. Medially it joins the lateral lamella of the lamina cribrosa to form a very thin, fragile junction, about one-tenth the thickness of the lateral skull base (Fig. 1.23). The vertical height between the cribriform fossa and the fovea ethmoidalis is variable, up to 17 mm, and may be asymmetrical. The medial slope of the roof may also be variable. The thin lateral lamella is at risk of penetration during ethmoid dissection.

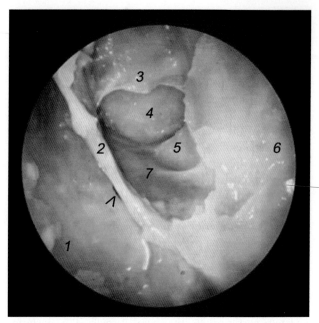

Figure 1.23   The left posterior ethmoid cells have been removed to show the skull base superiorly and the lamina papyracea laterally (6). Note the posterior ethmoid neurovascular bundle (3) as it traverses the skull base. Note the lamella (7) of the superior turbinate (2) traversing laterally from an anteromedial to a posterolateral direction. This posterior ethmoid cell is a small sphenoethmoid cell, at the apex of which is seen the optic nerve (5). The arrowhead is pointing to the sphenoid ostium. Also seen are the posterior nasal septum (1) and the fovea ethmoidalis (4).

MAXILLARY SINUS OSTIUM

Normally hidden from view by an intact uncinate process (Fig. 1.24), the maxillary sinus ostium is elliptical in shape and approximately 7–11 mm long and 2–6 mm high. It is located at the junction of the anterosuperior and posteroinferior aspects of the infundibulum (Figs 1.25 and 1.26). Removal of the uncinate process is necessary to visualize the opening (Figs 1.27 and 1.28).

The ostium lies in a slanted plane, almost 90° to the orientation of the hiatus semilunaris and may be as deep as 18–20 mm. It leads into a short canal that runs inferiorly and laterally into the maxillary sinus.

MAXILLARY WALL FONTANELLE

The anterior and posterior fontanelles are membranous areas in the lateral nasal wall, formed by a double layer of mucosa that fills in the gaps in the bony lateral nasal wall (Figs 1.29 and 1.30). The small anterior fontanelle is anterosuperior to the hiatus semilunaris inferioris. The larger posterior fontanelle is posteroinferior to the hiatus semilunaris and forms the medial wall of the antrum between the natural ostium and the vertical plate of the palatine bone. Often an accessory ostium is seen in this area (10–50 per cent).

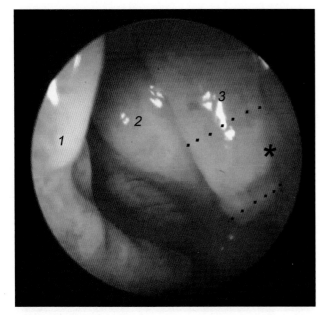

Figure 1.24   The left natural maxillary ostium lies in the ethmoid infundibulum and cannot be visualized on this endoscopic view without removing the uncinate process. The black asterisk shows the location of the natural maxillary ostium and the dotted lines indicate the portion of the uncinate process that has to be removed to visualize the ostium. Also seen are the middle turbinate (1), bulla ethmoidalis (2) and the uncinate process (3).

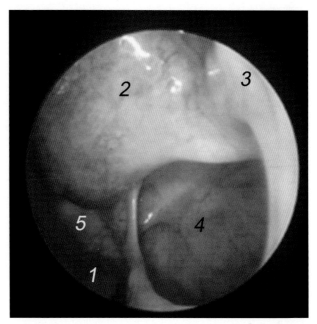

Figure 1.26   A wide middle meatal antrostomy has been created on the left side. The bulla ethmoidalis (2) is still intact. Note the middle turbinate (1), basal lamella (5), posterior wall of the maxillary sinus (4) and the lamina papyracea (3).

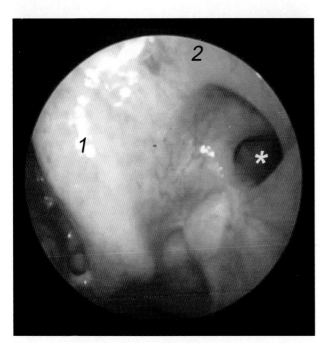

Figure 1.25   Endoscopic view of the left middle meatus. The uncinate process has been removed to show the maxillary ostium (white asterisk). Note that the natural maxillary ostium is a short three-dimensional channel rather than a two-dimensional structure. Also seen is the bulla ethmoidalis (1). Removal of the uncinate process opens the ethmoid infundibulum, the lateral boundary of which is the lamina papyracea (2).

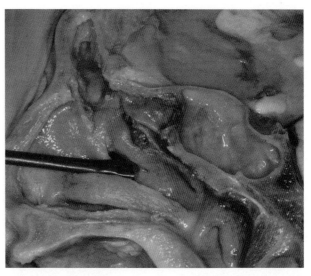

Figure 1.27   A reverse cutting forceps has been engaged in the ethmoid infundibulum to remove the lower part of the uncinate process and expose the natural maxillary ostium which opens in the ethmoid infundibulum.

FRONTAL RECESS

The frontal recess is a complex anatomical area leading from the anterior ethmoids superiorly to the frontal ostium (Figs 1.31–1.36). Its anatomical boundaries are formed by the agger nasi cell anteriorly, the anterior ethmoid artery posteriorly, the anterior portion of the middle turbinate medially, and the lamina papyracea laterally.

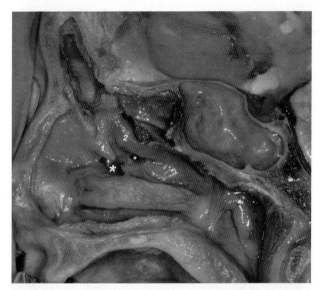

Figure 1.28   The lower part of the uncinate process has been removed, exposing the natural maxillary ostium (large white asterisk). The upper part of the uncinate process is still intact (1). Another ostium (small white asterisk) seen inferior to the bulla ethmoidalis (2) is an accessory ostium located in the posterior fontanelle.

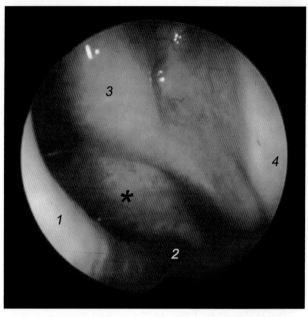

Figure 1.29   Endoscopic view of the left nasal cavity. Note the middle turbinate (1) curving laterally to form the basal lamella (asterisk). Also seen are the posterior insertion of the middle turbinate (2), the bulla ethmoidalis (3) and the posterior fontanelle (4).

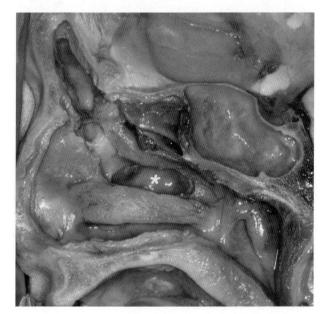

Figure 1.30   A large middle meatal antrostomy (asterisk) has been created by removing the posterior fontanelle.

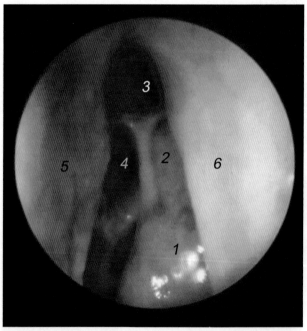

Figure 1.31   Endoscopic view of the left frontal recess. Note the insertion of the bulla ethmoidalis (1) onto the skull base. The bulla lamella divides the superior recess into the frontal recess anteriorly (3) and the retrobullar recess (4) posteriorly. Also seen are the middle turbinate (5) and the uncinate process (6).

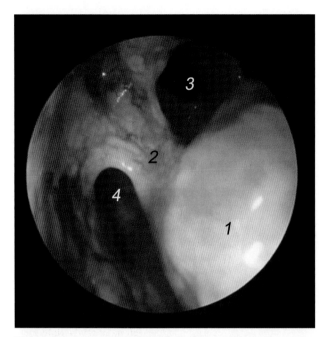

Figure 1.32 Close-up view of the insertion of the bulla ethmoidalis on the left side (1) onto the skull base (2). Seen anteriorly is the frontal recess (3) and posteriorly the retrobullar recess (4).

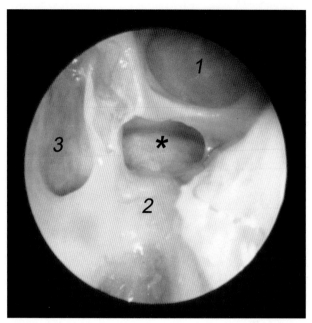

Figure 1.33 View of the left frontal recess (asterisk) with the bulla ethmoidalis (2) intact. Note the relationship of the agger nasi (1) with the frontal recess. The medial boundary of the frontal recess is formed by the middle turbinate (3).

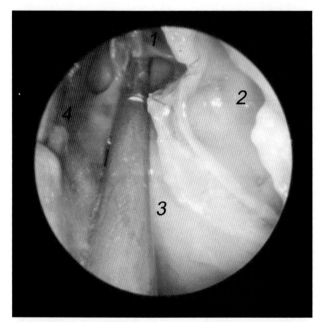

Figure 1.34 A curette has been passed into the left frontal sinus through the frontal recess. Removing the posterior and superior wall of the agger nasi (1) provides direct access to the frontal sinus in the absence of any frontal cells. Keeping the bulla intact (3) for the identification of the frontal recess protects the anterior ethmoid artery and the skull base during this manoeuvre. The medial boundary of the frontal recess is the middle turbinate (4) and laterally it is the lamina papyracea (2).

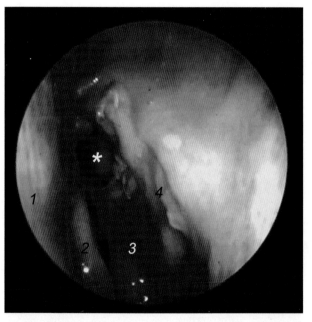

Figure 1.35 Endoscopic view of the left frontal recess (asterisk) with the bulla ethmoidalis (3) intact. Note the nasal septum (1), middle turbinate (2) and the lamina papyracea (4).

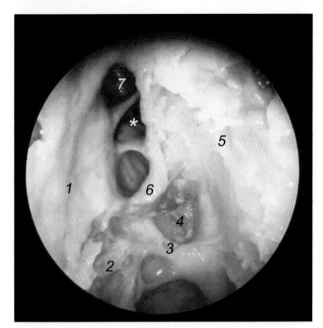

Figure 1.36 Removal of the left bulla ethmoidalis exposes the skull base (2) and the anterior ethmoid artery (3), which usually traverses the skull base obliquely in a posterolateral to anteromedial direction. Note the first fovea of the ethmoid roof (4). Structures 2, 3 and 4 are posterior to the insertion of the bulla ethmoidalis onto the skull base (6). Also seen are the middle turbinate (1) and the lamina papyracea (5). The asterisk is showing the frontal recess and the agger nasi cell (7) is also visible.

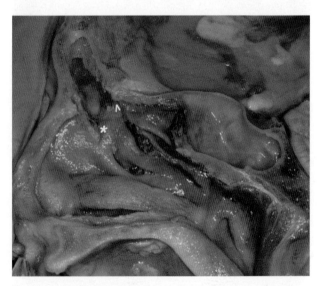

Figure 1.37 The recess has been opened to show the frontal recess drainage pathway, which traverses lateral to the removed middle turbinate and medial to the uncinate process (still intact). The asterisk is showing the superior part of the uncinate process inserting laterally onto the lamina papyracea to form the terminal recess. The arrowhead is pointing to the insertion of the bulla onto the skull base.

The superior attachment of the uncinate process determines the drainage pattern of the frontal sinus (Figs 1.37–1.39).

In 86 per cent of patients the uncinate process is attached to the lamina papyracea and the infundibulum ends superiorly, against the lamina papyracea, as the recessus terminalis. In such cases the frontal recess drains into the space between the uncinate and the middle turbinate. In 14 per cent of cases the uncinate either attaches superiorly to the skull base, or laterally to the middle turbinate. In

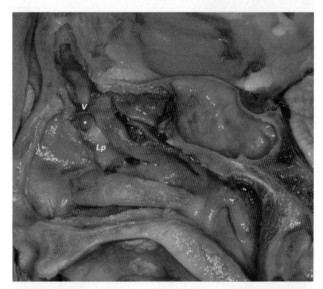

Figure 1.38 The upper part of the uncinate process has been removed, opening the ethmoid infundibulum. Note the lateral wall of the ethmoid infundibulum formed by the lamina papyracea (Lp). Note the superior attachment of the uncinate process (arrowhead) inserting laterally onto the lamina papyracea and separating the frontal recess from the ethmoid infundibulum. The ethmoid infundibulum ends superiorly into a terminal recess (asterisk).

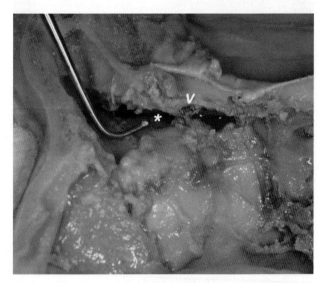

Figure 1.39 The frontal recess has been opened. Note the large supraorbital cell (asterisk). The arrowhead is pointing to the anterior ethmoid artery, which forms the posterior limit of the frontal recess.

these configurations the frontal sinus will drain directly into the infundibulum.

The agger nasi cell forms the anterior limit of the frontal recess. It is approximately in the same coronal plane as the nasolacrimal duct. An enlarged agger nasi cell may impinge on the frontal sinus, narrowing the frontal recess. Frontoethmoidal cells, as described and classified by Kuhn, are also anterior ethmoid cells that are located superior to the agger nasi. When present, they can cause further narrowing of the frontal recess from anteriorly. Frontoethmoidal cells are classified as types 1 to 4 (see Table 12.1, p. 106).[1]

The anterior ethmoid artery, a branch of the ophthalmic artery, lies in the roof of the ethmoid sinus and forms the posterior limit of the frontal recess (Figs 1.39 and 1.40). This artery is in the same coronal plane as the anterior aspect of the bulla ethmoidalis, or just behind. Therefore, the anterior wall of the bulla may be considered as the posterior extent of the frontal recess. After leaving the orbit through the anterior ethmoid foramen, the anterior ethmoid artery crosses the anterior ethmoid complex in a medial and anterior direction and exits the ethmoid complex, to run anteriorly in the olfactory groove. It then passes through a slit by the side of the crista galli and returns through the cribriform plate to re-enter the nasal cavity.

SPHENOID SINUS

The size of the sphenoid sinus is variable, depending on the degree of pneumatization. There are three commonly described patterns (Table 1.1). The sinus ostium is located high in the sphenoethmoid recess, on the anterior sphenoid wall, and at the level of the superior turbinate (Fig. 1.41).

The anterior sphenoid wall has a variable degree of obliquity, and runs in an anteromedial to posterolateral direction. In the presence of a sphenoethmoidal (Onodi) cell the anterior wall of the sphenoid sinus will not extend to the skull base (i.e. the sphenoethmoid or Onodi cell is superior and lateral to the sphenoid sinus) (Fig. 1.42).

The roof of the sphenoid is level anteriorly with the skull base. It is fairly flat and is called the planum sphenoidale. The junction of the planum sphenoidale and posterior sphenoid wall is thickened to form the tuberculum sella. The optic chiasm is about 2–7 mm posterior to the tuberculum sella. Inferior to the tuberculum sella, the posterior wall forms the anterior wall of the sella turcica (Fig. 1.43). The pituitary gland is located within the sella turcica. Inferiorly, the posterior wall separates the clivus.

The lateral sphenoid wall may have two prominences. The anterosuperior prominence is formed by the optic nerve and the posteroinferior prominence is formed by the

Table 1.1   Patterns of pneumatization of the sphenoid sinus

Type	Amount of pneumatization	Description
Sellar	76 per cent	Pneumatization beyond anterior sellar wall
Presellar	21 per cent	Pneumatization to sellar wall
Conchal	3 per cent	Poorly pneumatized

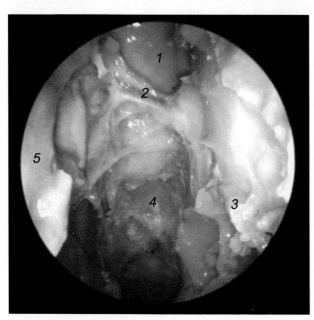

Figure 1.40   The left bulla ethmoidalis, the basal lamella, and the posterior ethmoid cells have been removed, exposing anterior ethmoid artery (2) and skull base (4). Note how the posterior table of the frontal sinus (1) slopes posteriorly to become the skull base. Laterally the lamina papyracea (3) has been identified and exposed. Also seen is the middle turbinate (5).

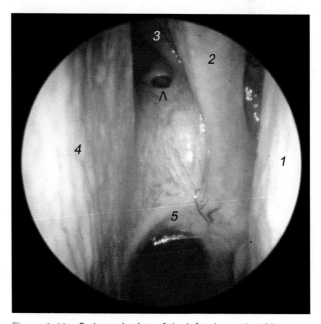

Figure 1.41   Endoscopic view of the left sphenoethmoid recess. The recess is bounded medially by the nasal septum (4) and laterally by the superior turbinate (3). The sphenoid ostium (arrowhead) is usually located in this recess about 1.5 cm superiorly to the posterior choana (5). Also seen are the inferior (1) and middle (2) turbinates.

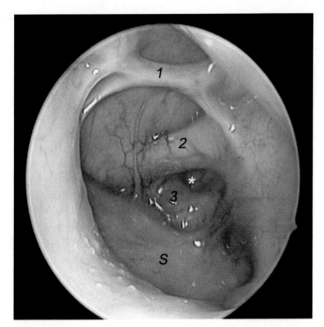

Figure 1.42   View of a large sphenoethmoid (Onodi) cell. Note the carotid artery (3) and the optic nerve (2) are dehiscent at the apex of this cell. The sphenoid sinus (s) has been displaced inferiorly and medially by this pneumatization process. Note the dehiscent posterior ethmoid artery (1) traversing the skull base. The asterisk is pointing to the left optico-carotid recess (see also Fig. 1.44).

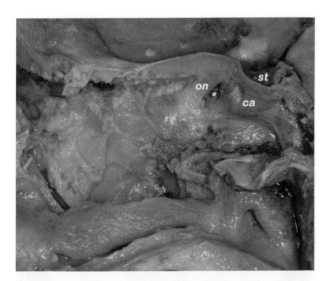

Figure 1.43   The bone overlying the structures on the lateral wall of the sphenoid has been removed. The medial layer of the cavernous sinus has been exposed. The anterosuperior prominence on the lateral wall is the optic nerve (on) and the posteroinferior prominence is the cavernous carotid artery (ca), which is the most medial structure in the cavernous sinus. Note a recess (asterisk) between the two structures. This is termed the optico-carotid recess. The pituitary gland lies in the sella turcica (st). Note the intimate relationship of the cavernous carotid artery with the sella turcica.

cavernous carotid artery (Fig. 1.44). In a well-pneumatized specimen, these structures may be dehiscent (optic nerve in 4–5 per cent, carotid in up to 20 per cent). A small recess, the infraoptic recess, also called the optico-carotid recess, may occupy the space between the two, and laterally the maxillary branch of the trigeminal nerve may be seen (Fig. 1.45).

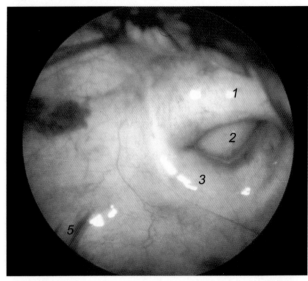

Figure 1.44   Intrasphenoid endoscopic view of the left lateral wall of the sphenoid sinus showing the optic nerve (1), optico-carotid recess (2) and the carotid artery (3). Also seen are the tuberculum sella (4) on the posterior wall and the anterior wall of the sella (5).

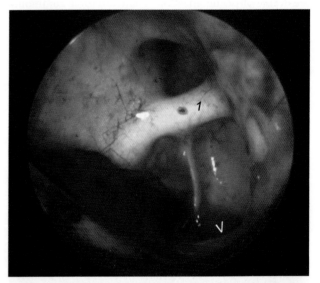

Figure 1.45   Endoscopic (70°) view of the left lateral recess of a well-pneumatized sphenoid sinus. Note the second branch of the trigeminal nerve (1), as it traverses the lateral recess. This nerve is superiorly and laterally located to the vidian nerve, which runs inferiorly (arrowhead).

REFERENCE

1. Bent P, Cuilty-Siller C, Kuhn FA. The frontal cell as a cause of frontal sinus obstruction. *Am J Rhinol* 1994; **8**: 185–91.

2

Making sense of symptoms

NICHOLAS JONES

CATARRH AND POSTNASAL DRIP

The term 'catarrh' means different things to different patients and you need to be particular in finding out what a patient might mean when they use this term. The key questions to ask are:

- Do you blow much out?
- Please can you point with one finger the area where you feel it?
- Does it make you sniff, snort, dry swallow or hawk?
- Is it clear, yellow or green and is that mainly first thing in the morning?
- Is it at the level of [the palate] or at the [cricoid cartilage]? (The surgeon should point to these two regions rather than use the exact terms.)

The rationale behind these questions is outlined below.

If the patient has a coexisting anterior nasal drip (which is unusual), they are either experiencing overproduction of thin mucus, such as in severe allergic rhinitis, or an autonomic rhinitis where the cilia cannot cope with the quantity of mucus. Interestingly, only a few patients with chronic rhinosinusitis present with an anterior discharge as ciliary function can normally cope and remove the mucus posteriorly. When there is an anterior discharge in chronic rhinosinusitis it may be caused by an infection where the bacterial toxins paralyse the cilia, or by abnormal mucus such as in cystic fibrosis, or primary ciliary dyskinesia.

If the patient's symptoms primarily consist of a posterior nasal discharge, then more detective work is needed to establish whether the patient has become hyperaware of normal mucus, or whether they do have overproduction of mucus. There are many reasons why the lining of the nose

can produce more mucus and these essentially include all the causes of chronic rhinosinusitis. However, chronic rhinosinusitis is only found in a minority of patients who complain of postnasal drip. It is important that these problems are differentiated from those associated with habitual snorting or clearing of the throat as medical treatment in this group will prove to be useless.

Several groups of patients complain of catarrh or postnasal mucus in the absence of any excessive or abnormal mucus production. One of the most common groups is of the snorers whose uvula is oedematous and who complain of a sensation of 'something' around the soft palate, and after further enquiry may complain of a collection of thick 'wallpaper paste' like mucus collecting in their throat in the morning (Fig. 2.1). They may try

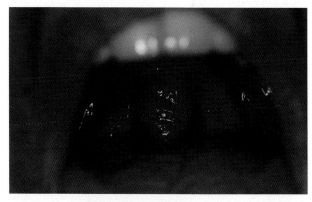

Figure 2.1 An oedematous uvula that is a sign of snoring. Some of these patients complain of 'bringing up' discoloured mucus and believe it is due to sinusitis; however, it is due to stagnant mucus collecting in the nasopharynx overnight. They have no discoloured mucus during the day.

to hawk up the mucus. They may snort, causing further vibration of the palate; indeed this can be an isolated habit that appears to sensitize the palate to feel normal postnasal mucus. Snorers often have mucus that dries up as they mouth breathe and snore; this mucus becomes more tenacious as it collects in the nasopharynx and oropharynx during the night. Some patients believe that it is unhealthy to swallow this mucus so they try to regurgitate it by hawking.

Another group consists of those patients with globus pharyngeus who instead of complaining of a 'lump' in the throat complain of catarrh, and they have a sensation of 'something' or mucus at the level of the cricoid cartilage. These patients often have a habit of throat clearing or dry swallowing and this seems to help perpetuate these symptoms.

Features differentiating pathological mucus from normal mucus

If a patient is unable to blow anything out into their handkerchief or says, 'My nose is dry, I can't blow anything out', it is unlikely they have abnormal mucus production (an exception is with an atrophic lining or where the cilia have been damaged by excessive surgery or disease – but these patients will usually complain of crusting). Ask the patient about the colour of the mucus. Is it clear, yellow, or green, or does it vary in colour? Many patients who mouth breathe when they sleep, wake up with some discoloured mucus that has collected in their naso- or oropharynx; the mucus becomes discoloured with oropharyngeal commensals. It is therefore important to ask patients who complain of discoloured mucus if it is just in the morning or whether it is throughout the day. It is useful to ask them to blow their nose into a handkerchief and see whether they have any discoloured mucus to confirm that is the case. If they do blow out purulent mucopus into their handkerchief, or it can be seen tracking down the nasopharynx (Fig. 2.2), or at endoscopy (Fig. 2.3) they

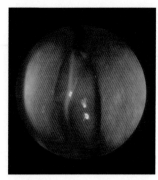

Figure 2.3   Endoscopic view of purulent secretions in the right middle meatus. Endoscopy is better than computed tomography in diagnosing sinusitis.

probably have chronic infective rhinosinusitis. If mucus becomes infected its viscosity increases and its viscoelastic properties make it even less liable to drip.[1] These patients need treatment in the form of douching, antibiotics and topical anti-inflammatory sprays, but this diagnosis is relatively unusual. Patients with allergic rhinitis or nasal polyposis often produce a lot of yellow-stained mucus, which is due to the presence of eosinophils, and this discoloration does not necessarily mean that it is infected.

In the context of the large number of people with allergic rhinitis and an increase in their production of mucus, few complain of excessive postnasal mucus. It is far more common for patients to have a hyperawareness of normal postnasal mucus and through repeated clearing of their throat or snorting to have 'sensitized' these areas to the 20–40 mL of nasal mucus and around 1000 mL of saliva we swallow each day (Fig. 2.4).[2]

Patients with primary ciliary dyskinesia, cystic fibrosis or immunodeficiency will present with discoloured secretions that they can blow out into a tissue, or that can be seen with an endoscope in the middle meatus (Fig. 2.5) or tracking down from the sphenoethmoid recess. Surgery is disappointing in these groups as it does not address the underlying pathology.

Surgery can help reduce the discoloration of postnasal mucus in patients with genuine chronically infected rhinosinusitis when medical treatment fails to aid drainage. They may need to douche regularly if the cilia are not functioning or in cystic fibrosis. In patients with

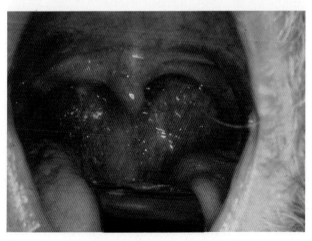

Figure 2.2   Discoloured mucopus tracking down from the nasopharynx indicating infective bacterial rhinosinusitis.

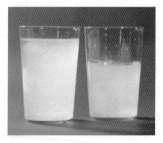

Figure 2.4   Most people swallow 20–40 mL of nasal mucus, the same amount from the lower respiratory tract and around 1000 mL of saliva each day.

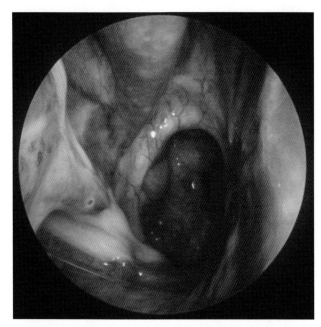

Figure 2.5 Endoscopic view of mucopus tracking down the right posterior choana. If this does not respond to antibiotics consider immunodeficiency, an atypical infection or, if the patient has lower respiratory tract problems, primary ciliary dyskinesia.

idiopathic nasal polyposis who often have associated late-onset asthma, it is important not to promise the patient a 'cure', as mucus secretion is part of their systemic mucosal disease. Because of this, ongoing medical treatment is often important. Patients with asthma can expect at least a temporary improvement in their lower respiratory symptoms after sinus surgery and it is worth taking time to explain to the patient the connection between inflammation of the upper and lower respiratory tract.

Physiology of mucus production and qualifying the term "postnasal drip"

There is no objective investigation to confirm the diagnosis and there is a lack of specificity and sensitivity of symptoms and/or signs that make the diagnosis. The nasal mucus is normally tenacious and it cannot drip like tap water.[3] Postnasal drip syndrome (PNDS) appears to have become more of a label than a useful term to describe underlying nasal pathology. Indeed, a recent review on the subject describes PNDS as a 'dustbin' label.[4] Otorhinolaryngology clinics are well frequented by patients with habitual 'throat clearing', 'catarrh', 'something dripping down the throat' or a sore throat. The vast majority of these patients have no demonstrable nasal disease. Any of these symptoms could imply the presence of an underlying PNDS to the non-specialist.

The term 'drip' is a misnomer and implies that mucus can drip from the soft palate or nasopharynx into the larynx or hypopharynx. This does not happen because of the rheological properties of mucus: namely, its cohesional

forces, spinnability and adhesiveness.[4] The label of PNDS should be replaced by the more accurate diagnoses of rhinitis and rhinosinusitis in the small subgroup when this is a cause for secretions. In the remaining patients, non-specific pharyngeal symptoms, on their own, which have previously been attributed to 'PNDS' are usually not an indication of intranasal disease. They usually have a hyperawareness of their normal mucus and saliva. A strategy to break the cycle of repetitive throat clearing, dry swallowing and hawking is to advise the patient to strictly avoid all these for 1 week and instead swallow ice cold water that will stimulate the back of the throat and take away the desire to do so. The patient must be disciplined about doing this and ensure they have enough bottles of ice-cold water in the fridge all the time and also keep some by their bedside. An explanation that the secretions that they have are healthy and can be swallowed without causing any problems also helps. An audit of this strategy has shown it works well in a large proportion of patients with these symptoms.[5]

FACIAL PAIN

Sinus headache

The term 'sinus headache' is almost an oxymoron. The vast majority of patients who present with a symmetrical frontal or temporal headache, sometimes with an occipital component, have tension-type headache. Unilateral episodic headaches are often vascular in origin. Sinusitis rarely causes headache, let alone facial pain, except when there is an acute bacterial infection and the sinus in question cannot drain – and it is usually unilateral and like a 'boil' in the sinus cavity. These patients usually have a history of a viral upper respiratory infection immediately before this and they have pyrexia with unilateral nasal obstruction. The vast majority of patients with acute sinusitis respond to antibiotics. More than two episodes of genuine bacterial sinusitis in 1 year should be investigated for evidence of poor immunity. Patients with chronic bacterial sinusitis rarely have any pain unless the sinus ostia are blocked and then the symptoms are the same as in acute sinusitis. There are texts that report that an isolated sphenoid sinusitis can cause headaches. However, it should be borne in mind that first, this is extremely rare, and, second, most of these patients respond to antibiotics.

Patients with a headache often make a self-diagnosis of 'sinusitis' as they know that some sinuses lie within the head. With the advent of nasal endoscopy and computed tomography (CT), along with the finding that many patients' symptoms of headache or facial pain persist after sinus surgery it has become apparent that this is not the case.[6,7] It is also relevant that over 80 per cent of patients with purulent secretions visible at nasal endoscopy have no headache or facial pain.[8] Even when patients with intermittent symptoms of headache or facial pain, who believe that it is due to infection, are asked to attend the clinic when they are symptomatic the majority are found not to have any evidence of infection and another neurological cause for their pain is often responsible.

Over 90 per cent of self-diagnosed and doctor-diagnosed sinus headaches meet the International Headache Society criteria for migraines and yet 61 per cent receive an antibiotic prescription.[9] One study of 100 patients who believed that they suffered from sinus headache found that 52 per cent had migraine, 11 per cent had chronic migraine associated with medication overuse, 23 per cent had probable migraine, 1 per cent cluster headache, 1 per cent hemicrania continua, 3 per cent secondary to rhinosinusitis, 9 per cent were nonclassifiable.[10] Over 46 per cent of migraine sufferers have at least one unilateral nasal symptom of congestion or rhinorrhoea or ocular lacrimation, redness or swelling during an attack.[11]

Patients with headache or facial pain secondary to genuine sinusitis usually have endoscopic signs of disease,[12] and they almost invariably have coexisting symptoms of nasal obstruction, hyposmia and/or a purulent nasal discharge.[13] An article on the management of sinogenic pain advises using 'significant caution when considering surgery in these patients because of high long-term failure rates and the eventual identification of other causes of the pain in many cases'.[14]

Cady and Schreiber[15] reported that nearly 90 per cent of their participants with self-diagnosed or doctor-diagnosed sinus headache met the International Headache Society[16] criteria for migraine-type headache and responded to triptans. These authors note that during a migrainous episode there is engorgement and erythema of the nasal mucosa along with rhinorrhoea, and after subcutaneous administration of sumatriptan there is resolution of both the symptoms and the endoscopic signs. Others have found that migraine often affects the face and can be misinterpreted as being due to sinusitis, particularly as symptoms can last 48 hours and vascular changes in the lining of the nose can also produce nasal obstruction through vasodilatation of the vascular turbinate tissue.[17,18] An interdisciplinary consensus group recently agreed that 'the majority of sinus headaches can actually be classified as migraines' and that 'unnecessary diagnostic studies, surgical interventions, and medical treatments are often the result of the inappropriate diagnosis of sinus headache'.[19]

Seventy to eighty per cent of the population have headaches and 50 per cent have at least one a month, 15 per cent once a week and 5 per cent daily.[20] The Copenhagen group on tension-type headache postulates that central sensitization of the trigeminal nucleus resulting from prolonged nociceptive input from a peripheral injury, surgery, inflammation, pericranium or from myofascial nociceptive input, along with psychological or neurological factors that can reduce supraspinal inhibition, can contribute to tension-type headache.[21,22]

Sinogenic pain

Acute sinusitis usually follows an acute upper respiratory tract infection and is mostly unilateral, intense and associated with pyrexia and unilateral nasal obstruction, and there may be a purulent discharge. Chronic sinusitis is, however, usually painless, with episodes of pain occurring during acute exacerbations, which are often precipitated by an upper respiratory tract infection or when there is obstruction of the sinus ostia by polyps, when pus is present.[13] An increase in the severity of pain on bending forward is traditionally thought to be diagnostic of sinusitis, but this is non-specific as many types of facial pain and headache are made worse by this movement.

The key points in the history of sinogenic pain are: an exacerbation of pain during an upper respiratory tract infection, an association with rhinological symptoms and a response to medical treatment. Examination of the face is often normal in patients with chronic sinusitis. Visible facial swelling is usually due to other pathology, such as dental sepsis (Fig. 2.6). If a diagnosis of sinusitis has been made and the patient has not responded to treatment, nasal endoscopy is very helpful, if not essential, in making the diagnosis of sinusitis. No evidence of middle meatal mucopus makes a diagnosis of sinogenic pain most unlikely.

There is poor evidence that a vacuum within a blocked sinus can cause protracted pain. Transient facial pain in patients with other symptoms and signs of rhinosinusitis can occur with pressure changes when flying, diving or skiing, but this resolves as the pressure within the sinuses equalizes through perfusion with the surrounding vasculature. Patients who repeatedly experience these symptoms when there is a pressure change are often helped by surgery to open the sinuses. Chronic pain is rarely the result of a blocked sinus. For example, silent sinus syndrome, which is due to a blocked sinus with resorption of its contents such that the orbital floor

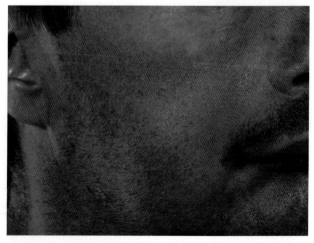

Figure 2.6   Swelling of the cheek is nearly always due to dental disease.

prolapses into the maxillary sinus, causes no pain. As has already been mentioned in the previous section, isolated sphenoid sinusitis is very rare but can cause headache and the majority respond to antibiotics and topical decongestants. Nasal endoscopy and CT are essential in making a diagnosis.

Midfacial segment pain

A relatively recently described condition, which affects about a third of patients with facial pain seen in ENT clinics, is midfacial segment pain. This is a version of tension-type headache that affects the midface, although 60 per cent have a coexisting headache, and has been shown not to be related to sinusitis.[23] The features of midfacial segment pain include the following.

- It is a symmetrical sensation of pressure or tightness – some patients may say that their nose feels blocked even though they have no nasal airway obstruction.
- It involves the areas of the nasion, under the bridge of the nose, on either side of the nose, the peri- or retro-orbital regions, or across the cheeks (Fig. 2.7). The symptoms of tension-type headache often coexist.
- There may be hyperaesthesia of the skin and soft tissues over the affected area.
- Nasal endoscopy is normal (Fig. 2.8).
- CT tomography of the paranasal sinuses is normal (note a third of asymptomatic patients have incidental mucosal changes on CT).
- The symptoms may be intermittent (<15 days/month) or chronic (>15 days/month).
- There are no consistent exacerbating or relieving factors.

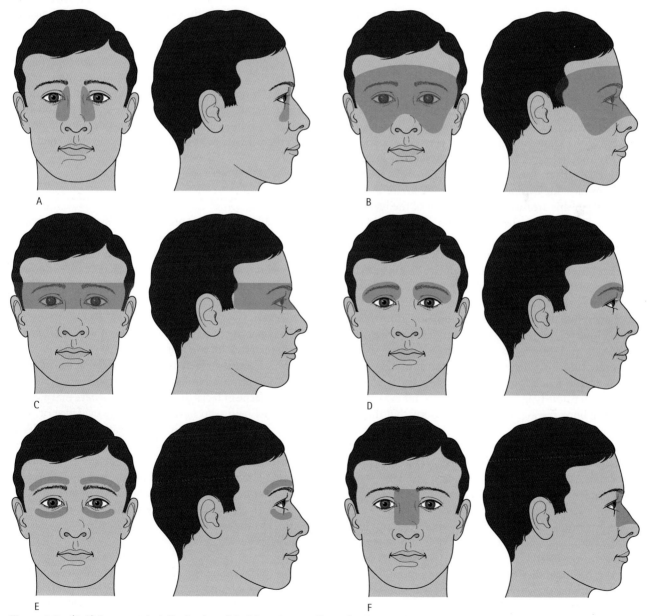

Figure 2.7 (A–F) A symmetrical distribution of facial pressure or discomfort is part of the clinical picture of midfacial segment pain.

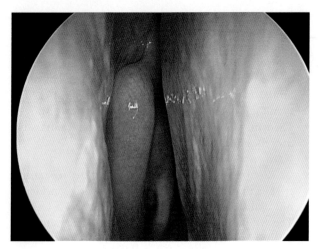

Figure 2.8   If nasal endoscopy is normal then any facial pain is unlikely to be due to sinusitis.

- There are no nasal symptoms (note that approximately 20 per cent of most populations have intermittent or persistent allergic rhinitis, which may occur incidentally in this condition).

Thus midfacial segment pain has all the characteristics of tension-type headache with the exception that it affects the midface. The forehead and occipital region may also be affected at the same time in about 60 per cent of patients. Patients often take a range of analgesics but they have no, or minimal, effect. Patients may be convinced that their symptoms are due to sinusitis as most are aware that the sinuses lie in this area with the exception of the bridge of the nose. They may have been treated for a long period with antibiotics and topical nasal steroids and a few patients have had some transient response on occasions that may be related to the placebo effect or cognitive dissonance, but these are inconsistent. Patients often describe tenderness on touching the areas of the forehead or cheeks, leading them to think there is underlying inflammation of the bone. However, on examination there is hyperaesthesia of the skin and soft tissues in these areas (see list above), and gently touching these is enough to cause discomfort similar to the tender areas over the forehead and scalp seen with tension-type headache. There is no evidence of underling bony disease. The patient may say that the skin of the infraorbital margin region or cheeks swells up, but there are no objective signs – this symptom may relate to an alteration in sensation in this area. Nasal endoscopy is normal. As approximately 1 in 3 asymptomatic people have incidental changes on CT, this may confuse the picture.

The majority of patients with this condition respond to low-dose amitriptyline, but usually require up to 6 weeks of 10 mg (occasionally 20 mg) of the drug at night before it works. It should then be continued for 6 months before stopping it, and the 20 per cent whose symptoms return when they stop it need to restart it if the pain returns. It is our practice to inform patients that amitriptyline is also used in higher doses for other conditions, such as nocturnal enuresis and depression, but its effectiveness in midfacial segment pain is unrelated to its analgesic properties. The analgesic effect of amitriptyline is much more rapid and usually requires 75 mg. It is often reassuring for patients to know the dose used for depression is some seven or more times the dose used in tension-type headache or midfacial segment pain. Other serotonin reuptake inhibitors are not effective (again as in tension-type headache). If the patient does not respond to amitriptyline, then relief may be obtained from gabapentin or pregabalin.

Septal or sinus surgery for midfacial segment pain makes no difference in approximately a third of patients who undergo this treatment and makes the symptoms worse in another third. In the remaining third it helps the pain but only for a few weeks and rarely more than for a few months. It is as though the surgical stimulus alters the 'balance' of neuronal activity in the trigeminal caudal nucleus for a short time. It is possible that the placebo effect or cognitive dissonance may also be responsible for a temporary symptomatic improvement. These effects cannot explain the benefit achieved with amitriptyline, as the placebo effect usually subsides within months.

The term midfacial segment pain avoids the use of the term 'tension', which helps as the mention of tension often results in a long and relatively unproductive discussion with the patient about the role of stress in their condition.

Headaches

Almost all patients who present with a symmetrical frontal or temporal headache have a tension-type headache. Unilateral, episodic headaches are often vascular in origin, and include variations of migraine, hemicrania continua, periodic migrainous neuralgia or paroxysmal hemicrania – although the latter two are more of periorbital pain than headache.

The majority of patients who present with headache to otorhinolaryngologists believe they have 'sinus or nasal trouble'. There is an increasing awareness that neurological causes are responsible for a large proportion of patients with headache or facial discomfort. We believe that patients with facial pain who have no objective evidence of sinus disease (endoscopy negative, CT negative) are most likely not to be helped by nasal or sinus surgery, particularly in the medium and long term. A comprehensive examination (including nasal endoscopy) is highly desirable if medical nasal treatment has failed to help symptoms of facial discomfort or headache. Only if there are neurological signs, or the discomfort is progressive, are further investigations warranted.

Failure to respond to the treatment for tension-type headache, migraine or midfacial segment pain should make the doctor question the diagnosis, as the treatment is successful in the majority of patients with the condition.

'BLOCKAGE' WITHOUT AIRWAY OBSTRUCTION

Some patients, rather than complaining of facial discomfort, pressure, heaviness or pain, complain of a sensation of blockage when their airway is good. Several conditions can cause this symptom and it is important to make sure that you make the correct diagnosis as the treatments vary a great deal.

To be able to feel airflow, receptors within the nose need to register a change in humidity and temperature. If the lining is dry the sensation of airflow is reduced. Patients with this condition often sniff in order to enhance the sensation of airflow and this in turn may exacerbate the problem by causing secondary nasal valve collapse. Sniffing menthol helps at the time this is done as it stimulates the receptors and relieves the lack of sensation. A lack of sensation with a dry lining is not uncommon in patients who have had a lot of nasal surgery and in particular turbinate surgery of any kind (Fig. 2.9). At a glance little may appear to be abnormal but on closer examination the septal mucosa does not have any moisture on it. Sometimes there will be obvious crusting but the patient may have cleared any debris before attending. Management simply involves giving the patient an explanation that this is the problem along with advice about regular douching and, most importantly, that the prolonged application of petroleum jelly over several months may be needed to allow the mucosa to recover. The petroleum jelly should not be applied with a cotton bud as it is abrasive but placed on the little finger first, then put inside the nostril and, finally, sniffed and 'milked' up by squeezing the nostrils.

Other patients may express their feeling of heaviness or pressure under the bridge of the nose as 'blockage'. These patients have a good airway, normal mucosa at endoscopy, and they often have a mild form of midfacial segment pain (see above for description).

The nasal valve can cause nasal obstruction but often when it is blamed as the cause it is secondary to other factors. The external valve is made of the ala, the skin of the vestibule, the nasal sill and the contour of the medial crus of the lower lateral cartilage, and it has a tendency to collapse at high flow rates even in normal individuals. The nasal valve area and internal nasal valve are two entities that should not be confused. The nasal valve area is the narrowest portion of the nasal passage (Fig. 2.10). It is bounded medially by the septum and the tuberculum of Zukercandle, superiorly and laterally by the caudal margin of the upper lateral cartilages, its fibro-adipose attachment to the pyriform aperture, the anterior end of the inferior turbinate and inferiorly it is made of the floor of the pyriform aperture. The nasal valve, on the other hand, is the specific slit-like segment between the caudal margin of the upper lateral cartilage and the septum and it is measured in degrees at approximately 15°.

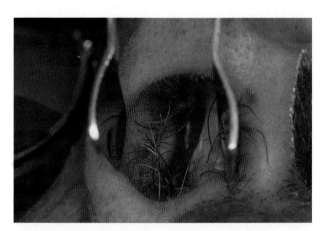

Figure 2.10 The nasal valve area is the narrowest portion of the nasal passage.

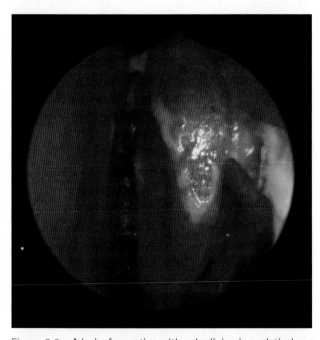

Figure 2.9 A lack of sensation with a dry lining is a relatively common cause of complaints about nasal obstruction when the airway is good.

The mucosal soft tissue changes that affect the inferior turbinate and septum are the commonest causes of narrowing of the nasal valve area and in turn this can cause secondary collapse of the nasal valve. Cartilaginous abnormalities of the upper lateral cartilages are subdivided into those that are medialized, absent, thickened, deflected or twisted, and those in which the distal end is elongated, scrolled or weak.[24] Nasal valve problems occur primarily following excessive resection of the lower lateral cartilages, or they can be due to a long returning of upper lateral cartilages, an inherent concave shape of the lower lateral cartilages, no overlap between the upper and lower lateral cartilages, inherently weak upper and lower lateral cartilages, soft tissue stenosis, a narrow pyriform aperture or facial nerve palsy affecting the dilator muscles. However, valve collapse more commonly occurs secondary to a septal deviation or turbinate hypertrophy and this is termed secondary valve collapse. It is important to distinguish primary from secondary valve collapse as treating the valve in secondary collapse usually gives a poor result. The most common cause of nasal valve collapse without the secondary influence of turbinate hypertrophy is a previous rhinoplasty.

A diagnosis of nasal valve dysfunction can be made by simple inspection and watching the patient breathe at rest (Fig. 2.11). Inspection during increasing rates of inspiration can reveal various degrees of collapse of the nasal valve. There are no objective measurements as the insert in acoustic rhinometry splints the lower lateral cartilages open and the tape used in active anterior rhinomanometry has the same effect. A Jobson–Horne probe may be used to gently support the upper lateral cartilage and ask the patient if it provides symptomatic benefit (Fig. 2.12). The appearance of an inverted 'V' over the middle third of the nose is in keeping with collapse of the upper lateral cartilages (Fig. 2.13). This may be secondary to trauma when the upper lateral cartilages are detached from the nasal bones or secondary to nasal surgery where the same injury is caused injudiciously or when an excessive amount of the upper lateral cartilages is resected. If artificially supporting the nasal valve, or opening the soft tissues of the alar region along with the nasal valve with a Jobson–Horne probe, does not provide good subjective improvement in airflow, it is worthwhile excluding mucosal hypertrophy or dry mucosa as the cause for the patient's symptoms. Cottle's sign, which involves distracting the nasal valve by pulling on the soft tissues of the cheek (Fig. 2.14), is a non-specific sign that often provides symptomatic improvement in most primary and secondary causes affecting the nasal valve and is of little diagnostic use.

It is important not to overlook these problems as surgery elsewhere will be unhelpful.

TENDERNESS AND/OR FACIAL SWELLING WITHOUT ANY OBJECTIVE SIGNS

It is not uncommon for patients to say that their cheeks swell when they have facial discomfort when there are no objective signs, even when they are symptomatic. They often turn to their partner for corroboration, who agrees that their face swells yet there are no objective signs. We have already mentioned that patients with facial pain that is migrainous or vascular in origin have pain that is not uncommonly associated with some ipsilateral nasal congestion and the release of some neuropeptides in the vascular distribution of their pain. This may be responsible for some sensation of facial swelling and they may have a coexisting facial flush. Another explanation in patients who

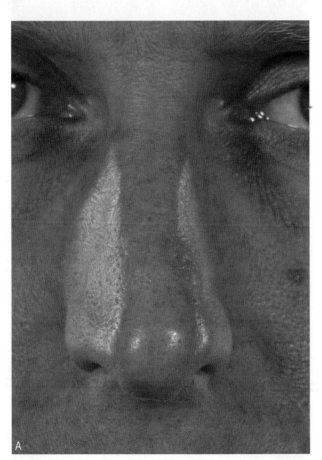
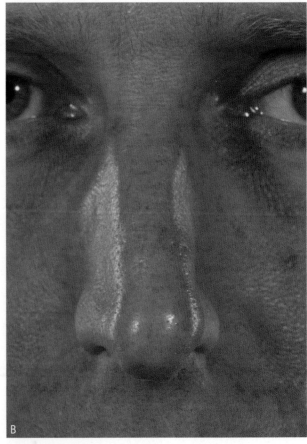

Figure 2.11   The patient (A) at rest and (B) after gently breathing, demonstrating primary valve collapse.

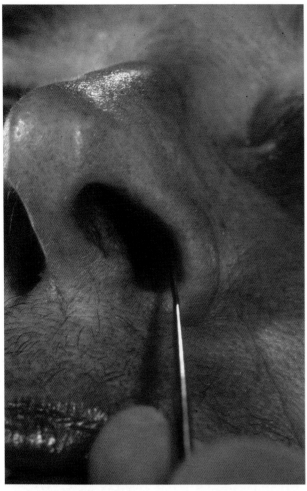

Figure 2.12   A Jobson–Horne probe supporting the upper lateral cartilage to elucidate whether this provides symptomatic benefit.

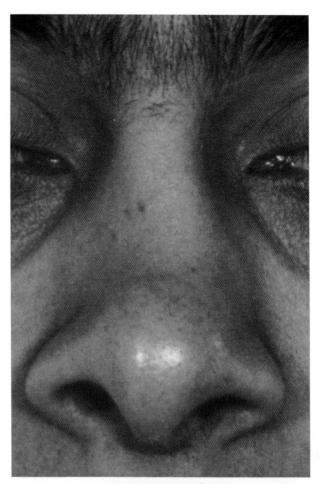

Figure 2.13   The appearance of an inverted 'V' over the middle third of the nose often indicates collapse of the upper lateral cartilages.

complain of facial swelling without any signs, particularly when it is bilateral, is that they have an alteration in sensation in the affected area. This can go hand in hand with the hyperaesthesia that many of these patients feel and is often part of midfacial segment pain. Some workers have described mechanisms that can produce central sensitization through an alteration in neural plasticity and endeavoured to explain the phenomenon of hyperalgesia and how dysaesthesia or even pain can persist.[25,26]

Facial swelling, and in particular swelling of the cheek, is unusual with infective rhinosinusitis, except where accompanied by periorbital cellulitis. The most common causes of swelling of the cheek are of dental origin. In patients with maxillary mucocoeles, tumours, or who have dehiscence in the wall of the maxillary sinus, acute sinusitis can cause facial swelling – but this is unusual. Infective rhinosinusitis rarely causes swelling of the cheek.

INCAPACITATING SNEEZING

Any irritant such as dust, smoke, odours, chemical irritants and allergens can initiate a sneezing bout but more than four sneezing bouts a day is indicative of allergic rhinitis. The best treatment for this is non-sedative antihistamines, which usually work well, and a topical nasal steroid provides supplementary help in many patients, although a minority find that a nasal spray can initiate a sneezing bout. Sprays that contain benzalkonium chloride as a preservative tend to initiate sneezing bouts more than those that do not.

A small minority of patients have incapacitating sneezing bouts that can last for hours. Most of these patients are young adolescents or children and psychogenic factors play a major role.[27,28] Cognitive behaviour therapy, addressing the patient's wider issues about anxiety or suggestion therapy with isotonic saline can help.

STEROID RESISTANT RHINITIS

Many studies claim that topical nasal steroids produce a significant improvement in allergic rhinitis. The patient's view may differ. If the patient's symptoms for nasal obstruction were, let us estimate, 8 out of 10 for severity and after they took their treatment their symptoms decreased

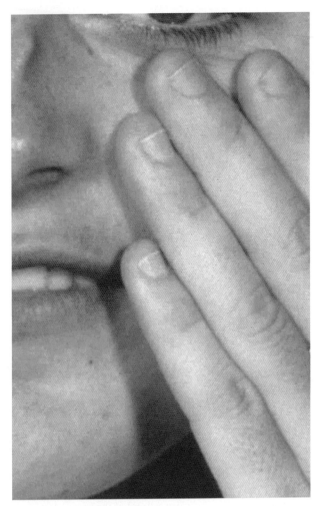

Figure 2.14   Cottle's sign.

disappointing. Although at 6 months many patients still have an improved airway, after 12 months this is rarely the case. These patients, when they return with the same symptoms, rarely want to repeat the intervention that they have had. This suggests that it was not worth the discomfort that they underwent. So what can you do to help these patients? A frank explanation that surgery is not a cure, that it will provide only temporary relief but at the cost of some discomfort, and that it is best avoided, is wise. Should the patient insist that they would rather have the treatment you might succumb but you will not need to be on the defensive about the inadequacy of your result. After several years you may share my disillusionment as regards any turbinate procedure.

'CLICKING' SINUSES

This is not a common symptom but it has a similar significance as the sensation of the ears popping. The fact that that the sinuses do click may indicate that the pressure is equalizing as the sinus ostia open. This may indicate some minor mucosal hypertrophy or some increase in secretions but it is rarely associated with significant sinus disease. As an isolated symptom it does not warrant intervention and as part of a collection of symptoms it should be ignored other than to explain to the patient that it is not a cause for concern.

NOT BEING ABLE TO 'BLOW MY NOSE'

As a solitary symptom, not being able to blow the nose is not associated with any pathology. Often patients who complain of this have a coexisting awareness of 'something' at the back of the soft palate and they may snort or dry swallow. This is akin to the hyperawareness of mucus described above. If not being able to 'blow my nose' is associated with crusting, an atrophic lining may be responsible and occasionally sarcoid or a vasculitis, and these should be considered in the differential diagnosis.

LETHARGY AND DARK RINGS UNDER THE EYES

Lethargy and dark rings under the eyes are non-specific symptoms that are not associated with sinusitis. These symptoms are more frequently associated with midfacial segment pain (see above).

PAROSMIA, ANOSMIA AND OLFACTORY HALLUCINATIONS (TABLE 2.1)

Hyposmia is the commonest disorder of smell and is usually caused by any inflammation of the nasal lining

to 6 out of 10 then it might be claimed that the patient has had a 'significant response'. From the patient's point of view their remaining symptoms are far from cured and very significant. In treating patients with rhinosinusitis of most causes, as well as those that have unknown causes, be careful not to raise a patient's expectations too much.

Having qualified the degree of improvement that some patients will obtain after treatment for either allergic or idiopathic rhinitis, some will have a minimum response to topical nasal or even systemic steroids. It is tempting for the surgeon to reach for the knife/laser/diathermy, especially as the patient is keen to obtain some improvement. Under these circumstances, it is important to ensure that there is no other pathology affecting nasal sensation, as surgery, if undertaken, will complicate the picture even more. The conditions that can feign blockage are a dry lining, valve collapse and mild midfacial pain, as has been described above. If these have been excluded and maximum medical treatment (this may include oral and topical nasal steroids, a non-sedative antihistamine, allergen avoidance, especially where there is single sensitivity to house dust mite) has been tried and failed the question is what to do next. In the medium and, in particular, the long term, results of turbinectomy, laser turbinate ablation and diathermy are

Table 2.1   Parosmia, anosmia and olfactory hallucinations

Olfactory dysfunction	Definition
Total anosmia	Inability to detect any qualitative olfactory sensation
Partial anosmia	Ability to detect some, but not all, qualitative olfactory sensation
General or total hyposmia	Decreased sensitivity to all odorants
Hyposmia	Decreased sensitivity to some, but not all, odorants
Specific anosmia	Many individuals lack the ability to detect specific odorants that can be smelled by others
Dysosmia, parosmia or cacosmia, phantosmia	Distorted odour perception: either the perception of an unpleasant odour when a normal odour is presented or the perception of an odour in the absence of an olfactory stimulus
General, total hyperosmia or multiple chemical sensitivity	Increased sensitivity to odours, a doubtful entity
Partial hyperosmia	Increased sensitivity to only some odours
Olfactory agnosia	Inability to classify, contrast, or identify an odour sensation verbally, even though the ability to distinguish between odorants or to recognize them may be normal

of any cause ranging from a cold, severe allergic rhinitis, chronic rhinosinusitis, to sarcoid or a vasculitis. Partial anosmia (an ability to detect some, but not all, qualitative olfactory sensations) usually follows when there has been some damage to the olfactory mucosa or bulb, and this may follow an influenza-like illness where the virus is neuropathic to the olfactory apparatus or following trauma such as a head injury or after nasal surgery. The extreme end of this spectrum is anosmia. What we do not know is that in a cohort of people who have had a neuropathic virus or head injury causing severe damage to their olfactory mucosa how many recover and after what length of time. In secondary care we see individuals whose sense of smell has only partially returned or failed to return and these may represent the minority who have not recovered as many may have done so in the first few weeks. It is difficult to predict the outcome in any individual and there are reports of an individual's sense of smell returning up to 7 years after these events, even though the basal cells which replace the neuroepithelium do so approximately every 40 days. Frontal blows are a common type of trauma that results in olfactory loss, but occipital blows, in themselves much less common, are much more likely to result in total anosmia. Amnesia for greater than 24 hours is an indicator of a poorer prognosis. Although it is often premature to dismiss the possibility that some or all of the patient's sense of smell may return, it is unwise to predict that it will improve, as recovery occurs in fewer than 10 per cent, with most occurring within 6 months.

Congenital anosmia is present in some females with Turner's syndrome and in individuals with premature baldness, vascular headaches, and other abnormalities. It presents remarkably late as the individual knows no difference. Patients with anosmia or severe hyposmia need to be advised about using smoke alarms. They may become fastidious about cleaning both themselves and their surroundings and avoid fragrances for fear of overuse.

Parosmia or cacosmia, from the Greek *kakos* (bad) *osme* (smell), can be even more disturbing than anosmia. These patients may also have had an influenza-like illness or head trauma resulting in the disruption of the neuronal pathways to the glomeruli in the olfactory bulb. Typically a particular substance such as coffee, perfume or smoke will initiate another sense of smell such as a chemical-like sensation, or, even more distressingly, a smell of faeces. In some individuals all olfactory substances induce the same sensation. It is important to exclude other causes such as anaerobic organisms in the paranasal sinuses, diseased teeth and, occasionally, organisms within the vestibular hairs.

The risk of mild hyposmia and anosmia following nasal surgery is about 30 per cent and 1 per cent, respectively.[29] Nasal and paranasal surgery can affect the olfactory pathway by direct trauma to the olfactory epithelium on the middle or superior turbinate, septum or cribriform plate, or by obstructing the olfactory cleft with adhesions. The olfactory mucosa should be preserved if at all possible, as to remove it will significantly affect an individual's quality of life (see Chapter 17).

OLFACTORY HALLUCINATIONS OR PHANTOSMIA

Olfactory hallucinations and phantosmia are both terms that apply to the perception of an odour in the absence of an olfactory stimulus. Olfactory hallucination can be a symptom of various non-nasal conditions such as head injury, epilepsy, migraine, cluster headache, schizophrenia, depression, bipolar mood disorders, eating disorders, substance misuse, iatrogenic, cerebral aneurysm and tumours.[30] Migrainous olfactory hallucinations are rare and there is usually a clear temporal relationship between episodes of headache and olfactory hallucination.

Epileptic olfactory auras are rare. Electroencephalogram (EEG) changes during the olfactory hallucination indicate an epileptic origin of the aura. Phantosmia following head injury is uncommon. Iatrogenic olfactory hallucination is sometimes seen in epileptic patients in the early stages of dopaminergic therapy and these patients frequently also have a synchronous visual hallucination. Olfactory hallucination is relatively rare in psychotic patients. The presence of olfactory hallucination along with psychosis indicates serious psychopathology with a poor prognosis.

Various modalities of treatments for idiopathic olfactory hallucinations have been reported in the literature and include surgical extirpation of the olfactory neuroepithelium,[31] ablation of the olfactory bulb[29] and sodium valproate.[30] Rhinosinusitis, viral infection of the upper respiratory tract and head injury with cribriform plate fracture have all been reported to be associated with phantosmia and sometimes with simultaneous parosmia. Nordin et al. found that 90 per cent of patients with chronic rhinosinusitis in their survey had experienced phantosmia.[32] Successful treatment of rhinosinusitis often alleviates olfactory symptoms of parosmia.

PROFUSE CLEAR RHINORRHOEA

Unilateral clear rhinorrhoea should be investigated to exclude a cerebrospinal fluid (CSF) leak. A specimen of the discharge must be sent for analysis of β_2 transferrin by immunofixation; this test has a high specificity and has superseded all other diagnostic techniques.[33] Unilateral autonomic rhinitis can appear very much like CSF rhinorrhoea, and it is essential that fluid is sent for β_2 transferrin analysis before surgery is contemplated.[34] Other causes that can feign a CSF leak are mucous retention cysts bursting regularly and nasal secretions pooling in the maxillary or another sinus and draining when the head is placed in a certain position.

Clear rhinorrhoea is typically caused by allergic rhinitis and it is a symptom that responds well to antihistamines. Topical nasal steroids can also help. If these measures are not enough, an ipratropium nasal spray applied four times a day along with an antihistamine and steroid spray will often suffice. Vidian neurectomy has been advocated but its effect only lasts for 6–9 months, even if fragments of bone are placed in the vidian canal.

CHRONIC COUGH

Upper respiratory tract infections are the commonest cause of an acute cough that, by definition, should have resolved within 2 months.[4] Patients with a cough lasting longer than this period are defined as having a chronic cough. Studies about the aetiology of chronic cough suggest that approximately 95 per cent of symptoms in immunocompetent, non-smoking patients with a normal or near-normal chest radiograph are caused by postnasal drip syndrome (PNDS), asthma, gastro-oesophageal reflux disease (GORD), chronic bronchitis, bronchiectasis, eosinophilic bronchitis or the use of an angiotensin-converting enzyme (ACE) inhibitor.[35] Less common causes such as bronchogenic carcinoma, left ventricular failure, sarcoidosis and tuberculosis may explain the remaining 5 per cent.

Physiologically, cough is a defence mechanism protecting the tracheobronchial tree. Afferent receptors are believed to be innervated through the vagus nerve via the pharyngeal, superior laryngeal and pulmonary branches. The tracheobronchial region has been suggested to have as great a role in the generation of cough as the larynx, as evidenced by the poor or absent cough of lung–heart transplant recipients with absent pulmonary vagal innervation. The glossopharyngeal and trigeminal nerves are also thought to carry cough impulses from receptors in the pharynx, nose and paranasal sinuses. Stimulation of the vagus can also initiate cough whether it is by stimulating the external auditory canal or by instilling acid into the lower third of the oesophagus.

No diagnostic test is said to define those who are diagnosed as having PNDS other than a response to a first-generation antihistamine. Examining the available evidence suggests that mechanical stimulation of the pharynx by mucus is not an adequate theory for the production of cough. Inflammatory mediators in the lower airways are raised in PNDS, cough variant asthma and GORD and the theory that an inflammatory process is affecting 'one airway' is a plausible one. Nasal disease is more likely to result in cough through the coexisting involvement of the lower airways through an as yet undefined pathway, and eosinophil – and mast cell – mediation appears a probable mechanism. Studies have shown that 60–78 per cent of asthmatic people also have rhinosinusitis.[36,37]

GASTRO-OESOPHAGEAL REFLUX DISEASE

Although symptoms elicited in the history such as heartburn, dysphagia, dysphonia, globus, acid regurgitation and a bitter taste in the mouth are helpful in suggesting a diagnosis, GORD has been shown to be asymptomatic or 'silent' in between 40 per cent and 75 per cent of patients with GORD-induced cough. Patients with laryngopharyngeal reflux when upright can have a chronic cough, dysphonia, globus, throat clearing, dysphagia and excessive throat mucus. It is best to consider GORD as a cause of chronic cough only after excluding PNDS and asthma, primarily by a failure to respond to treatment for these conditions. It has been suggested that chronic cough from any cause may precipitate GORD and thus commences a self-perpetuating cycle. This may be one explanation why GORD is often diagnosed in combination with another cause of chronic cough. How GORD triggers cough is not entirely clear. The two potential pathophysiological mechanisms are aspiration of gastric contents irritating the larynx or tracheobronchial tree, and second, an oesophago-bronchial reflex via the vagus nerve.

REFERENCES

1. Boat TF, Cheng PW, Leigh MW. Biochemistry of mucus. In: Takishima T, Shimura S, eds. *Airway secretion: lung biology in health and disease.* New York: Dekker, 1973:217–82.
2. Jones N. The nose and paranasal sinuses physiology and anatomy. *Adv Drug Deliv Rev* 2001; **51**: 5–19.
3. Quraishi MS, Jones NS, Mason J. The rheology of nasal mucus: a review. *Clin Otolaryngol* 1998; **23**: 403–13.
4. Morice AH. Post-nasal drip syndrome – a symptom to be sniffed at? *Pulm Pharmacol Ther* 2004; **17**: 343–5.
5. Acharya AN, Mirza S, Jones NS. Ice cold carbonated water: a therapy for persistent hyperawareness of pharyngeal mucus and throat clearing. *J Laryngol Otol* 2007; **121**: 354–7.
6. West B, Jones NS. Endoscopy-negative, computed tomography-negative facial pain in a nasal clinic. *Laryngoscope* 2001; **111**: 581–6.
7. Jones NS, Cooney TR. Facial pain and sinonasal surgery. *Rhinology* 2003; **41**: 193–200.
8. Clifton N, Jones NS. The prevalence of facial pain in 108 consecutive patients with paranasal mucopurulent discharge at endoscopy. *J Laryngol Otol* 2007; **121**: 345–8.
9. Tepper SJ. New thoughts on sinus headache. *Allergy Asthma Proc* 2004; **25**: 95–6.
10. Clifton N, Jones NS, Abu-Bakra M *et al.* The prevalence of nasal contact points in a population with facial pain and a control population. *J Laryngol Otol* 2001; **115**: 629–32.
11. Barbanti P, Fabbrini G, Perare M. Unilateral cranial autonomic symptoms in migraine. *Cephalagia* 2004; **22**: 256–9.
12. Hughes R, Jones NS. The role of endoscopy in outpatient management. *Clin Otolaryngol* 1998; **23**: 224–6.
13. Fahy C, Jones NS. Nasal polyposis and facial pain. *Clin Otolaryngol* 2001; **26**: 510–13.
14. Stewart MG. Sinus pain: is it real? *Curr Opin Otorhinolaryngol Head Neck Surg* 2002; **10**: 29–32.
15. Cady RK, Schreiber CP. Sinus headache: a clinical conundrum. *Otolaryngol Clin North Am* 2004; **37**: 267–88.
16. Headache Classification Committee of the International Headache Society. International Classification of Headache Disorders, 2nd edn. *Cephalgia* 2004; **24** Suppl 1: 1–151.
17. Daudia A, Jones NS. Facial migraine in a rhinological setting. *Clin Otolaryngol* 2002; **27**: 521–5.
18. Schreiber CP, Hutchinson S, Webster CJ. Prevalence of migraine among patients with a history of self-reported or physician diagnosed 'sinus' headaches. *Arch Intern Med* 2004; **13**: 164, 1769–72.
19. Levine HL, Setzen M, Cady RK *et al.* An otolaryngology, neurology, allergy, and primary care consensus on diagnosis and treatment of sinus headache. *Otolaryngol Head Neck Surg* 2006; **134**: 516–23.
20. Spierings ELH. Acute, subacute, and chronic headache. *Otolaryngol Clin North Am* 2003; **36**: 1095–107.
21. Bendtsen L. Central sensitization in tension-type headache – possible pathophysiological mechanisms. *Cephalagia* 2000; **20**: 486–508.
22. Jensen R, Olesen J. Tension-type headache: an update on mechanisms and treatment. *Curr Opin Neurol* 2000; **13**: 285–9.
23. Jones NS. Midfacial segment pain: implications for rhinitis and rhinosinusitis. *Clin Allergy Immunol* 2007; **19**: 323–33.
24. Wustrow TP, Kastenbauer E. Surgery of internal nasal valve. *Facial Plast Surg* 1995; **11**: 213–27.
25. Ren K, Dubner R. Central nervous system plasticity and persistent pain. *J Orofac Pain* 1999; **13**: 155–63.
26. Sessle BJ. Acute and chronic craniofacial pain: brainstem mechanisms of nociceptive transmission and neuroplasticity, and other clinical correlates. *Crit Rev Oral Biol Med* 2000; **11**: 57–91.
27. Lin TJ, Maccia CA, Turnier CG. Psychogenic intractable sneezing: case reports and a review of treatment options. *Ann Allergy Immunol* 2003; **91**: 575–8.
28. Fochtmann LJ. Intractable sneezing as a conversion symptom. *Psychosomatics* 1995; **36**: 103–12.
29. Kimmelman CP. The risk to olfaction from nasal surgery. *Laryngoscope* 1994; **104**: 981–8.
30. Majumdar S, Jones NS, McKerrow W *et al.* The management of idiopathic olfactory hallucinations. *Laryngoscope* 2003; **113**: 879–881.
31. Leopold DA. Successful treatment of phantosmia with preservation of olfaction. *Arch Otolaryngol Head Neck Surg* 1991; **117**: 1402–6.
32. Nordin S, Murphy C, Davidson T. Prevalence and assessment of qualitative olfactory dysfunction in different age groups. *Laryngoscope* 1996; **106**: 739–44.
33. Nandapalan V, Watson ID, Swift AC. Beta-2-transferrin and cerebrospinal fluid rhinorrhoea. *Clin Otolaryngol* 1996; **21**: 259–64.
34. Bateman N, Jones NS. Rhinorrhoea feigning cerebrospinal fluid leak: nine illustrative cases. *J Laryngol Otol* 2000; **114**: 462–4.
35. Irwin RS, Madison JM. The persistently troublesome cough. *Am J Respir Crit Care Med* 2002; **165**: 1469–74.
36. Poe RH, Israel RH, Utell MJ *et al.* Chronic cough: bronchoscopy or pulmonary function testing? *Am Rev Respir Dis* 1982; **126**: 160–2.
37. Poe RH, Harder RV, Israel RH *et al.* Chronic persistent cough – experience in diagnosis and outcome using an anatomic diagnostic protocol. *Chest* 1989; **95**: 723–8.

3

Medical management of rhinosinusitis

JEFFREY D SUH, JAMES N PALMER

INTRODUCTION

Rhinosinusitis affects an estimated 16 per cent of the adult population in the USA, translating to almost US$5.8 billion of direct healthcare costs in 1996. Most of these patients present to their primary care physician, resulting in approximately 18 million office visits a year. In a study analysing the epidemiology and health impact of sinusitis, Anand reported a total of 73 million restricted activity days.[1] There is also a marked impairment in quality of life, comparable with other chronic diseases such as chronic obstructive lung disease, angina and back pain.[2]

Rhinosinusitis is defined as symptomatic inflammation of the paranasal sinuses and nasal cavity. In 2007, the Task Force on Rhinosinusitis of the American Academy of Otolaryngology – Head and Neck Surgery (AAO-HNS) established definitions and classified the various types of rhinosinusitis. Table 3.1 gives the Task Force definitions of rhinosinusitis. These classifications are critical to understanding the variety of treatments of rhinosinusitis in adults.

The vast majority of cases of rhinosinusitis are acute, self-limiting viral events that follow an episode of the common cold. Fewer than 2 per cent of colds in adults and 30 per cent in children progress to bacterial rhinosinusitis. Chronic rhinosinusitis has been shown to be a much more complex disease and often has a multifactorial aetiology.

Table 3.1   Classification of sinusitis

	Duration
Acute sinusitis	<4 weeks
Subacute sinusitis	4–12 weeks
Chronic sinusitis	>12 weeks

The treatments described in this chapter are based on a number of factors including the type and the cause of the rhinosinusitis present, concurrent medical comorbidities, symptom severity and response to previous medical treatments. Rhinosinusitis may be viral, bacterial, fungal, anatomical, genetic or allergic in origin. The goals of medical management of rhinosinusitis include resolution of infection, resolution of mucosal disease, establishment of an open sinus ostium and prevention of medical complications.[3] It is important to note that although there are many potential strategies for medical management of rhinosinusitis, there is no standardized recommendation that defines 'maximal medical management'. It is estimated that 200 000 adults in the USA eventually undergo sinus surgery each year for chronic sinusitis that has not responded to medical management.

ACUTE SINUSITIS

In contrast to chronic rhinosinusitis (CRS), acute rhinosinusitis is most often thought to be caused by an infectious agent. Bacterial sinusitis is usually preceded by a viral upper respiratory tract infection (URTI). Other common conditions that can predispose a patient to acute sinusitis are cigarette smoke, anatomical factors such as nasal septum deformities and immune deficiencies. More than 200 different viruses are known to cause the symptoms of the common cold. The most frequently detected viruses include rhinovirus, respiratory syncytial virus, influenza virus and parainfluenza virus. Rhinovirus is the most common virus, causing an estimated 30–35 per cent of adult colds. There are more than 110 distinct rhinovirus types, and these are most active in early autumn, spring and summer.

Viral infection can promote acute bacterial rhinosinusitis (ABRS) by inducing oedema at the sinus ostia, which can lead to obstruction of sinus drainage. Mucus stasis can then provide favourable conditions for growth of bacteria. Nose blowing during an URTI has been implicated as another way that bacteria could be introduced into the sinuses.[4] Once the sinus drainage pathways are obstructed, there is a drop in the pH and oxygen content in the sinuses, which results in decreased mucociliary clearance of pathogens, and an environment for acute infection. Approximately 2 per cent of viral rhinosinusitis progresses to bacterial rhinosinusitis in adults.

The 2007 AAO-HNS Foundation guidelines serve to assist clinicians in differentiating acute viral rhinosinusitis (VRS) from ABRS.[5] Many of the symptoms of the two can be similar, but viral rhinosinusitis is usually self-limiting and the symptoms last for less than 10 days. Bacterial rhinosinusitis should be suspected if symptoms last longer than 10 days after the onset of the URTI, or if symptoms worsen after initial improvement. Past recommendations of applying major and minor symptoms such as fever, cough, fatigue, hyposmia, anosmia, maxillary dental pain, ear fullness/pressure to aid in the diagnosis of rhinosinusitis have fallen out of favour due to a lack of validated studies.[6] Fever has been shown to have a sensitivity and specificity of only about 50 per cent for ABRS.

While the initial diagnostic evaluation for acute rhinosinusitis should include a detailed physical examination, the only physical examination finding to have diagnostic value is purulence seen in the nasal cavity or posterior pharynx.[6] Purulent nasal drainage positively predicts the presence of bacteria on antral aspiration and radiographic evidence of ABRS.[5] Pain in the maxillary teeth is also a specific symptom of ABRS but is present in only 10 per cent of cases.

The AAO-HNS guidelines also discourage the use of radiographic imaging for the routine diagnosis of acute sinusitis. Imaging modalities such as plain films, computed tomography (CT) and magnetic resonance imaging (MRI) all show mucosal inflammation in the acute setting. Because sinus mucosal thickening is common in viral URTIs, it is impossible to distinguish bacterial from viral rhinosinusitis on imaging alone. Gwaltney *et al.* showed that the vast majority of patients undergoing CT during an acute episode of viral rhinosinusitis had improvement or resolution of findings on follow-up imaging 2 weeks later.[7]

Treatment of acute sinusitis

The goals of treating acute sinusitis are to reduce mucosal swelling, restore normal sinus function, relieve symptoms and prevent complications. Commonly prescribed treatments for acute sinusitis include watchful waiting, saline irrigation, decongestants, antihistamines, corticosteroids, mucolytics and antibiotics. Topical spray decongestants, such as oxymetazoline, ephedrine and phenylephrine, are helpful in relieving acute symptoms. Patients should be instructed not to use these topical

decongestants for longer than 3–4 consecutive days due to the risk of rhinitis medicamentosa. Saline irrigation is a simple and inexpensive means of softening viscous secretions and providing relief from congestion, and should be a first-line treatment. Ipratropium bromide nasal spray may be used for the symptomatic relief of rhinorrhoea associated with the common cold. Antihistamines have not been shown to be effective for the treatment of bacterial rhinosinusitis, and they can cause excessive dryness and sedation. Many of these treatments will be discussed in more detail in the treatment of chronic sinusitis below.

Antibiotics for acute sinusitis

The most commonly isolated bacteria from patients with acute bacterial sinusitis are *Streptococcus pneumoniae* (25–43 per cent), *Haemophilus influenza* (22–35 per cent) and *Moraxella catarrhalis* (2–10 per cent). Other less frequently seen bacterial pathogens include *Staphylococcus aureus* and anaerobic bacteria. The prevalence of antibiotic resistance to these bacteria is increasing with approximately 25 per cent of *Strep. pneumoniae* being penicillin resistant. Interestingly, *Strep. pneumoniae* also has high rates of resistance to other drugs: a third are resistant to trimethoprim/sulfamethoxazole and macrolides, a fifth to doxycycline and a tenth to clindamycin.

The AAO-HNS Task Force recommends that when antibiotics are given for the treatment of bacterial sinusitis, the first-line treatment should be amoxicillin. Amoxicillin is safe, affordable and effectively reaches high concentrations in sinus fluid. However, β-lactamase production can be found in up to 40 per cent of isolates of *H. influenzae*, *M. catarrhalis* and some strains of *Strep. pneumoniae*. Therefore, while we continue to use amoxicillin as a first-line treatment, we have a very low threshold for moving to other classes of antibiotics. In such treatment failures, we prescribe a fluoroquinolone or high-dose penicillin with a β-lactamase inhibitor.

CHRONIC SINUSITIS

Treatment of CRS is intended to reduce symptoms, improve the quality of life and prevent disease progression or recurrence. Medical management should be considered the cornerstone of treatment for acute and chronic rhinosinusitis. Surgery should be considered for medical failures or for patients with complications.

Medical therapies for chronic sinusitis

Medical management can be broken down into three large groups: antimicrobial, anti-inflammatory and mechanical (Fig. 3.1). It is helpful to break down treatments from each group, and combine them when appropriate into a

Maximal medical management

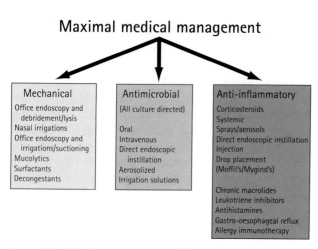

Figure 3.1   Medical management of chronic sinusitis.

comprehensive treatment plan. Also, the side effects of each therapy should be kept in mind, and weighed against the patient's symptom severity and other medical conditions. It is important to be cognizant that many therapies are time consuming and not all patients will be willing to invest the time necessary. Therefore, medical management of CRS must be tailored to each individual patient.

ANTIMICROBIAL TREATMENT

Oral antibiotics

Due to the multiple resistances and broad spectrum of flora in CRS, we believe antimicrobials should be given in a culture-directed fashion. After the correct antibiotic is chosen, there are multiple ways to deliver it, including oral, intravenous and topical. Antibiotic therapy for CRS has traditionally been aimed at a variety of aerobic and anaerobic bacteria. Studies have described a mix of bacteria, the most common anaerobes include *Peptostreptococcus*, *Prevotella*, *Fusobacterium*, *Actinomyces* and *Propionibacterium*. The most common aerobes include *Staph. aureus*, *Strep. pneumoniae*, *Pseudomonas aeruginosa*, *Moraxella catarrhalis*, *Strep. viridans* and *H. influenzae*. Antibiotics play a role in the management of CRS to decrease bacterial load and to treat acute bacterial exacerbations of CRS. In contrast to antibiotic therapy for acute sinusitis, antibiotics should be used for at least 3–4 weeks, as this will maximize their anti-inflammatory effect by lowering the bacterial load in the sinuses. Antimicrobials should not be used as a sole modality of therapy in CRS, as this is a disease of inflammation, not solely infection. Adjunctive therapy may include intranasal corticosteroids, saline irrigation, short courses of oral steroids and the other treatments discussed in this chapter.

Oral itraconazole is an antifungal that has been shown to be of benefit to patients with allergic bronchopulmonary aspergillosis (ABPA). It is hypothesized that itraconazole may similarly benefit patients with allergic fungal sinusitis, a disease similar to ABPA. Typical treatment of allergic fungal

sinusitis includes the use of nasal steroid sprays, oral steroids, and, occasionally, immunotherapy. Many patients require long courses of oral steroids to control their disease. Rains and Mineck[8] reviewed 137 patients with allergic fungal sinusitis treated with high-dose itraconazole (400 mg/day × 1 month, 300 mg/day × 1 month, 200 mg/day × 1 month, or until clear by endoscopy). This study concluded that itraconazole reduced the need for oral steroids and repeat surgical debridement. In another study of 16 patients with recurrent allergic fungal sinusitis, in 12 patients oral steroids could be stopped or the dose reduced after initiation of itraconazole therapy. Eleven of the 16 patients were recurrence free at 15.7 months. Known complications of itraconazole use include elevated liver enzymes, congestive heart failure, nausea, rash, headache, malaise, fatigue and oedema. We rarely use itraconazole, but in cases of suspected allergic fungal sinusitis with persistent mucosal oedema, we prescribe a 6-week course of 200 mg twice a day, with liver function testing at the beginning and end of therapy.

Topical antibiotics

Topical antibiotics have the theoretical advantage of high local levels of drug with minimal systemic absorption, lower costs and decreased morbidity. Vaughan and Carvalho[9] used 3-week courses of culture-directed topical antibiotics and demonstrated improvements in posterior nasal discharge, facial pain/pressure, a longer infection-free period and improved endoscopic appearance. There were no major side effects, and minor side effects were usually benign and self-limiting.

A study from the Cleveland Clinic found encouraging data on the use of topical mupirocin nasal irrigations as an alternative to intravenous antibiotics in the treatment of acute exacerbations of CRS due to meticillin-resistant *S. aureus* (MRSA).[10] Patients using mupirocin in sinus irrigations showed improved symptoms and reduced MRSA recovery on subsequent cultures. A more recent study has found that twice-a-day nasal irrigation with 0.05 per cent mupirocin in Ringer's solution improved endoscopic findings in 93 per cent of patients, while 75 per cent had symptom improvement.[11]

In theory, postsurgical patients are better candidates for the widespread delivery of topical antimicrobials than non-surgical patients. Kobayashi and Baba[12] demonstrated that in non-surgical patients concentrations of antibiotics used in irrigation did not reach sufficient levels in the maxillary sinus. However, in a review of topical antimicrobials for chronic sinusitis, Lim et al.[13] found studies showing efficacy in both surgical and non-surgical patients, but with higher levels of evidence for postsurgical patients.

ANTI-INFLAMMATORY TREATMENTS

Steroids

Topical nasal steroids and oral steroids are the cornerstone of medical treatment in CRS. Corticosteroids stabilize mast cells against mediator release, block formation of inflammatory mediators and inhibit chemotaxis of inflammatory cells. Clinically, steroids decrease mucosal inflammation, and can improve the sense of smell in the short term. Oral corticosteroids have also been shown to be effective in allergic rhinitis and allergic fungal sinusitis and reduce nasal polyps. Systemic corticosteroids are widely used in clinical practice for patients with CRS and nasal polyps. A double-blind, placebo-controlled trial of prednisolone, 50 mg daily for 14 days versus placebo, demonstrated improvement of sinonasal polyposis and symptoms as measured by the 31-item Rhinosinusitis Outcome Measure (RSOM-31) questionnaire, nasal endoscopy, and pre- and post-treatment MRI scans.[14] Woodworth *et al.* treated 21 patients with CRS with nasal polyps with 60 mg oral prednisone tapered over 3 weeks.[51] The study found that oral steroids decreased all measured chemokines and cytokines compared with placebo, along with improvement in 20-item Sinu-Nasal Outcome Test (SNOT-20) scores and the endoscopic examination for the patient population.

A number of studies have demonstrated the efficacy of intranasal steroids in the management of CRS. Nasal corticosteroids have been shown to inhibit both immediate and late phase reactions to antigenic stimulation in allergic rhinitis. In general, nasal steroids are poorly absorbed through the nasal mucosa and do not cause hypothalamic–pituitary–adrenal suppression when used at recommended doses. Table 3.2 lists some of the commonly used nasal steroids. Common adverse effects of nasal steroids include nasal irritation, mucosal bleeding and crusting. In a review of the use of intranasal steroids in CRS, Joe *et al.*[15] found that intranasal steroids were most beneficial in the treatment of CRS with polyps. The benefit of steroid nasal sprays for non-polypoid CRS has been harder to demonstrate. When combined with antibiotic use, efficacy in symptom reduction has been found during acute exacerbations.[16] Placement of drops at home can be done by the patient kneeling and then placing the forehead on the floor (Moffat's position) or with the head hanging off the bed (Mygind's position) (Fig. 3.2). For better frontal sinus penetration, an eyedropper can be used to instil approximately 0.25 mL of standard nasal steroid spray solution in either position, and the patient should remain in place for 5–15 minutes. This treatment regimen can have dramatic results (Fig. 3.3).

Table 3.2   Commonly used nasal steroids

Generic name	Brand name	Pregnancy class*
Triamcinolone	Nasacort	C
Fluticasone	Flonase, Veramyst	C
Mometasone	Nasonex	C
Rhinocort	Budesonide	B
Beclomethasone	Beconase	C

*WHO classification: A, always usable; B, broadly usable; C, caution/counselling; D, do not use.

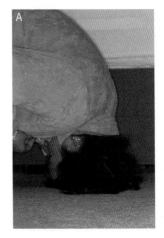
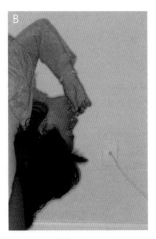

Figure 3.2   Nasal steroid drop instillation in (A) Moffat's position and (B) Mygind's position. Moffat's is best used in the preoperative patient, while Mygind's is best used in the postoperative patient.

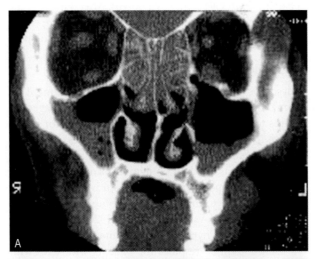
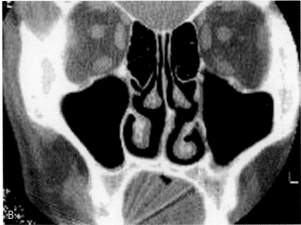

Figure 3.3   Same patient as in Figure 3.2. Computed tomography (CT) scans of the sinuses obtained: (A) after 1 year of topical intranasal steroids applied in the conventional upright spray manner; and (B) 3 months after nasal steroid drops applied in Moffat's position and held for 10 minutes twice daily. Patient symptoms had resolved.

Macrolide antibiotics

The use of long-term macrolide therapy originated in Japan, where it reduced the mortality rate of panbronchiolitis and concomitantly improved sinus symptoms. The theory of success with low-dose, long-term macrolide therapy is based more on the drugs' anti-inflammatory properties than antimicrobial properties. Macrolides have been found to inhibit inflammatory mediators such as interleukin (IL)-1 β, IL-8 and intercellular adhesion molecule-1.[17] Other effects include protecting bioactive phospholipids, reducing the number of neutrophils by accelerated apoptosis and increasing mucociliary transport.[18] In a double-blind, randomized placebo-controlled clinical trial of low-dose roxithromycin or placebo for 3 months in 64 subjects with CRS there were significant improvements in the SNOT-20 score, appearance at nasal endoscopy, saccharine transit time and IL-8 levels in lavage fluid in the macrolide group. A correlation was noted between improved outcome measures and low IgE levels.[19] In another study, erythromycin or clarithromycin was given to patients with CRS with nasal polyps. After 3 months the IL-8 level in nasal lavage was significantly decreased, which corresponded to a decrease in the size of the nasal polyps.[20]

Budesonide

Budesonide is used for the maintenance treatment of asthma and as prophylactic therapy in children aged 12 months to 8 years. Although it is not approved for use in sinusitis in the USA, use of budesonide respules (Pulmicort Respules; AstraZeneca LP, Wilmington, Delaware) in patients with nasal polyps or significant mucosal oedema has been gaining popularity. A recent study of patients with chronic sinusitis found that use of budesonide 0.25 mg once a day for 30 days improved SNOT-20 scores without suppression of the hypothalamic–pituitary–adrenal axis.[21] We use budesonide respules for patients with CRS with severe mucosal oedema or polyps, who do not respond to nasal corticosteroids. Dosing is one half respule per side once a day or twice a day, titrated based on endoscopic findings and clinical symptoms (Fig. 3.4).

Leukotriene inhibitors

Leukotriene inhibitors are systemic medications that are used for the treatment of asthma and allergic rhinitis (Table 3.3). They block leukotrienes that cause contraction of smooth muscle, chemotaxis and increased

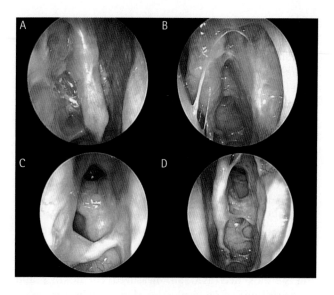

Figure 3.4   Same patient as in Figures 3.2 and 3.3, treated by nasal steroid spray only. (A, B) Treated with 1 month of budesonide respules delivered in Mygind's position, with no other changes to treatment regimen (C, D).

vascular permeability. A few studies have demonstrated some effect on reducing sinonasal symptoms and nasal polyps.[22] Leukotriene inhibitors have not been studied rigorously for CRS, and at this time are not considered as replacement for systemic corticosteroids. They may be considered as an adjunctive therapy in ASA (Samter's triad of asthma, salicylate intolerance and nasal polyps) triad cases of CRS. Recently the US Food and Drug Administration (FDA) has reported neuropsychiatric events with the use of leukotriene inhibitors including cases of agitation, aggression, hallucinations, depression, insomnia, irritability, restlessness, suicidal thinking and behaviour (including suicide) and tremor.

Antihistamines

Antihistamines work by competitive inhibition of histamine receptor sites on respiratory mucosal cells. Histamine type 1 (H1) blockers are most effective for atopic patients with symptoms of watery rhinorrhoea, sneezing and facial itching. Antihistamines are relatively ineffective in relieving chronic nasal congestion. Treatment guidelines from the Joint Task Force and World Health Organization (WHO) recommend that antihistamines, both topical (e.g. azelastine) and oral second-generation

Table 3.3   Leukotriene inhibitors

Name	Brand name	Pharmacology	Indications	Pregnancy class*
Montelukast	Singulair	Leukotriene receptor antagonist	Asthma, allergic rhinitis	B
Zafirlukast	Accolate	Leukotriene receptor antagonist	Asthma	B
Zileuton	Zyflo	Leukotriene synthesis inhibitor	Asthma	C

*WHO classification: A, always usable; B, broadly usable; C, caution/counselling; D, do not use.

(e.g. loratadine, desloratadine, fexofenadine, or cetirizine and levocetirizine) should be used as first-line therapy for allergic rhinitis.[23] Second-generation antihistamines have a higher affinity for the histamine receptor, with less of the sedating anticholinergic effect. Antihistamines have also been shown to block leukotriene and kinin release, and inhibit monocyte and lymphocyte chemotaxis.[24] Azelastine is a topical nasal second-generation antihistamine that has also demonstrated anti-inflammatory and mast cell stabilizing properties.[25,26] The effect of azelastine lasts at least 12 hours, thus allowing for a once or twice daily dosing regimen.

No clinical studies support the use of antihistamines in the treatment of patients with acute bacterial rhinosinusitis or CRS.[27] The anticholinergic effects of the first-generation antihistamines can cause excessive drying and impair mucus clearance by thickening mucus, which can cause more crust formation in the sinuses.

Immunotherapy

Although allergy has not been fully shown to be a contributing factor in CRS, most believe that allergy can play a role. At minimum, allergic rhinitis causes symptoms of nasal congestion, the most prevalent symptom of CRS. Therefore treatment of allergic rhinitis may help with symptom improvement in CRS. Allergy is considered to affect the sinuses through a combination of hypersecretion and obstruction of the ostiomeatal complex by mucosal oedema. The mechanism of immunotherapy is not completely understood. Immunotherapy most probably modifies the immune response to produce less IgE and more IgG. This mechanism involves the switching from Th2 response (allergic response) in favour of Th1 response (non-allergic response).[27] A Cochrane review concluded that injection immunotherapy is a safe and valid treatment for allergic rhinitis.[28] Injection immunotherapy is effective in improving symptoms and reducing the need for medication in patients with seasonal allergic rhinitis and improves disease-specific quality of life in these subjects.[28]

Mechanical treatments

IRRIGATION

Several randomized clinical trials report improved nasal symptoms with isotonic or hypertonic saline solutions. Patients with persistent inflammation should be instructed to perform nasal irrigations with saline at home. However, there is some evidence that irrigation may increase the frequency of Gram-negative organisms on culture. Therefore patients performing irrigations should be instructed to use sterile saline and regularly clean or dispose of the irrigation bottles or bulbs. Mucociliary clearance times improve after irrigation, especially for buffered hypertonic saline.[29] The method of irrigation does not seem to matter in symptom improvement.

Heatley et al. compared a bulb syringe to a nasal irrigation pot and found no difference in outcome and no difference in bacterial colonization rates.[30]

Tomooka et al. found that patients who used nasal irrigation for sinus problems reported significant improvements in 23 of 30 symptoms after 6 weeks of use.[31] The symptoms included nasal congestion, postnasal drip, seasonal/perennial allergies and nasal discharge. Compliance during this time period was 92 per cent. Unal et al. compared Ringer's lactate solution to isotonic saline and found patients who used Ringer's solution as irrigation after surgery had a significantly better mucociliary transport time than the patients using isotonic saline solution.[32]

Saline irrigation may be efficacious for secondary prevention of rhinosinusitis. In one unblinded trial, daily hypertonic saline nasal irrigation improved disease-specific quality of life after 6 months.[33] With adherence to therapy of 87 per cent, side effects were minimal and included: nasal irritation, epistaxis, nasal burning, tearing and headaches. In a follow-up study, a subset of patients reported reduced sinus symptoms and sinusitis-related medication use for an additional 12 months.[34]

Patient education on nasal irrigations is most effective when instruction includes patient participation to achieve proficiency in performing this technique. We routinely have our clinic staff teach patients proper technique during appointments. Clinicians should work with patients to develop strategies that facilitate incorporating saline nasal irrigations as part of routine sinus care. We believe it is more important for a patient to irrigate with any method than not irrigate at all. When able to choose, we prefer a large-volume, low-pressure squirt bottle that is easily cleaned.

MUCOLYTICS

Mechanical drainage can also be improved with a mucolytic. Guaifenesin is the most commonly used mucolytic to thin secretions and improve nasal and sinus drainage. There has only been one double-blind study of guaifenesin for rhinosinusitis, in human immunodeficiency virus (HIV)-positive patients who reported improved secretion drainage at doses of 2400 mg/day at 3 weeks. The guaifenesin group also reported less nasal congestion and thinner postnasal drainage compared with the placebo group.[35] It is important to inform patients about the possible side effect of nausea when using this drug in doses greater than 1200 mg/day.

SURFACTANTS

Chiu et al.[36] demonstrated the efficacy of 1 per cent baby shampoo nasal irrigations in patients with chronic rhinosinusitis. The patients were treated with twice-a-day sinus irrigation with 1 per cent baby shampoo, which led to improvement in SNOT-22 scores for nearly 50 per cent of patients who remained symptomatic despite surgical and conventional medical management. The greatest improvements were reduced thickened nasal secretions and postnasal drainage. Baby shampoo nasal irrigation has promise as an inexpensive, well-tolerated adjuvant therapy to conventional medical therapies for symptomatic patients after functional endoscopic sinus surgery (FESS).

DECONGESTANTS

Decongestants are α-adrenergic agonists that induce the release of noradrenaline (norepinephrine) from sympathetic nerves, leading to vasoconstriction of the nasal vasculature. Common adverse effects are insomnia, heart palpitations and hypertension. These side effects are more common with oral decongestants than nasal sprays due to less systemic absorption. They are used for relief of nasal congestion, but no studies have demonstrated quicker resolution of sinusitis with topical decongestants. Table 3.4 lists some of the commonly used oral and topical decongestants.

In patients with stable hypertension, decongestants have not been shown to seriously increase blood pressure. Decongestants should be used with caution in patients with ischaemic heart disease, glaucoma or prostatic hypertrophy.[37] Decongestants should not be combined with monoamine oxidase (MAO) inhibitors. Decongestants such as pseudoephedrine, considered class B for pregnancy, carry a small risk of vasoconstriction of the uterine arteries and have been associated with the development of gastroschisis. This theory is debatable as evidence suggests that this effect is negligible at typical dosages.[38] Symptoms are improved with topical decongestants, but reduced mucosal blood flow may increase inflammation[39] and increase ciliary loss.[40] Decongestants should not be used for longer than 3 days to avoid rebound vasodilation.

ALTERNATIVE MEDICINE

The use of alternative therapies to treat health conditions has been gaining increasing attention from both patients and healthcare providers. It is estimated that 40 per cent of Americans use a form of complementary medicine with an estimated cost of US$21 billon annually.[41] In the past 20 years, there has been an expansion of the use of complementary and alternative therapies among patients.

Acupuncture has been used as a complementary therapy for a variety of medical conditions including rhinosinusitis.[42] Acupuncture is the placement of disposable, single-use needles at specific points to elicit a specific therapeutic action. Research has demonstrated replicable physiological effects, including changes in plasma levels of endorphins and enkephalins, and stress-related hormones, such as adrenocorticotropic hormone.[43] Pothman and Yeh demonstrated a favourable effect of acupuncture in the treatment of children and young adults with chronic maxillary sinusitis.[44] Acupuncture has been found to have beneficial effects on sinusitis-related pain,[45] postoperative nausea and vomiting, postoperative pain, analgesic requirements and opioid related side effects.[46] Complications related to acupuncture are rare, making it a safe alternative treatment avenue, although it has little literature backing its efficacy in the treatment of CRS.[47]

Heatley et al.[30] compared CRS patients treated with nasal irrigation with patients who received daily reflexology massage. They found that daily reflexology massage was as effective as saline irrigation in improving symptoms of CRS in over 70 per cent of subjects. Because the usage of alternative medicine is increasing in the general population, rhinologists should be aware of its potential positive and negative impacts on rhinosinusitis.

WHAT IS MAXIMAL MEDICAL THERAPY?

To date, there is no consensus on 'maximal medical therapy' for CRS. Chronic rhinosinusitis has a multifactorial aetiology, and therefore its treatments are diverse and often patient specific. The exact medical regimen chosen will vary from individual to individual and must take into account previous treatments and known contributing factors.

Our treatment regimen for primary CRS in a patient who has never had surgery includes a combination of 3–4 weeks of culture-directed antibiotics, oral steroid burst (prednisone 60 mg × 3 days, 40 mg × 3 days, 20 mg × 3 days, then 10 mg once daily × 3 doses) and daily isotonic nasal irrigation. Re-evaluation by endoscopy, symptoms and possible CT imaging is performed at 4–6 weeks before entertaining the thought of surgical intervention. Another round of medical treatment including antibiotics and oral steroids is always an alternative to surgery. In the setting of prior surgery and new/recalcitrant symptoms, we will first

Table 3.4   Commonly used decongestants

Decongestants	Medication	Dosage
Oral	Pseudoephedrine	60 mg every 6 hours or 120 mg every 12 hours
Topical	Phenylephrine (Neo-Synephrine)	2 sprays every 4 hours
	Oxymetazoline (Afrin)	2 sprays every 12 hours NB Should not be used for more than 3 days

perform a new history and examination before choosing medical therapies.

The European Position Paper on Rhinosinusitis and Nasal Polyps (EP3OS) consensus document provides a summary that complements this chapter.[48]

SELECTED CASES

Acute exacerbation of chronic sinusitis

The treatment of a typical acute exacerbation of CRS usually entails a shorter course of oral antibiotics (1–3 weeks), nasal irrigation, and an oral steroid taper. Antibiotics should be culture directed or provide broad spectrum coverage. Commonly used antibiotics in this scenario include amoxicillin/clavulanate potassium 875 mg twice daily or levofloxacin 500 mg once a day for 1–3 weeks. Alternatives include sulfamethoxazole/trimethoprim double strength twice daily or clindamycin 150 mg thrice daily, depending on the culture and sensitivity. A common prednisone taper is 60 mg × 3 days, 40 mg × 3 days, 20 mg × 3 days, followed by 10 mg once daily × 3 doses. The taper is adjusted for body habitus, medical comorbidities and treatment response. Nasal irrigation is especially useful in the postoperative patient and should be done at least twice a day. Additives such as baby shampoo or mupirocin will be considered. Imaging is not routinely performed if there is a good endoscopic appearance.

Nasal polyps

Severe nasal polyps are usually treated surgically to reduce the bulk of the disease. Following surgery, patients usually continue prednisone (usually 0.2 mg/kg/day then 0.1 mg/kg/day) until there is endoscopic evidence of decreased oedema. The dose is approximately 20 mg/day then 10 mg/day in a 70 kilogram patient. These patients will also be placed on nasal steroid sprays or Pulmicort respules (high-dose budesonide). As mentioned above, Pulmicort is not approved by the FDA for the treatment of CRS, thus in the USA, patients must be made aware of this off-label use. Following irrigation with nasal saline, one-half Pulmicort respule (0.5 mg/2 mL of budesonide) is used in each nostril for 10–12 minutes in the head hanging position. Over time, the dose of Pulmicort is decreased to 0.25 mg/2 mL and then once daily depending on treatment response (see Fig. 3.4). While we routinely use antibiotics after sinus surgery, they are not continued after the first postoperative visit unless there is evidence of infection.

PREOPERATIVE REGIMEN

Patients with severe nasal polyps are usually given a course of oral steroids prior to surgery. Sieskiewicz *et al.* showed that in patients with severe nasal polyps treated preoperatively with steroids (prednisone 30 mg × 5 days) there was a better surgical field and better endoscopic visualization than in patients not treated with steroids.[49] Although intraoperative blood loss was similar between the steroid and control groups, the authors also found that surgical time was reduced when steroids were used. Wright and Agrawal found that sinus surgery was rated to be more difficult in patients not given preoperative steroids when compared with patients given steroids (prednisone 30 mg × 5 days).[50] We also use steroids preoperatively, using a prednisone taper (60 mg × 3 days, 40 mg × 3 days, 20 mg until surgery) and taper postoperatively. Also, when possible, total intravenous anaesthesia with propofol–remifentanil is used with controlled hypotension to reduce intraoperative blood loss and to improve visibility in the surgical field. A standard immediate postoperative regimen includes prednisone 20 mg/day tapered at 1 month, 2 weeks of culture-directed antibiotics or empirical antibiotics (sulfamethoxazole and trimethoprim double strength twice daily × 2 weeks, and clindamycin 150 mg thrice daily × 2 weeks) and isotonic nasal saline irrigations twice daily.

CONCLUSION

Medical therapy of CRS is best individualized for each patient, with special attention given to identifying at least one treatment modality from each of the categories of antimicrobial, anti-inflammatory and mechanical cleansing. While 'maximal medical management for CRS' has not been rigorously defined, at minimum it includes prolonged antimicrobial therapy and aggressive anti-inflammatory treatment, such as oral prednisone. Only when these medical modalities have been attempted and identified as unsuccessful should surgery be considered as a treatment option.

REFERENCES

1. Anand VK. Epidemiology and economic impact of rhinosinusitis. *Ann Otol Rhinol Laryngol* 2004; **193** Suppl: S3–S5.
2. Glikilich RE, Metson R. The health impact of chronic sinusitis in patients seeking otolaryngologic care. *Otolaryngol Head Neck Surg* 1995; **113**: 104–9.
3. Kennedy DW, Gwaltney JM, Jones JG. Medical management of sinusitis: educational goals and management guidelines. The International Conference on Sinus Disease. *Ann Otol Rhinol Laryngol* 1995; **167** Suppl: 22–30.
4. Gwaltney JM Jr, Hendley JO, Phillips CD *et al.* Nose blowing propels nasal fluid into the paranasal sinuses. *Clin Infect Dis* 2000; **30**: 387–91.
5. Rosenfeld RM, Andes D, Bhattacharyya N *et al.* Clinical practice guideline: adult sinusitis. *Otolaryngol Head Neck Surg* 2007; **137** Suppl 3: S1–31.

6. Pearlman A, Conley D. Review of current guidelines related to the diagnosis and treatment of rhinosinusitis. *Curr Opin Otolaryngol Head Neck Surg* 2008; **16**: 226–30.

7. Gwaltney JM Jr, Phillips CK, Miller RD *et al.* Computed tomographic study of the common cold. *N Engl J Med* 1994; **330**: 25–30.

8. Rains BM 3rd, Mineck CW. Treatment of allergic fungal sinusitis with high-dose itraconazole. *Am J Rhinol* 2003; **17**: 1–8.

9. Vaughan WC, Carvalho G. Use of nebulized antibiotics for acute infections in chronic sinusitis. *Otolaryngol Head Neck Surg* 2002; **127**: 558–68.

10. Solares CA, Batra PS, Hall GS *et al.* Treatment of chronic rhinosinusitis exacerbations due to methicillin-resistant *Staphylococcus aureus* with mupirocin irrigations. *Am J Otolaryngol* 2006; **27**: 161–5.

11. Uren B, Psaltis A, Wormald PJ. Nasal lavage with mupirocin for the treatment of surgically recalcitrant chronic rhinosinusitis. *Laryngoscope* 2008; **118**: 1677–80.

12. Kobayashi T, Baba S. Topical use of antibiotics for paranasal sinusitis. *Rhinology* 1992; **14** Suppl: 77–81.

13. Lim M, Citardi MJ, Leong JL. Topical antimicrobials in the management of chronic rhinosinusitis: a systematic review. *Am J Rhinol* 2008; **22**: 381–9.

14. Hissaria P, Smith W, Wormald PJ *et al.* Short course of systemic corticosteroids in sinonasal polyposis: a double-blind, randomized, placebo-controlled trial with evaluation of outcome measures. *J Allergy Clin Immunol* 2006; **118**: 128–33.

15. Joe SA, Thambi R, Huang J. A systematic review of the use of intranasal steroids in the treatment of chronic rhinosinusitis. *Otolaryngol Head Neck Surg* 2008; **139**: 340–7.

16. Statham MM, Seiden A. Potential new avenues of treatment for chronic rhinosinusitis: an anti-inflammatory approach. *Otolaryngol Clin North Am* 2005; **38**: 1351–65.

17. Shinkai M, Henke MO, Rubin BK. Macrolide antibiotics as immunomodulatory medications: proposed mechanisms of action. *Pharmacol Ther* 2008; **117**: 393–405.

18. Lund VJ. Maximal medical therapy for chronic rhinosinusitis. *Otolaryngol Clin North Am* 2005; **38**: 1301–10.

19. Wallwork B, Coman W, Mackay-Sim A *et al.* A double-blind, randomized, placebo-controlled trial of macrolide in the treatment of chronic rhinosinusitis. *Laryngoscope* 2006; **116**: 189–93.

20. Yamada Y, Fujieda S, Mori S *et al.* Macrolide treatment decreased the size of nasal polyps and IL-8 levels in nasal lavage. *Am J Rhinol* 2000; **14**: 143–8.

21. Sachanandani NS, Piccirillo JF, Kramper MA *et al.* The effect of nasally administered budesonide respules on adrenal cortex function in patients with chronic rhinosinusitis. *Arch Otolaryngol Head Neck Surg* 2009; **135**: 303–7.

22. Parnes SM. The role of leukotriene inhibitors in patients with paranasal sinus disease. *Curr Opin Otolaryngol Head Neck Surg* 2003; **11**: 184–91.

23. Bousquet J, van Cauwenberge PB, Khaltaev N *et al.* Allergic rhinitis and its impact on asthma: ARIA workshop report. *J Allergy Clin Immunol* 2001; **108**: S147–S334.

24. Nalebuff DJ. Allergic rhinitis. Chapter 36. In: Cummings CW, Fredrickson JM, Harker LA, eds. *Otolaryngology – head and neck surgery.* St Louis: CV Mosby, 1986:651–62.

25. Horak F. Effectiveness of twice daily azelastine nasal spray in patients with seasonal allergic rhinitis. *Ther Clin Risk Manag* 2008; **4**: 1009–22.

26. Bernstein JA. Azelastine hydrochloride: a review of pharmacology, pharmacokinetics, clinical efficacy and tolerability. *Curr Med Res Opin* 2007; **23**: 2441–52.

27. Benninger MS, Anon J, Mabry RL. The medical management of rhinosinusitis. *Otolaryngol Head Neck Surg* 1997; **117**: S41–9.

28. Calderon MA, Alves B, Jacobson M *et al.* Allergen injection immunotherapy for seasonal allergic rhinitis. *Cochrane Database Syst Rev* 2007; 1–24.

29. Talbott AR, Herr TM, Parsons DM. Mucociliary clearance and buffered hypertonic saline solution. *Laryngoscope* 1997; **107**: 500–3.

30. Heatley DG, McConnell KE, Kille TL *et al.* Nasal irrigation for the alleviation of sinonasal symptoms. *Otolaryngol Head Neck Surg* 2001; **125**: 44–8.

31. Tomooka LT, Murphy C, Davidson TM. Clinical study and literature review of nasal irrigation. *Laryngoscope* 2000; **110**: 1189–93.

32. Unal M, Görür K, Ozcan C. Ringer-lactate solution versus isotonic saline solution on mucociliary function after nasal septal surgery. *J Laryngol Otol* 2001; **115**: 796–7.

33. Rabago D, Zgierska A, Mundt M *et al.* Efficacy of daily hypertonic saline nasal irrigation among patients with sinusitis: a randomized controlled trial. *J Fam Pract* 2002; **51**: 1049–55.

34. Rabago D, Pasic T, Zgierska A *et al.* The efficacy of hypertonic saline nasal irrigation for chronic sinonasal symptoms. *Otolaryngol Head Neck Surg* 2005; **133**: 3–8.

35. Wawrose SF, Tami TA, Amoils CP. The role of guaifenesin in the treatment of sinonasal disease in patients infected with the human immunodeficiency virus (HIV). *Laryngoscope* 1992; **102**: 1225–8.

36. Chiu AG, Palmer JN, Woodworth BA *et al.* Baby shampoo nasal irrigations for the symptomatic post-functional endoscopic sinus surgery patient. *Am J Rhinol* 2008; **22**: 34–7.

37. Scheid DC, Hamm RM. Acute bacterial rhinosinusitis in adults: part II. Treatment. *Am Fam Physician* 2004; **70**: 1697–704.

38. Black RA, Hill DA. Over-the-counter medications in pregnancy. *Am Fam Physician* 2003; **67**: 2517–24.

39. Bende M, Fukami M, Arfors KE *et al.* Effect of oxymetazoline nose drops on acute sinusitis in the rabbit. *Ann Otol Rhinol Laryngol* 1996; **105**: 222–5.

40. Min YG, Kim HS, Suh SH *et al.* Paranasal sinusitis after long-term use of topical nasal decongestants. *Acta Otolaryngol* 1996; **116**: 465–71.

41. Eisenberg DM, Davis RB, Ettner SL *et al.* Trends in

alternative medicine use in the United States, 1990–1997: Results of a follow up national survey. *JAMA* 1998; **280**: 1569–75.

42. Pletcher SD, Goldberg AN, Lee J *et al.* Use of acupuncture in the treatment of sinus and nasal symptoms: results of a practitioner survey. *Am J Rhinol* 2006; **20**: 235–7.

43. Kaptchuk TJ. Acupuncture: theory, efficacy, and practice. *Ann Intern Med* 2002; **136**: 374–83.

44. Pothman R, Yeh HL. The effects of treatment with antibiotics, laser and acupuncture upon chronic maxillary sinusitis in children. *Am J Chin Med* 1982; **10**: 55–8.

45. Lundeberg T, Laurell G, Thomas M. The effect of acupuncture on sinus pain and experimentally induced pain. *Ear Nose Throat J* 1988; **67**: 565–9.

46. Agarwal A, Ranjan R, Dhiraaj S *et al.* Acupressure for prevention of pre-operative anxiety: a prospective, randomised, placebo controlled study. *Anaesthesia* 2005; **60**: 978–981.

47. Ernst E. Acupuncture – a critical analysis. *J Intern Med* 2006; **259**: 125–37.

48. Fokkens W, Lund V, Kaplan AP *et al.* EP3OS. 2007: European position paper on rhinosinusitis and nasal polyps. *Rhinology* 2007; **45**(2): 97–101.

49. Sieskiewicz A, Olszewska E, Rogowski M *et al.* Preoperative corticosteroid oral therapy and intraoperative bleeding during functional endoscopic sinus surgery in patients with severe nasal polyposis: a preliminary investigation. *Ann Otol Rhinol Laryngol* 2006; **115**: 490–4.

50. Wright ED, Agrawal S. Impact of perioperative systemic steroids on surgical outcomes in patients with chronic rhinosinusitis with polyposis: evaluation with the novel Perioperative Sinus Endoscopy (POSE) scoring system. *Laryngoscope* 2007; **117** Suppl 115: 1–28.

51. Woodworth BA, Joseph K, Kaplan AP *et al.* Alterations in eotaxin, monocyte chemoattractant protein-4, interleukin-5, and interleukin-13 after systemic steroid treatment for nasal polyps. *Otolaryngol Head Neck Surg* 2004; **131**(5): 585–9.

4

Technical advances and the endoscopically assisted bimanual technique

DANIEL B SIMMEN

INTRODUCTION

The bimanual technique has expanded the range of surgery and it allows more precise surgery to be carried out with better visibility. In classical endoscopic sinus surgery, the endoscopic surgeon holds the endoscope with one hand while carrying out the surgical procedure with the other hand. The surgeon will spend a lot of time sucking blood out, removing the sucker, inserting the surgical instrument and then they have to repeat the process when blood has recollected. From the ergonomic viewpoint this way of working is inefficient. With only one free hand for surgery, as the other has to hold the endoscope, it is also difficult to retract any structure out of the way, or for tension to be placed on any tissue that needs to be cut (Fig. 4.1).

The indications for endoscopic surgery of the paranasal sinuses are expanding, so that now not only complex

procedures of the frontal sinuses and anterior wall of the maxillary sinus can be done, but tumours of the skull base and pterygopalatine fossa can also be removed. It is difficult to conduct these expanded operations using the classical 'one-handed' technique. Removal of bone and tumour tissue and controlling bleeding at the same time is particularly difficult to accomplish with only one hand available to hold either an instrument or a sucker. Increasingly it helps if the surgeon can operate with both hands. The bimanual technique requires a second surgeon to hold and direct the video endoscope, enabling the endoscopic surgeon to use both hands while operating. With this technique the leading surgeon can apply microsurgical principles by dissecting, manipulating, cutting or punching tissue delicately. This method can also improve interdisciplinary cooperation. It helps that two surgeons can interact and do specific parts of the operation according to their skills and the demands of the different surgical steps (Fig. 4.2).

CONVENTIONAL ENDOSCOPIC SINUS SURGERY

Chronic rhinosinusitis has an incidence of 3–5 per cent, making it one of the most prevalent diseases.[1,2] Many patients with chronic rhinosinusitis do not respond adequately to pharmacological therapy. Endoscopic surgery of the paranasal sinuses offers a therapeutic option although it is usually necessary to combine it with medical treatment.[3] Since endoscopic sinus surgery was first described over 30 years ago there have been impressive advances in operative techniques.[4–7] Better endoscopes,

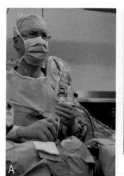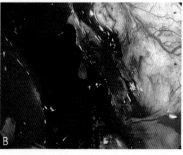

Figure 4.1 Classical endoscopic sinus surgery. The surgeon (A) holds the endoscope with one hand, (B) while carrying out the surgical procedure with the other hand, and spends a lot of time sucking blood out.

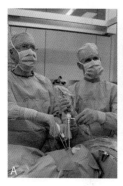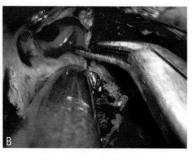

Figure 4.2 The bimanual technique requires (A) a second surgeon to hold and direct the video endoscope enabling (B) the endoscopic surgeon to follow microsurgical principles.

video cameras, and improved operating instruments have made it possible to see every crevice in great detail and remove tissue to within a millimetre.

As mentioned at the start of this chapter, in the classical technique, the surgeon holds the endoscope in one hand and uses the other hand to perform the operation. This one-handed technique has its limitations. It is particularly difficult to remove bone and tumour tissue and control bleeding with just one hand. The use of powered instrumentation has helped to allow suction to take place at the same time as surgery as it also means that some traction is placed on loose tissue through suction before a sharp jaw of the shaver cuts the tissue that has been aspirated into it.[8] This technique helps to remove nasal polyps efficiently but it cannot be used near the periorbita, pterygopalatine fossa or vital structures such as the carotid artery or optic nerve, as it can all too easily cause damage.

The indications for endoscopic sinus procedures are constantly being expanded. Technological advances, especially in computed tomography (CT)/magnetic resonance imaging (MRI)/merged scans and image-guided surgery have improved the surgeon's concept of the anatomy in relation to both benign and malignant diseases of the paranasal sinuses and skull base.

ADVANTAGES OF THE ENDOSCOPICALLY ASSISTED BIMANUAL OPERATING TECHNIQUE

Operating with both hands

The difficulties mentioned above mean that it is very useful for the endoscopic surgeon to be able to use both hands while operating.[9,10] In this bimanual technique an assistant holds the video endoscope, thus freeing both of the surgeon's hands so that he or she can deal more effectively with severe bleeding or dissecting tissue planes (see Fig. 4.2A). The assistant is responsible for directing the endoscope and keeping a steady image of the operative field displayed on the video monitor. This technique not only allows the operative field to be kept clearer of blood

but it also means that the surgeon can retract with one instrument and cut tissue with the other. Cutting tissue is far more exact than tearing it and this can only be done cleanly when the tissue is under tension.

The bimanual technique differs from procedures done under a microscope. Although the microscope allows surgeons to operate with both hands, the endoscopic technique has the advantage of providing a more magnified view that is unencumbered by the walls of the nasal passages. It also eliminates the problem of loss of light caused by instruments in the path of the microscope light beam, since the endoscopic light source is always delivered to the exact site. The endoscopically assisted bimanual technique thus combines the advantages of the endoscopic technique with the key advantage of the operating microscope, namely the ability to operate with both hands (Fig. 4.3). The endoscopically assisted bimanual technique was first described by May et al. in 1990.[9] Despite the advantages of the bimanual technique, the classical one-handed technique is still practised more widely. The main reason for this is that the bimanual technique requires an extra assistant. However, the advantages of the bimanual technique, especially the improved visualization of the operative field due to the constant presence of a suction tip, make it possible to perform more complex procedures on the paranasal sinuses with greater safety and precision. This particularly applies to the more severe

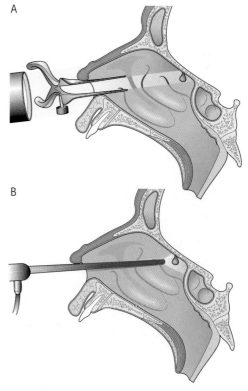

Figure 4.3 (A) The microscope allows the surgeon to operate with both hands but the main disadvantage is the lack of a close-up view through the narrow nostril and the loss of light. (B) The endoscope allows close-up and angled views with optimal illumination.

forms of chronic rhinosinusitis with polyposis, revision procedures and tumour resection. Moreover, a recent study has documented a reduction in operating time when the bimanual technique is used.[11] The shorter operating time leads to lower costs, and this saving more than offsets the added costs for the extra assistant.

Suction tip stays in the operative field resulting in fewer instrument changes

Surgical procedures on inflamed mucosa and vascular tumours cause relatively heavy bleeding, which may obscure the surgeon's view of the operation site. Clear visualization of the operative site is essential for anatomical orientation, and therefore the blood should be removed as rapidly as possible. In the classical one-handed technique, the surgeon must frequently remove and exchange the operating instrument for a suction device. These frequent instrument changes not only prolong the operation but also increase the likelihood that the distal lens of the endoscope will become soiled or smeared. With the bimanual technique, the surgeon can keep the suction tip in the operative field at all times while having the other hand free for cutting tissue (Fig. 4.4). In this way the operative field remains largely free of blood, resulting in better visualization and anatomical orientation and less frequent instrument changes. This is the major reason why the operating time is approximately 20 per cent shorter with the bimanual technique than with the one-handed technique. The ability to keep the suction tip in the operative field also facilitates bone removal with a drill or bur as it allows irrigation fluid to be aspirated as well.

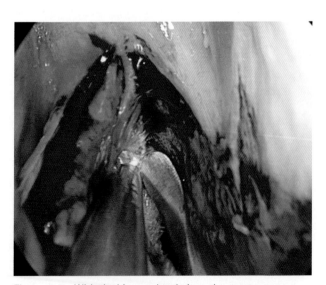

Figure 4.4   With the bimanual technique the surgeon can keep the suction tip (left hand) in the operating field at all times and dissect at the same time (dissection of a skull base tumour along the skull base). Reproduced with permission from *Chemical Senses*.[12]

Optimum exposure

The bimanual technique allows better operative exposure since the second instrument can be used to retract tissue (Fig. 4.5). For example, the suction tip can be used to gently push the middle turbinate medially towards the nasal septum, making it easier to see into the ethmoid sinuses and help access. In the resection of tumours it is often necessary to retract tissue that is obscuring other structures in order to find or create a tissue plane, and this is better done with the bimanual technique.

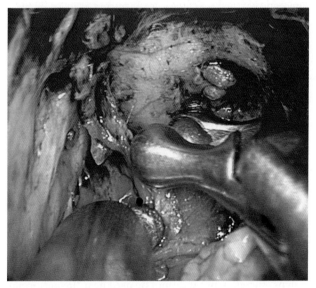

Figure 4.5   Better operative exposure by pressing tissue down from the skull base and making it easier to access narrow areas.

Holding and cutting

The bimanual technique allows for greater precision in manipulating and cutting tissue. For example, the surgeon

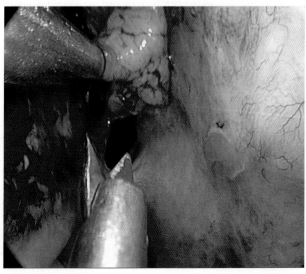

Figure 4.6   Greater precision is achieved by holding and cutting tissue at the same time.

can use the suction tip to hold the tissue in place while simultaneously removing it by cutting it off from the surrounding tissue with scissors (Fig. 4.6). A precise cut produces a smaller wound and less bleeding than if the tissue is avulsed. The 'hold-and-cut' technique eliminates the danger of removing too much tissue by avulsing tissue with a grasper.

Teamwork

The endoscopically assisted bimanual technique requires an assistant who *actively* participates in the procedure by controlling the camera position. This may be an advantage as it offers a constant opportunity to discuss the intraoperative situation 'as a team'. For example, the assistant may focus attention on critical anatomical structures that the surgeon might otherwise be too busy to notice (Fig. 4.7). By promoting an ongoing mutual exchange of information this team approach has the potential to improve the quality of the operation. Furthermore an interdisciplinary team can carry out a procedure, with individual members sharing their ideas and knowledge about the approach and method used to remove the tumour. Each step of the operation can be done by the individual whose expertise is best suited to that aspect of the operation. This team approach has the potential to improve the quality of the operation.

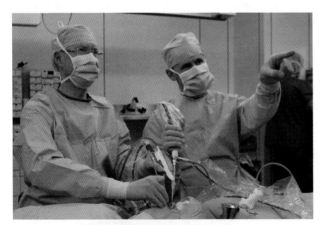

Figure 4.7   The endoscopically assisted bimanual technique requires a second surgeon who actively participates in the procedure and discusses the intraoperative situation as a team.

Training

The bimanual technique is ideal for training purposes. The experienced surgeon can assist an inexperienced colleague and can take over the procedure at any time. This is an added benefit to having two surgeons involved in the case during the whole operation (Fig. 4.8).

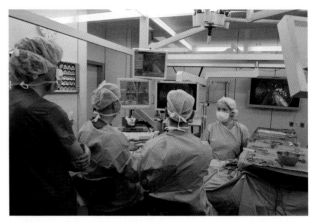

Figure 4.8   Bimanual technique is ideal for training and teaching purposes.

THEATRE SET-UP

The essential part of the equipment for the endoscopically assisted bimanual operating technique is a video camera attached to the endoscope and a video monitor of good size and quality, which provides the surgeon with the necessary image. The assistant holds the endoscope and is responsible for maintaining an optimum visual display of the operative field (Fig. 4.9). Separating the two tasks – keeping the operative field on the camera screen and carrying out the operation – requires good communication between the surgeon and the assistant. The surgeon instructs the assistant which part of the operative field to focus on. This requires some degree of training and learning together between the two operators, but we know from experience that smooth and effective teamwork can be quickly established.

Several years of experience with this technique have shown that coordination between surgeon and assistant runs like clockwork and that communication during the operation focuses almost entirely on the details of the operation itself, rather than on issues of coordination.

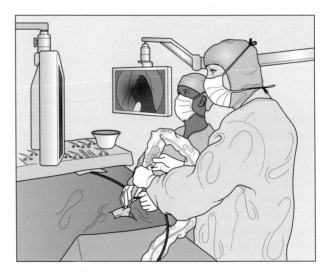

Figure 4.9   Theatre set-up for the bimanual assisted technique.

Theatre layout

The surgeon and assistant sit or stand next to each other. The video monitor is placed on the opposite side so that the operators can watch it without having to turn their heads. This makes it easier to operate for an extended period of time without experiencing neck strain. A nurse keeps the surgical instruments ready near the foot of the table next to the video monitor so that they can be passed during the procedure (Fig. 4.10). It is best if the surgeon does not need to look away from the screen when the instrument is passed. This means that the assistant should learn how to place the instrument in the surgeon's hand so that it is ready to use. Whenever possible, an extra video monitor should be set up so that the nurse can follow the procedure more closely and anticipate the need for particular instruments.

The anaesthetic equipment should be placed at the foot of the operating table to leave space at the head of the table for the operating team, which includes the scrub nurse, operating instruments and additional technical equipment (video cart, navigation unit).

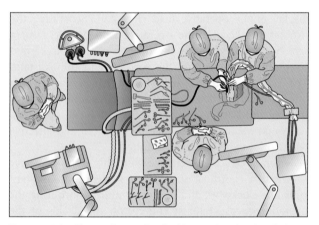

Figure 4.10   Theatre layout for the bimanual assisted technique.

PRACTICAL HINTS

Ergonomic handling of the endoscope

The endoscope may be held with one or both hands, depending on which is more comfortable for the second surgeon. The flexible cold light cable should be brought out of the top or side of the operative area so that it will not interfere with the surgeon and the passage of instruments. This also applies to the connecting cable for the video camera (Fig. 4.11). Placing the patient's head in a slightly hyperextended position will make it easier to control the endoscope and will also create some additional room for the surgeon, particularly when accessing the frontal sinus.

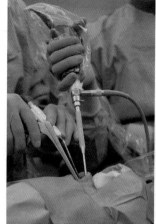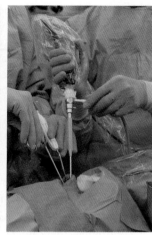

Figure 4.11   Ergonomic handling of the video endoscope with (A) one or (B) both hands, depending on the second surgeon's preference.

Stabilizing the endoscope in the nasal vestibule

A stable position for the endoscope is essential in maintaining a good image. This is achieved by gently bracing the endoscope against the apex of the nasal vestibule (Fig. 4.12). In this way the assistant can direct the endoscope more precisely and reduce shake. The surgeon can help the insertion of the endoscope by using both instruments to gently spread open the tissue at the narrowest point in the nasal vestibule, the nasal valve. This will also prevent smearing of the lens during insertion of the endoscope. This 'one nostril approach' is the workhorse for most endonasal rhinosurgical and rhino-neurosurgical procedures.

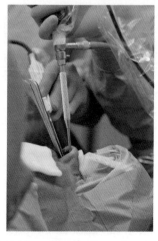

Figure 4.12   A stable position for the endoscope is essential for a good image, and at the same time, allowing enough space in the inferior part of the nose for the surgeon.

Cleaning the endoscope

If the endoscope lens is slightly soiled, it can be cleaned by rinsing it with water and it does not need to be withdrawn. This is most easily done by directing irrigating fluid along the shaft of the endoscope and removing the fluid with the suction tip which, in the bimanual technique, is always present in the field. In this way the lens can be cleaned and the operation can be continued without delay. If the lens is more heavily soiled it should be withdrawn and cleaned mechanically by an assistant.

Holding and cutting

By working with both hands, the surgeon is able to fix the targeted tissue with one instrument (a suction tip or grasper) and cut it with a second instrument. This allows high surgical precision. It results in a smaller wound surface than when tissue is removed by traction with a grasping instrument, and there is less blood loss. This technique also reduces the danger of removing too much tissue (Fig. 4.13).

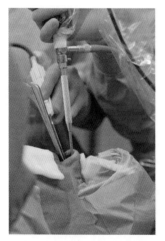

Figure 4.13   Holding and cutting at the same time resulting in a smaller wound surface.

Retraction of tissue

One difficulty in operating on the paranasal sinuses is the tight confines of the anatomical passages. Inflammatory mucosal changes or tumour tissue will often restrict the space that is available to the surgeon. With the bimanual technique, one instrument (e.g. the suction tip) can be used for tissue retraction. This improves visualization and increases surgical precision. In our experience, careful retraction of the middle turbinate toward the nasal septum also makes it easier to work in the ethmoid sinuses (Fig. 4.14).

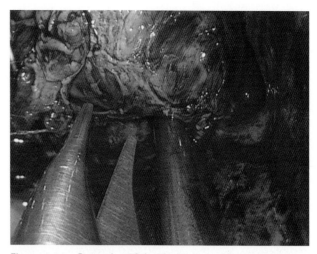

Figure 4.14   Retraction of tissue with the suction to improve visualization and improve the surgical precision of removing the tumour.

Drilling and suction

An endoscopic drill or bur is frequently used to remove bone. With the bimanual technique the suction tip can remain in the operative field and it is always on standby for clearing the field of irrigating fluid and drilling debris. This improves visualization and reduces soiling of the lens. Even prolonged drilling in the frontal sinus or sphenoid sinus can be done without difficulty. It is important for the assistant to position the endoscope carefully so that the lens is not damaged by the drill (Fig. 4.15).

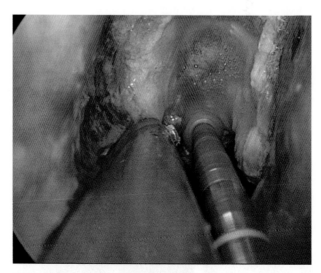

Figure 4.15   Drilling and suction at the same time helps to irrigate and clear the operating field.

Coagulation and suction

Heavy bleeding is not uncommon in sinus operations, particularly when operating near the branches of the sphenopalatine artery. This arterial bleeding should be controlled by electrocoagulation. With the bimanual technique, the suction tip is constantly available to keep extravasated blood from pooling in the operative field. The bleeding vessel can be cauterized with a conventional monopolar or bipolar instrument. The bimanual technique also eliminates the possible problem of a cautery instrument with a built-in suction channel becoming clogged by coagulated blood. It also helps bipolar diathermy to work more effectively as suction removes blood away from the area of the forceps to allow current to pass between the diathermy tips (Fig. 4.16).

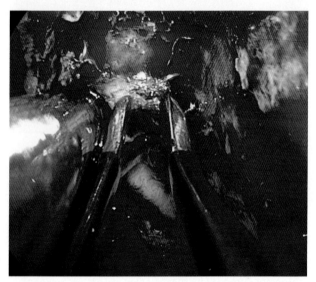

Figure 4.16   Coagulation and suction at the same time controls the operating field from excessive pooling of blood.

Navigation and drilling

The endoscopically assisted bimanual operating technique also works well in conjunction with a navigation system. The suction tip, for example, may function as the tracking

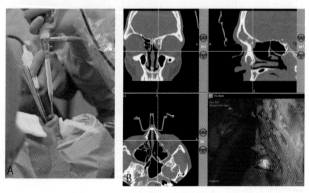

Figure 4.17   (A) Navigation and suction by the surgeon's left hand with an electromagnetic system. The suction tip may function as (B) the tracking instrument, and at the same time keeps the operating field free of blood.

instrument for surgical navigation. We know from experience that the suction tip spends a lot of the time in the operative field, making it an excellent navigation sensor for all phases of the operation (e.g. drilling at anatomically challenging sites such as the frontal sinus and sphenoid sinus) (Fig. 4.17).

MODIFICATION OF THE STANDARD 'ONE NOSTRIL APPROACH'

Surgical teams involved in skull base and rhino-neurosurgery have developed various modifications to meet their specific needs. In the posterior skull base resection of the posterior part of the septum, a so-called 'two nostril approach' has been developed to allow one channel to be used for guiding the endoscope and the other pathway to be used by the surgeon. This set-up is ideal for interdisciplinary work and more extensive skull base procedures that extend intracranially. For anterior skull base operations and for the frontal sinus a septal window is needed to carry out a two nostril approach. The advantage of this modification is the expanded angle and ability to cross the midline and reach areas that are much more difficult to reach with the ipsilateral approach (Fig. 4.18).

Another modification is when the two surgeons sit opposite one another so they both have full freedom in moving and handling instruments and each surgeon

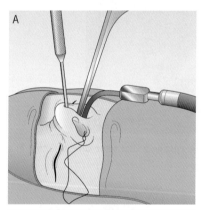

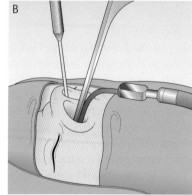

Figure 4.18   Various modifications have been developed to help different surgical situations. (A) The classic one nostril approach and (B) the two nostril approach to improve access to the posterior skull base. With this method the posterior septal plate is resected to gain access.

has their own monitor to work from. Comfortable posture is needed for both surgeons so they can perform bimanual work and guide the endoscope for long periods if necessary. There is not just one set-up for the bimanual assisted technique – each team can work out what suits them best. This is a dynamic process that will always adapt to new technical developments. This surgery requires an open and flexible team that is able to change its set-up to a microsurgical technique if necessary in order to help improve patient safety and outcome when this is necessary.

CONCLUSION

The bimanual endoscopic sinus surgery technique combines the advantages of the endoscopic technique with the key advantages of being able to operate with both hands. The bimanual technique appears to confer more benefit in more complex cases such as the endoscopic removal of paranasal sinus tumours although this has yet to be quantified objectively. The patient may benefit from a shorter operation time and the surgeon has better visibility, which may in return reduce the incidence of complications. There may be potential economic benefits because of the more efficient use of operating theatre time.

REFERENCES

1. Hedman J, Kaprio J, Poussa T *et al.* Prevalence of asthma, aspirin intolerance, nasal polyposis and chronic obstructive pulmonary disease in a population-based study. *Int J Epidemiol* 1999; **28**: 717–22.

2. Jones NS. The prevalence of facial pain and purulent sinusitis. *Curr Opin Otolaryngol Head Neck Surg* 2009; **17**: 38–42.

3. Damm M, Quante G, Jungehuelsing M *et al.* Impact of functional endoscopic sinus surgery on symptoms and quality of life in chronic rhinosinusitis. *Laryngoscope* 2002; **112**: 310–15.

4. Kennedy DW. Functional endoscopic sinus surgery technique. *Arch Otolaryngol* 1985; **111**: 643–9.

5. Stammberger H. Endoscopic endonasal surgery–concepts in treatment of recurring rhinosinusitis. Part II. Surgical technique. *Otolaryngol Head Neck Surg* 1986; **94**: 147–56.

6. Rice DH. Basic surgical techniques and variations of endoscopic sinus surgery. *Otolaryngol Clin North Am* 1989; **22**: 713–26.

7. Simmen D, Jones N. *Endoscopic sinus surgery and extended applications.* New York, Stuttgart: Thieme, 2005.

8. Krouse JH, Christmas DA. Powered instrumentation in functional endoscopic sinus surgery. II: A comparative study. *Ear Nose Throat J* 1996; **75**: 42–4.

9. May M, Hoffmann DF, Sobol SM. Video endoscopic sinus surgery: a two-handed technique. *Laryngoscope* 1990; **100**: 430–2.

10. Arnholt JL, Mair EA. A 'third hand' for endoscopic skull base surgery. *Laryngoscope* 2002; **112**: 2244–9.

11. Briner HR, Simmen D, Jones N. Endoscopic sinus surgery: advantages of the bimanual technique. *Am J Rhinol* 2005; **19**: 269–73.

12. Zhao K, Scherer PW, Hajiloo SA, Dalton P. Effect of anatomy on human nasal air flow and odorant transport patterns: Implications for olfaction. *Chem Sens* 2004, **29**: 365–79.

5

Preoperative work-up and assessment

PETER-JOHN WORMALD, MARC A TEWFIK

CLINICAL ASSESSMENT

Prior to undertaking primary or revision functional endoscopic sinus surgery (FESS), patients with chronic rhinosinusitis (CRS) should be offered maximal medical therapy[1] (see Chapter 3 for a full discussion of medical therapy). Failure to respond to this therapy should be clearly documented in the patient's chart. The definition of maximal medical therapy is dependent on the subclass of CRS being treated, broadly divided by the presence or absence of nasal polyps. In either case, the clinician should attempt to elicit the patient's symptoms and classify them according to severity. The total severity can be classified by having patients answer the following question using a visual analogue scale (VAS) graded on a 10 cm scale: 'How troublesome are your symptoms of rhinosinusitis?' A VAS score of ≤3 corresponds to mild, >3–7 corresponds to moderate, and >7 corresponds to severe.[2] This will help to guide the clinician in deciding which medical treatments are most appropriate.

Sinonasal endoscopy is crucial in evaluating all patients presenting with symptoms of CRS. It may help identify structural variations, masses or secretions not seen on anterior rhinoscopy. The presence of a posterior fontanelle ostium and circular flow of mucus should be sought. This can be an important cause of recalcitrant maxillary sinus disease after surgery, and can often be seen with a 30° endoscope.

All CRS patients should undergo a 2-month course of topical corticosteroids and nasal saline irrigations. The patient should be given careful instructions regarding the importance of strict daily administration, with the aim of improving compliance. Patients with polyps receive a 3-week tapering dose of oral steroids, whereas patients with mucopurulence on examination should be given culture-directed antibiotics.[3]

Comorbidities affecting sinus disease

The goal of the medical work-up is to identify mucosal, systemic and environmental factors responsible for poor outcome. A history of underlying immune deficiency, connective tissue disorder, cigarette smoking, malignancies or a genetic disorder such as cystic fibrosis or primary ciliary dyskinesia should be sought. A complete immune work-up should include a neutrophil count and antibody titres to *Pneumococcus*, *Haemophilus* and tetanus and if they are low, response after a vaccine should be checked to rule out immune deficiency if suspected. Investigation is also helpful to rule out other systemic disorders such as Wegener's granulomatosis and sarcoidosis. Defects in the functional immune response not evident on static testing have been identified in certain patients who have refractory CRS. In the absence of response to all other therapies, a 6-month trial of intravenous immunoglobulin may be warranted.[4]

Based on similarities of underlying epidemiology, pathophysiology and histopathology, the links between CRS and asthma become evident supporting the one airway, one disease concept. Approximately 20 per cent of rhinosinusitis patients have asthma, which is up to four times the prevalence in the general population.[5] Numerous studies[6,7] have shown a positive effect on asthma following the treatment of CRS, with sinus surgery as the main focus of most of these. Outcomes measures have included symptom improvement, changes in lung function and decreased use of the medications to manage asthma. The management of CRS and asthma therefore go hand in hand, and the clinician should always remain alert to this interplay.

It is also important to consider the potential contribution of allergy to symptoms or disease. A total serum IgE level, as well as a haemogram with differential cell count to detect serum eosinophilia, may be useful to further characterize patients and may alert the surgeon to the possibility of Churg–Strauss syndrome. Allergy testing and management should be included in their care to minimize the contribution of allergy to the disorder. Allergen reduction or avoidance, medications and possibly immunotherapy may have a role in management.

Cigarette smoking has been associated with statistically worse outcomes after ESS based on disease-specific quality-of-life measures.[8] Exposure to cigarette smoke adversely affects mucosal ciliary function,[9] as well as sinus cilia regeneration following FESS.[10] A history of smoking should be elicited for all patients presenting with postoperative sinonasal complaints and smoking cessation encouraged, with an emphasis on the detrimental effects of cigarette smoke on nasal and sinus health.

Sinonasal non-Hodgkin's natural killer or T-cell lymphomas have an aggressive clinical course, and can present initially as severe rhinitis alone. Diagnosis is made based on a high index of clinical suspicion, in combination with multiple deep and adequately processed biopsies. The biopsies should be submitted fresh and unfixed, and the treating physician must insist on the application of immunohistochemistry in order to accurately make the diagnosis. Untreated sinonasal T-cell lymphomas are uniformly fatal; however, if chemotherapy and local radiation are initiated prior to dissemination, a 45 per cent 5-year survival rate can be achieved.

COMORBIDITIES AFFECTING THE SURGICAL FIELD

The surgical field is critically important to the safety and success of FESS. The minimization of intraoperative bleeding is a major factor in determining a clear surgical field, which allows the surgeon to safely remove disease, while decreasing the risk of complications. Several factors affecting the surgical field have been studied.[11–15] Important factors include reverse Trendelenburg positioning, and the application of topical and local vasoconstrictors.[12,15] In research performed at our institution, the ideal mean arterial pressure has been shown to be less than 60–75 mmHg and the ideal heart rate to be less than 60 beats/min.[11,14] This is best achieved through the use of total intravenous anaesthesia, which results in less vasodilation than with inhaled anaesthetic agents.[14,16]

Patient comorbidities causing increased surgical bleeding can be broadly divided into local and systemic processes. Local causes consist mainly of infection, such as in acute sinusitis or a purulent complication thereof, inflammatory processes including the granulomatous diseases, and excess local tissue trauma.

Systemic comorbidities that may increase the amount of surgical bleeding must also be sought and addressed. Individuals with underlying hypertension, and/or peripheral vascular disease should be clearly identified and optimized preoperatively, as controlled hypotension may be more challenging in this group of patients. Mitral valve stenosis can increase bleeding through increased venous pressure. Liver and renal diseases are important causes of clotting factor deficiency and platelet dysfunction, respectively. Chronic alcohol abuse, malnutrition, and vitamin deficiencies (most notably vitamin K), can also affect coagulation, and must be explored if suspected clinically.

Bleeding diatheses, such as haemophilia A or B, and von Willebrand's disease, require clotting factor replacement or specialized pharmacotherapy (1-desamino-8-D-arginine vasopressin [DDAVP], tranexamic acid or aminocaproic acid), and must be planned for. Inherited collagen and blood vessel abnormalities, including hereditary haemorrhagic telangiectasias and arteriovenous malformations, are other less common causes of profuse surgical bleeding.

MEDICATIONS AFFECTING THE SURGICAL FIELD

Aspirin irreversibly blocks cyclo-oxygenase-1, inhibiting platelet aggregation for the circulating lifetime of the platelet. Because this inhibitory effect may persist for 7–10 days, it is recommended to discontinue aspirin at least 1 week before surgery. Non-aspirin non-steroidal anti-inflammatory drugs (NSAIDs) act in a reversible fashion. Thus, withholding non-aspirin NSAIDs 2–3 days before surgery is reasonable, although their effect on mucosal wound healing has not been studied in humans. The highly selective cyclo-oxygenase-2 inhibitors (e.g. celecoxib) have no effect on platelet aggregation and bleeding time, even when given at supratherapeutic doses.

Patients on long-term warfarin therapy (including those with mechanical heart valves or atrial fibrillation) have an increased risk of intraoperative haemorrhage. It is recommended that patients stop taking warfarin 4 days prior to surgery, and resume the drug at the usual dose on the night of surgery, in consultation with their regular treating physician. Depending on their indication for anticoagulation, patients may need to be given low molecular weight heparin during this perioperative bridging period.

A number of herbal and alternative therapies can affect coagulation pathways, and the surgeon should be aware of these. Ginseng may cause irreversible platelet inhibition. Ginkgo appears to alter vasoregulation, as well as inhibit platelet-activating factor. Kava inhibits cyclo-oxygenase, which may interfere with platelet aggregation. Fish oil, which is among the most popular dietary supplements of the day, also has a significant anticoagulant effect. It is prudent for patients to discontinue all herbal and alternative medicines at least 7 days prior to surgery.

OPTIMIZATION OF THE SURGICAL FIELD

Systemic steroids may be beneficial in the preoperative period to reduce the size and vascularity of polyps in patients with significant nasal polyposis, thus reducing capillary bleeding during FESS. A preliminary study found that 30 mg of prednisone administered daily for 5 days preoperatively resulted in a significantly improved surgical field grading score during endoscopic sinus surgery.[17] This translated into a shorter operating time for the steroid treated group, although there was no difference in mean total blood loss. Empirical treatment regimens range from 30 mg to 50 mg of prednisone daily for between 5 and 7 days preoperatively. However, further studies are necessary to clarify the optimal dose of steroids, length of treatment and groups of patients that would benefit from this treatment.

Given that surgery on acutely infected and inflamed tissues invariably results in increased bleeding, it would follow that preoperative antibiotics in such situations would improve the surgical field. However, most patients undergoing FESS have had extended medical therapy, including numerous courses of antibiotics and oral steroids, and therefore rarely have an acute infection at the time of surgery. The usefulness of routine preoperative antibiotics in this elective surgical patient population remains to be determined. Randomized controlled studies are needed to determine which type of antibiotics should be used, the length of preoperative treatment, and the patient group most likely to benefit from its use. Currently, we do not routinely give patients antibiotics preoperatively.

THE COMPUTED TOMOGRAPHY SCAN

General assessment of the computed tomography scan prior to surgery

A computed tomography (CT) scan should be performed after maximal medical treatment. However, some patients are referred with a CT scan and if there is no change in the symptoms and the status of the nose and sinuses at endoscopy, these scans can be accepted as a likely reflection of the ongoing state of the sinuses. The initial CT assessment is done to assess the pattern of disease. The first question is whether there is enough disease to warrant surgical intervention. Patients who have isolated retention cysts are usually not considered for surgery. In patients with endoscopic documentation of recurrent attacks of acute sinusitis with pus, with normal CT scans between attacks, mini-FESS (uncinectomy and opening of the bulla ethmoidalis) may be considered. It is often wise to see these patients when they are symptomatic to check that they have genuine sinusitis as often it transpires that they have an atypical form of migraine. In all other patients, sinus surgery is not considered if there is no evidence of disease on the CT scan. If the major symptom in a patient is nasal obstruction in the absence of sinus disease, the septum and turbinates should be assessed. If nasal crowding and obstruction is seen on endoscopy, septoplasty and inferior turbinoplasty should be considered. If the patient has sufficient disease on the CT scan that warrants surgery then the CT should be further assessed particularly for signs of anatomical abnormalities that may predispose the patient to intraoperative complications.

The CT should be systematically reviewed using the acronym 'CLOSE' (proposed by Steve Floreani, Adelaide, Australia).

- C – stands for cribriform plate. The height of the cribriform plate should be assessed according to Keros' classification 1–3. The deeper the cribriform plate (Keros 2 and 3) the larger is the amount of thin bone forming the lateral wall of the olfactory fossa. Of particular importance is the angle that this lateral wall forms with the perpendicular. Most patients should have a vertical lateral lamina of the cribriform plate but in some patients this is tilted at an angle (Fig. 5.1), which exposes the thin lateral lamina to instruments working in the frontal recess and exposes the patient to a greater risk of skull base injury with cerebrospinal fluid (CSF) leak.
- L – stands for lamina papyracea. The entire lamina papyracea should be scanned, looking for dehiscences of the lamina and particularly for any orbital fat protrusion into the sinuses, the so-called 'blow-out' fracture (Fig. 5.2). If this is not picked up preoperatively then the patient is at significant risk of orbital damage during surgery if this region is entered. This is especially true if a microdebrider is used to enter the sinuses, as the suction and cutting elements in microdebriders result in very rapid removal of soft tissue, especially orbital fat.

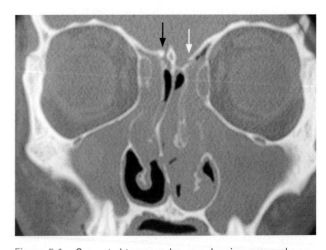

Figure 5.1   Computed tomography scan showing a normal vertical lateral wall of the olfactory recess (black arrow) and an angulated lateral wall (white arrow), putting it at risk during surgery in this region.

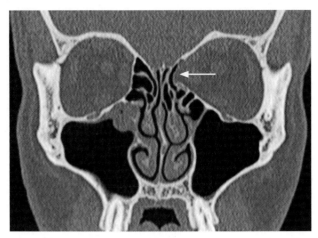

Figure 5.2   Orbital prolapse into the ethmoid complex (arrow), placing this area at risk during surgery.

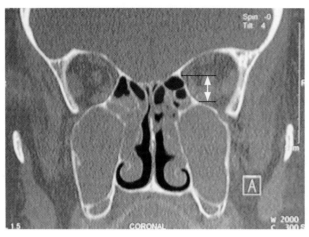

Figure 5.4   The height of the posterior ethmoids is indicated by the white arrow between the horizontal black lines.

- O – stands for optic nerve and Onodi cell. The posterior ethmoids and the sphenoid bone need to be assessed for the presence of an Onodi cell and whether the optic nerve is present in the posterior ethmoids. The best CT scan to check for the presence of an Onodi cell is the coronal scan. The transition from the posterior ethmoids to the sphenoid is determined by identifying the first coronal CT in which the posterior bony choanae can be seen. The cell directly above the bony choanae is the sphenoid sinus. If there is a horizontal septation above this cell, and this cell is in continuity with the posterior ethmoids, this cell is an Onodi cell (Fig. 5.3). The Onodi cell pneumatizes above and over the sphenoid sinus, creating the horizontal septations and bringing the optic nerve into the lateral wall of the cell. The position and pneumatization of the sphenoid also need to be assessed and if the anterior clinoid is pneumatized, this may place the optic nerve on a mesentery across the roof of the sphenoid.

- S – stands for skull base. It is important to assess the vertical height of the posterior ethmoids and therefore the height of the skull base relative to the lamina papyracea. In some patients this skull base can be very low with a very compressed vertical height (Fig. 5.4). If this is not recognized, the surgeon may inadvertently rapidly approach the skull base on entering the posterior ethmoids and breach the skull base. Recognition of the low skull base on CT scans may avoid this complication as the surgeon will expect to come across the skull base quickly.

- E – stands for the (anterior) ethmoid artery. The anterior ethmoid artery should be sought in all patients and can be identified on the CT scan. If the anterior ethmoid artery is on a mesentery and this is not recognized, the artery may be severed as the septations on the skull base are removed. The easiest way to identify the anterior ethmoid artery is to follow the curve of the lamina papyracea anteroposteriorly looking for the 'rose thorn' or 'nipple' appearance of the lamina as the artery tents the lamina when it leaves the orbit to enter into the skull base (Fig. 5.5).

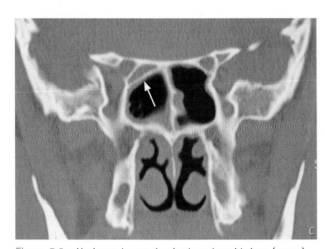

Figure 5.3   Horizontal septation in the sphenoid sinus (arrow) – the cell above this septation is the Onodi cell and the cell below it is the sphenoid sinus.

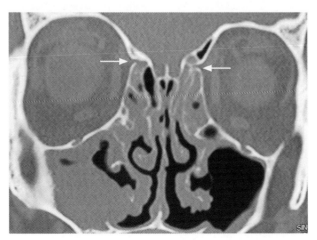

Figure 5.5   The anterior ethmoid arteries (arrows) are seen forming outpouching of the lamina papyracea.

EXTENT OF SURGERY

The extent of surgery is determined by assessing the extent of disease. Patients who only have disease in the ostiomeatal complex region or mild maxillary disease should undergo a mini-FESS (uncinectomy and opening of the bulla ethmoidalis). In patients who have disease in the frontal recess and frontal sinus, complete clearance of the frontal recess and exposure of the frontal ostium is indicated. In patients with disease of the posterior ethmoids, all posterior ethmoid cells should be completely removed. In patients with sphenoid disease, wide opening of the sphenoid is indicated.

The philosophy for all the sinuses is the same – if the sinus is diseased then the ostium of the sinus should be exposed by either widening of the ostium or removal of cells obstructing the ostium. This applies equally to the maxillary, frontal and sphenoid sinuses. In the past there has been hesitancy regarding dealing with the frontal sinus in the same way as dealing with the maxillary sinus, i.e. exposing the ostium if disease is present in the sinus on CT scan. There is no benefit of having one rule for the maxillary sinus and a different rule for the frontal sinus. It is also clear from the literature that among the most common causes for failed sinus surgery is residual cells obstructing sinus ostia (Fig. 5.6). However, by the same token, if the sinus is not diseased on CT scan, it is not operated on. It is important to also be aware that partial surgery, especially in the frontal recess, can be more harmful than no surgery. Partial removal of cells in the frontal recess will often lead to postoperative scarring as the drainage pathways around these cells are often narrow with closely applied mucosal surfaces. Partial surgery often creates raw surfaces that are closely applied to each other in these narrow confines resulting in adhesions and obstruction of the drainage pathways.

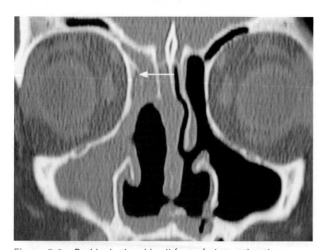

Figure 5.6   Residual ethmoid cell (arrow) obstructing the outflow tract of the frontal sinus.

PROGNOSTIC FACTORS

The major prognostic factors in the outcome of ESS are: first, the extent of the disease and the presence of polyps, eosinophilic mucus or fungus; and second, anatomical factors, of which the size of the frontal ostium is the most important. Chapter 12 describes the studies conducted by us and others which indicate that the more extensive the disease, the more radical is the surgery needed to achieve control and a good outcome. In these studies the only feature that clearly predicted a poor outcome was the presence of eosinophilic mucus. These factors are fully discussed in Chapter 12. Here, we concentrate on the anatomical factors, specifically the most important anatomical factor – the size of the frontal ostia. Patients who have large frontal ostia (Fig. 5.7) usually do much better than patients with narrow ostia (Fig. 5.8) as removal of the obstructive cells from the ostium results in sufficient ventilation and drainage of the sinus to keep the mucosa relatively healthy. In patients with narrow frontal ostia, there is a greater tendency for the ostia to stenose and in some cases fibrose, especially if there is ongoing significant inflammation. Small frontal ostia have a greater tendency to become progressively more oedematous with eventual obstruction of the sinus ostium and recurrence of disease and symptoms.

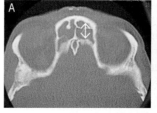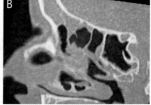

Figure 5.7   (A) Anteroposterior diameter of the frontal ostium on the axial computed tomography (CT) scan (see double-headed arrow). (B) The same distance seen in the parasagittal CT scan. The axial and parasagittal scans are the most useful for estimating the size of the frontal ostium.

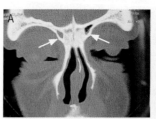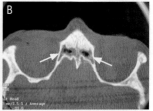

Figure 5.8   (A) Coronal computed tomography (CT) scan showing very small frontal ostia (white arrows). (B) Axial CT scan showing small frontal ostia (white arrows) with very limited anteroposterior span.

SURGICAL ANATOMY

The most important aspect of the preoperative assessment is reading the CT scans preoperatively and creating a three-dimensional (3D) picture of the anatomy of the region to be operated on, including the drainage pathways.[18–20] This should be done for both the frontal recess and the posterior ethmoids and sphenoid.[20] In patients who have had previous surgery, this may not be possible as the combination of previous surgery disrupting the anatomy and severe disease recurrence may obliterate cellular structure and make this technique impossible. In these cases the first step is to find the sphenoid, identify the roof of the sphenoid and follow this and the lamina papyracea forwards into the frontal sinus. This technique is, however, not recommended in previously unoperated patients. In this group, the cells and drainage pathways are clearly identified, and each cell is individually entered and recognized making the dissection precise and safe. The technique of finding the sphenoid first and then dissecting anteriorly along the skull base into the frontal ostium can result in much confusion as the frontal recess is approached. Identification of each individual cell in the frontal recess with this technique is difficult. Consequently surgery with this technique is largely dependent on experience and inexperienced surgeons may fail to completely clear the frontal ostium.

Three-dimensional reconstruction of the frontal recess and frontal sinus[20]

The first step is to identify the agger nasi cell on the coronal CT scans and find this cell on the parasagittal scans.[18–20] Once it is accurately identified, a building block is placed representing this cell. The next cell directly adjacent to the agger cell is identified first on the coronal

then on the parasagittal scan and further a building block is placed for this cell. Other cells, such as frontoethmoidal type 3 and 4 cells, intersinus septal cells and frontal bullar cells, are identified and blocks placed for them as well. The bulla ethmoidalis and if present, suprabullar cells, are also identified and blocks placed for these cells (Fig. 5.9). This process creates a comprehensive 3D understanding of the cells that make up the anterior ethmoid complex and frontal sinus. The next step is to view the axial scans starting high in the frontal sinus and progressing inferiorly following the drainage pathway of the frontal sinus. Once the frontal drainage pathway is fully assessed, the building blocks and pathway are put together to form a complete 3D picture of the anatomy (Fig. 5.10). This allows a comprehensive surgical plan to be made for the frontal recess before the patient is operated on.

The surgical plan for the frontal recess

If the patient has recognizable cells on CT, the frontal recess is always done first. The preferred technique is the axillary flap approach as this allows the agger nasi cell to be the first cell to be entered in the frontal recess. After the axillary flap is raised, the anterior face of the agger nasi cell is exposed. This is removed with a Hajek Koeffler punch and the agger nasi cell is visualized. The agger nasi cell is clearly and easily identified on the CT scan and on the 3D reconstruction. In addition now that the drainage pathway has been identified on the CT scans, the instrument (we prefer a malleable suction curette; Medtronic ENT), can be slid up the drainage pathway and the roof of the agger nasi cell fractured and removed. Viewing the 3D reconstruction in Figure 5.10, we can clearly see that the next cell is the type 1 frontoethmoidal cell and this is clearly visualized in the frontal recess. The suction curette can now be passed medial to the cell and the cell fractured

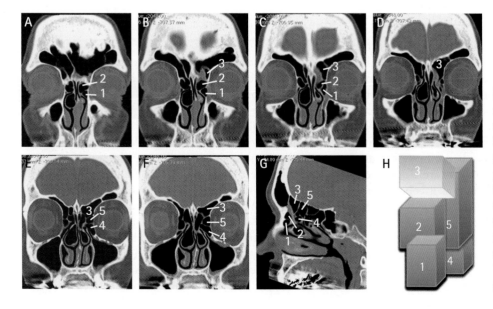

Figure 5.9 (A–H) The agger nasi cell is identified first in the series of coronal CT scans and indicated by the number 1. This cell is then identified on the parasagittal scan (G) and a building block placed for this cell. The same process is followed for the type 1 frontoethmoidal cell (2), frontal bullar cell (3), suprabullar cell (4) and bulla ethmoidalis (5). This creates a 3D picture of the anatomy of the left frontal recess.

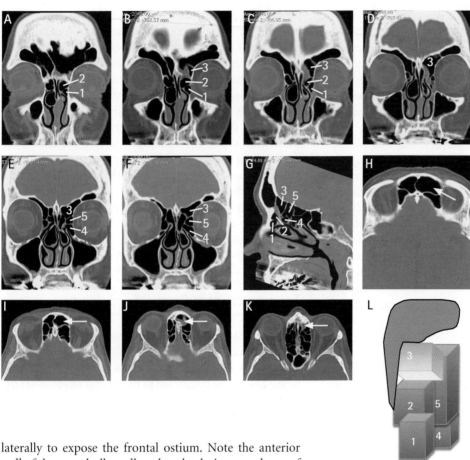

Figure 5.10   (A–L) To establish the frontal sinus drainage pathway in relation to the 3D picture, the axial CT scans (H–K) are viewed from the frontal sinus down into the ethmoid complex. Once the pathway is established (white arrows) it is drawn into the 3D picture, giving a complete understanding of the anatomy of the left frontal recess and allowing detailed surgical planning.

laterally to expose the frontal ostium. Note the anterior wall of the suprabullar cell pushes the drainage pathway of the frontal sinus anteromedially and partially obstructs the posterior region of the frontal ostium (Fig. 5.10). This can be entered and the wall removed fully to expose the frontal ostium. A clear and complete understanding of frontal recess anatomy allows, first, such careful planning of the dissection of the frontal recess before surgery is carried out and, second, safe and complete dissection of this area.

Three-dimensional reconstruction of posterior ethmoids and sphenoid sinus[20]

The principle of first doing a 3D reconstruction of the anatomy prior to surgery holds true for the posterior ethmoids as well as the anterior ethmoids. The first step is to identify the transition from the anterior to the posterior ethmoids.[20] This is done by seeking the first coronal CT scan in which the superior turbinate can be clearly seen (Fig. 5.11C). At this point the horizontal ground lamella can be identified and the superior meatus clearly seen. Once these two critical landmarks are clearly seen, that scan is in the posterior ethmoids as it is behind the vertical portion of the ground lamella. The cells from this point posterior can now be assessed both on the coronal and parasagittal scans. Once these cells have been clearly identified, building blocks are placed to represent these cells (Fig. 5.11). Next the sphenoid sinus is identified. Again the transition from posterior ethmoids to sphenoid

is seen in the first scan in which the posterior bony choanae are clearly seen (Fig. 5.11F). The cell directly above the posterior bony choanae is the sphenoid sinus. If there is a horizontal septation above this cell, an Onodi cell is present. Once a clear picture of the anatomy of the posterior ethmoids and sphenoid is obtained, a clear surgical plan can be developed.

The surgical plan for the posterior ethmoids and sphenoid sinus

After the bulla ethmoidalis has been removed, the vertical portion of the ground lamella and its transition into the horizontal portion is identified. At this transition point, a Blakesley or microdebrider blade is pushed through the ground lamella. The microdebrider is then used to open this space horizontally towards the lamella papyracea and medially onto the middle turbinate. The superior meatus should be directly behind this lamella and should be clearly identified as the lamella is removed. After the superior meatus is seen the anterior edge of the superior turbinate is sought in the medial region of the superior meatus. Once both these structures are clearly identified, the surgeon knows exactly where he or she is on the CT scan and can use the 3D reconstruction to enter each posterior ethmoid cell sequentially. If the sphenoid is to be entered, the lower

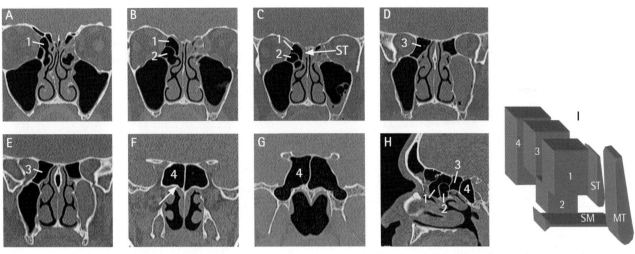

Figure 5.11   (A–I) A 3D reconstruction is performed for the posterior ethmoids. First the transition from the anterior to posterior ethmoids is found by identifying the middle turbinate (MT), superior meatus (SM) and the first scan (C) in which the superior turbinate (ST, white arrow) can be seen. The first cell seen in (A) is the bulla ethmoidalis (numbered 1). This migrates over the first posterior ethmoid cell (2). A second posterior ethmoid cell (3) sits directly behind this before the sphenoid (4) is reached. A building block is placed for each one of these cells to create a 3D picture that allows detailed planning of the surgical steps for this surgery.

third of the superior turbinate is resected and the natural ostium identified, entered and enlarged. The skull base in the sphenoid is identified and gives the level of the skull base to be cleared as the surgeon works anteriorly along the skull base. The suction curette is used to palpate the skull base between septations, and gently fracture these septations clearing the skull base until the entire skull base is clear from the frontal ostium into the sphenoid. If the anterior ethmoid artery is on a mesentery, care should be taken in this region not to injure it.

CONCLUSIONS

The first step of preparing a patient for surgery is to ensure that they were given proper medical treatment but without success. Second, abnormalities or anatomical structures that place the patient at additional risk during surgery need to be identified on the CT scan. The degree of difficulty of the case in relation to anatomy and disease severity needs to be recognized, and the surgeon needs to know their skill level and only operate on patients in whom they can deal with the disease and the anatomy. Once the decision to operate is made, the surgeon should read the CT scans to develop a complete 3D understanding of the anatomy and fully plan the surgery before surgery is started.

REFERENCES

1. Senior BA, Kennedy DW, Tanabodee J *et al*. Long-term results of functional endoscopic sinus surgery. *Laryngoscope* 1998; **108**: 151–7.

2. Fokkens W, Lund V, Mullol J. EP3OS 2007: European position paper on rhinosinusitis and nasal polyps 2007. A summary for otorhinolaryngologists. *Rhinology* 2007; **45**: 97–101.

3. Wallwork B, Coman W, Mackay-Sim A *et al*. A double-blind, randomized, placebo-controlled trial of macrolide in the treatment of chronic rhinosinusitis. *Laryngoscope* 2006; **116**: 189–93.

4. Chee L, Graham SM, Carothers DG *et al*. Immune dysfunction in refractory sinusitis in a tertiary care setting. *Laryngoscope* 2001; **111**: 233–5.

5. Jani AL, Hamilos DL. Current thinking on the relationship between rhinosinusitis and asthma. *J Asthma* 2005; **42**: 1–7.

6. Batra PS, Kern RC, Tripathi A *et al*. Outcome analysis of endoscopic sinus surgery in patients with nasal polyps and asthma. *Laryngoscope* 2003; **113**: 1703–6.

7. Ragab S, Scadding GK, Lund VJ *et al*. Treatment of chronic rhinosinusitis and its effects on asthma. *Eur Respir J* 2006; **28**: 68–74.

8. Briggs RD, Wright ST, Cordes S *et al*. Smoking in chronic rhinosinusitis: a predictor of poor long-term outcome after endoscopic sinus surgery. *Laryngoscope* 2004; **114**: 126–8.

9. Agius AM, Smallman LA, Pahor AL. Age, smoking and nasal ciliary beat frequency. *Clin Otolaryngol Allied Sci* 1998; **23**: 227–30.

10. Atef A, Zeid IA, Qotb M *et al*. Effect of passive smoking on ciliary regeneration of nasal mucosa after functional endoscopic sinus surgery in children. *J Laryngol Otol* 2008; **10**: 1–5.

11. Nair S, Collins M, Hung P *et al*. The effect of beta-blocker premedication on the surgical field during endoscopic sinus surgery. *Laryngoscope* 2004; **114**: 1042–6.

12. Wormald PJ, Athanasiadis T, Rees G *et al.* An evaluation of effect of pterygopalatine fossa injection with local anesthetic and adrenalin in the control of nasal bleeding during endoscopic sinus surgery. *Am J Rhinol* 2005; **19**: 288–92.

13. Athanasiadis T, Beule AG, Wormald PJ. Effects of topical antifibrinolytics in endoscopic sinus surgery: a pilot randomized controlled trial. *Am J Rhinol* 2007; **21**: 737–42.

14. Wormald PJ, van Renen G, Perks J *et al.* The effect of the total intravenous anesthesia compared with inhalational anesthesia on the surgical field during endoscopic sinus surgery. *Am J Rhinol* 2005; **19**: 514–20.

15. Cohen-Kerem R, Brown S, Villasenor LV *et al.* Epinephrine/lidocaine injection vs. saline during endoscopic sinus surgery. *Laryngoscope* 2008; **118**: 1275–81.

16. Eberhart LH, Folz BJ, Wulf H *et al.* Intravenous anesthesia provides optimal surgical conditions during microscopic and endoscopic sinus surgery. *Laryngoscope* 2003; **113**: 1369–73.

17. Sieskiewicz A, Olszewska E, Rogowski M *et al.* Preoperative corticosteroid oral therapy and intraoperative bleeding during functional endoscopic sinus surgery in patients with severe nasal polyposis: a preliminary investigation. *Ann Otol Rhinol Laryngol* 2006; **115**: 490–4.

18. Wormald PJ. Surgery of the frontal recess and frontal sinus. *Rhinology* 2005; **43**: 83–5.

19. Wormald PJ. Three dimensional building block approach to understanding the anatomy of the frontal recess and frontal sinus. *Oper Tech Otolaryngol* 2006; **17**: 2–5.

20. Wormald PJ. *Endoscopic sinus surgery: anatomy and 3-dimensional reconstruction and surgical technique*, 2nd edn. New York: Thieme, 2008:264.

6

Complications of sinus surgery

SCOTT M GRAHAM

OVERVIEW

Complications as a result of sinus surgery can occur in cases carried out by even the most experienced surgeons. A rate of serious complications in the order of 0.5 per cent is often quoted for sinus surgery.[1] The rate for an individual surgeon, in practised hands, may be a good deal lower but by its very nature is never zero. For this reason, a balanced analysis of potential complications is part of the informed consent process for any surgery.

The implementation of recent technological advances, particularly image-guided surgery and powered instrumentation, might be presumed to have the potential to alter the type and frequency of surgical complications. Image-guided surgery, indispensable in many of the extended applications of sinus surgery and in revision situations, appears not to have reduced complication rates. While an attractive conceptual argument can be made for image guidance to reduce complications, the reality seems otherwise. A variety of studies have shown similar complication rates in series of surgery utilizing image guidance compared with non-image-guided historical controls.[2] This would negate any consideration of image guidance as 'standard of care' for primary, non-complicated, surgery.

Powered instrumentation is now used as almost a matter of routine in modern sinus surgery. Indeed many advanced techniques would be incredibly tedious or frankly impossible without it. Powered instrumentation does not appear to have increased the incidence of complications in sinus surgery but it has altered the scale of adverse events.[3] The combination of the suction element with rapid efficient dissection can produce major complications in a very short time period. The challenge in using these instruments is to incorporate their great advantages into surgical practice while minimizing their potential for dramatically negative sequelae.

INTRACRANIAL COMPLICATIONS

Major advances have been made in the treatment of intracranial complications of sinus surgery. These complications include most commonly cerebrospinal fluid (CSF) leaks and also brain parenchymal injuries. Avoidance of intracranial injury starts with a detailed examination of the computed tomography (CT) scan. The configuration and integrity of the skull base needs to be reviewed on every single cut. Limited cut CTs, while offering some help in sinus diagnostics in the light of history and examination, have no place in preoperative planning, simply because of the extensive areas of skull base they leave unsurveyed.

At the very least the CT should be a coronal fine cut scan with images taken at intervals of 3 mm, or less. It is important to note the slope of the skull base and also the relative contributions of the very thin lateral lamella of the cribriform plate and the thicker orbital plate of the frontal bone. As a generalization the safest skull base configuration for intranasal surgery is that with a pronounced component of orbital plate of frontal bone. Statistically the most likely sites for intracranial penetration are the area at the lateral lamella of cribriform, anteriorly where the skull base is penetrated and weakened by the anterior ethmoid neurovascular bundle, and posteriorly where there may be confusion as to the exact relationship of the last posterior ethmoid cell and the sphenoid sinus. This is of particular concern in Onodi or sphenoethmoidal cells where the posterior ethmoid pneumatizes superior and lateral to the sphenoid. These cells show certain racial predilections and although they have classically been associated with optic nerve injury,[4] intracranial penetration is also a serious potential concern. (See also Chapter 5.)

Cerebrospinal fluid leaks tend to be diagnosed in four general scenarios. The first variety of CSF leak is diagnosed intraoperatively and occurs when, for example, the surgeon peels mucosa off a compromised skull base, producing a leak. In this situation the diagnosis is clear, the surgeon knows exactly what has happened and is aware of the exact location of the leak. In this circumstance the leak should be repaired intraoperatively in the same surgical setting.

The second CSF leak scenario also involves an intraoperative diagnosis of the leak. However, the surgeon in this situation is completely surprised by this finding. Perhaps this occurs in the face of considerable bleeding and he or she is unsure of the exact anatomical location of the leak. In this situation the conventional wisdom is that a CSF leak diagnosed intraoperatively should be repaired during the same anaesthetic session. Although this advice is almost always useful, there will be isolated instances where the state of surgical disorientation is such that attempting to repair a leak might result in further damage such as an orbital injury or brain parenchymal injury. In these cases the site of leakage can be packed and the patient referred to a tertiary care centre for a specialist rhinological opinion. Particular care must be exercised at the end of the anaesthesia, preventing bag ventilation by anaesthesia with its potential to increase the intranasal air pressure and cause pneumocephalus. The patient is counselled not to blow their nose or stifle sneezes until several days after the leak has been repaired.

Postoperatively, a CSF leak may become obvious in two general ways. A CSF leak may present with obvious, usually unilateral, clear watery rhinorrhoea. Postural provocation may produce fluid in the consulting room. Alternatively, a more subtle or intermittent postoperative CSF leak may first come to notice as a result of a complication of the leak, such as meningitis.

Cerebrospinal fluid leaks diagnosed intraoperatively require no special testing prior to repair. The majority of leaks that come to light in the postoperative period can be diagnosed with minimal testing by using thin cut CT scans (Fig. 6.1) and confirmatory β-transferrin testing.[5] Difficulties arise with the diagnosis of more subtle postoperative leaks (Fig. 6.2). Certainly β-transferrin and fine cut coronal CT scans should be the first tests performed. Intrathecal radioactive tracer studies or intrathecal contrast studies may be helpful in more difficult cases and where the leak is intermittent; intrathecal contrast studies offer the highest chance of success in cases in which the leak occurs in an area of the sinuses where the contrast might pool, such as the frontal or sphenoid.

Successful repair of CSF leaks depends on initial identification of the exact site of the leak. Image-guided surgery is helpful in this regard. We also use intrathecal fluorescein in conjunction with image-guided surgery.[6] Fluorescein is mixed with the patient's own CSF obtained via a lumbar drain, inserted shortly after anaesthetic induction at the time of planned repair. A dose of 0.1 mL of 10 per cent fluorescein suitable for injection measured in a tuberculin syringe is mixed with 10 mL of the patient's CSF. This is reinjected slowly over at least 10 minutes. In the USA, fluorescein is not approved by the Food and Drug

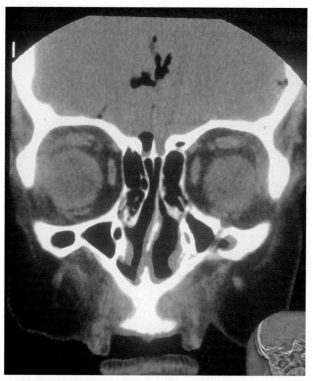

Figure 6.1   Coronal computed tomography (CT) scan demonstrating right skull base defect and pneumocephalus.

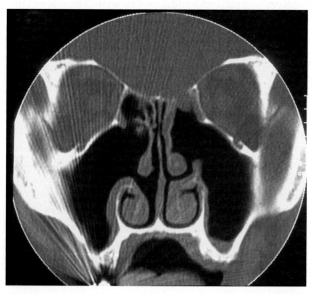

Figure 6.2   A small defect in the left fovea ethmoidalis caused by surgery.

Administration (FDA) for intrathecal use and separate consent is obtained. Most of the serious complications of fluorescein use such as status epilepticus or aseptic meningitis have been associated with the use of the wrong dose or variety of fluorescein or with fast bolus injection. A 'pencil point' 24-gauge epidural needle (Fig. 6.3) minimizes the possibility of a post-lumbar puncture headache and any fluorescein leaking and causing inflammation. In nearly all circumstances the light from the telescope is of

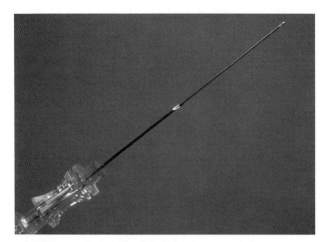

Figure 6.3   A 'pencil point' 24-gauge epidural needle.

sufficiently broad spectrum to identify fluorescein at the site of the leak (Fig. 6.4). Intrathecal fluorescein is helpful in diagnosing that a leak is present and in identifying its exact site, and in proving that the leak is closed at the end of the procedure.

There is no supporting evidence favouring one graft material for CSF leak repair over another or one technique over another. All materials and repair techniques work well for postoperative leaks. Successful repair rates of 90 per cent or better are quoted in most series. In general free grafts have been preferred to local flaps, although posterior septal flaps have become more popular recently. Graft material includes muscle, fat, fascia, mucosa and materials such as AlloDerm. Larger defects often require support with bone or cartilage, although large defects after endoscopic skull base surgery are now closed with soft tissue without more rigid support. Onlay or underlay techniques appear to work equally well. There is no literature to suggest that lumbar drains increase the rate of successful closure. It is, however, our practice to keep a lumbar drain, used initially for intrathecal fluorescein administration, in place for up to 5 days after surgery. Tissue glues may be of adjunctive use and we place a layer of Gelfoam under the repair to form a 'break layer' to isolate it from shearing trauma when the Merocel nasal pack is removed or alternatively the graft can be supported by oxidized cellulose that will resorb.

Powered instrumentation has changed the scale of intracranial complications.[3] With the use of non-powered instrumentation, CSF leaks with an excellent chance of endoscopic closure occurred most often. Brain

parenchymal injury is now more likely to occur because of the suction element associated with the microdebrider. These patients may present with neurological symptoms and their assessment includes imaging of the intracranial arterial circulation. Brain parenchymal injuries may result in vascular trauma with pseudoaneurysm formation requiring work-up with either an MRI angiogram or catheter angiogram. Neurosurgical advice is often critical in managing this patient group.

Orbital injury

The term 'lamina papyracea' well describes the thin bony separation of the ethmoid sinus and orbit. In the majority of circumstances injury to the lamina and underlying periorbita is the route of orbital penetration. The orbit may also be transgressed in its floor during maxillary sinus surgery or through its roof during, for example, open procedures on the frontal sinus.

Orbital penetration results in a variety of events ranging from simple exposure of periorbital fat (Fig. 6.5), and ecchymosis (Fig. 6.6) through venous or arterial bleeding and direct injury to intraorbital structures (Fig. 6.7). The clinical sequelae of these injuries can range from a striking but innocuous periorbital ecchymosis all of the way through to blindness (Fig. 6.8).

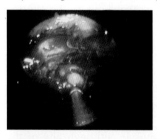

Figure 6.5   Exposed left periorbital fat captured from a video of the procedure. The fat was left untouched and the patient was asked not to blow their nose or stifle sneezes.

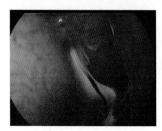

Figure 6.4   Intrathecal fluorescein, visible in the nose, demonstrating the site of a CSF leak.

Figure 6.6   Ecchymosis caused by traversing the periorbital tissue.

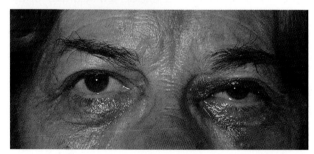

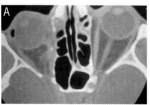
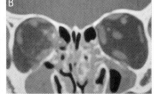

Figure 6.7   (A) Axial and (B) coronal computed tomography (CT) scans showing damage to the right medial rectus.

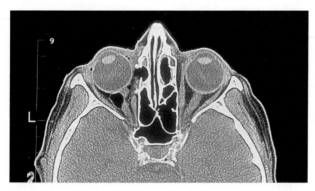

Figure 6.8   An axial CT scan demonstrating a defect in the left lamina and resection of the medial rectus muscle near its point of insertion on the globe. (Reproduced with permission from *Laryngoscope*[7]).

Powered instrumentation, now widely used in endoscopic sinus surgery, has also changed the scale of orbital complications. In the era of 'non-powered dissection', breach of the lamina and periorbita was by no means an unknown event. Gentle ballottement of the eye would produce noticeable transmitted movement of the orbital contents in the operative field. Simple exposure of orbital fat, providing it was promptly recognized, usually produced no remarkable clinical sequelae. Indeed a good deal of dissection could still be carried out on the affected side. No nasal packing was placed on the injured side so as not to prevent egress of any oozing blood. Powered instrumentation has of course changed all of this.

With the dissecting barrel of the powered dissection revolving perhaps 3000 or 5000 times a minute, substantial inadvertent intraorbital dissection can occur in a very short period of time. This most commonly results in injury to the medial rectus muscle, although any of the intraorbital structures are at risk[7] (Fig. 6.7). Usually a substantial portion of the muscle is drawn by suction into what are very sharp dissecting blades, as new blades are used for every patient. The powerful suction force compounds the extent of injury by potentially drawing tissue beyond the site of transgression into the blades. Management of this injury is further complicated by the fact that there is no 'good treatment' for medial rectus injury. Although muscle-balancing surgery may restore fused vision in primary gaze, diplopia returns if the patient looks to the right or left.

An orbital haematoma may occur slowly as a result of venous ooze, often compounded by occlusive packing, or more rapidly from arterial haemorrhage. Arterial haemorrhage most often takes the form of injury to the anterior ethmoid artery in the nose with transection and retraction of the severed end into the orbit. The anterior ethmoid artery also has an intracranial course and retraction with intracranial bleeding requiring craniotomy can occur. Usually, however, the bleeding is intraorbital. A haematoma can develop rapidly and dramatically on

the operating table. The diagnosis of the haematoma is facilitated by routinely leaving the eye untaped to permit easy assessment of the orbit.

Treatment of an orbital haematoma resulting from surgery conducted under general anaesthesia is hampered by the lack of the single most vital piece of clinical information – the patient's visual acuity. We know from our experience in treating maxillofacial trauma that not every patient with an orbital haematoma requires surgical intervention. If the vision is normal the patient can often be observed closely. Without knowledge of the patient's visual acuity the surgeon has to guess as to the most likely outcome. With this in mind most surgeons will identify the least favourable visual outcome of blindness as a real and likely possibility and proceed with surgical intervention on this basis.

Ipsilateral packing should be promptly removed if packing is in the nose when a haematoma develops. The initial treatment of an haematoma is similar to the treatment of an expanding haematoma anywhere in the body. Counterintuitively this involves application of firm pressure to the globe. This is done in the hope of tamponading the bleeding. Firm four finger pressure is applied to the orbital contents for 1–2 minutes, stopping if the globe becomes rock hard.[7]

An ophthalmological opinion and assistance should be immediately sought. The ophthalmologist will probably palpate the globe, view the retinal circulation and measure the intraocular pressure using tonometry. Intraocular pressures less than 30 mmHg are usually associated with a good visual outcome and consideration can be given to waking up the patient, closely observing their vision and employing ancillary treatments such as mannitol, steroids and β-blocker eyedrops. As a practical matter, an ophthalmologist may not be immediately available or their expertise may be in fields other than orbital surgery. Regardless, the patient's treatment should not be delayed.

A lateral canthotomy and inferior cantholysis can be carried out (Fig. 6.9). This involves a lateral canthal incision followed by release of the inferior crus of the lateral

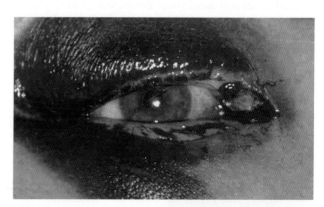

Figure 6.9   Left lateral canthotomy and inferior cantholysis to decompress the orbit. The wound does not need to be sutured as it heals of its own accord with little sign of any scar.

canthal tendon. A successful procedure allows the surgeon to grasp the lid in a pair of forceps and lay it on the cheek. The upper lid can be released in a similar way (see Fig. 7.5, page 62). More definitive treatment of the haematoma involves formal orbital decompression. The medial wall can be removed via an external ethmoidectomy approach, or by endoscopic decompression,[8] or approached via the transcaruncular route.[9] The choice between techniques is immaterial and depends on the surgeon's previous experience as well as the extent of prior dissection when the haematoma is observed. The orbital floor can also be decompressed. Bone is removed and the periorbita incised.

How quickly does the orbit need to be decompressed? No studies in humans have been carried out to answer this question; however, animal (monkey) studies from our own institution suggest that 90 minutes may elapse before permanent retinal ischaemia occurs. More recent work has suggested that this time may be longer in elderly, atherosclerotic hypertensive monkeys.[10] This apparent paradox has been partially explained by possible ischaemic preconditioning.

Injury to the lacrimal apparatus is usually the easiest to deal with of any of the complications of endoscopic sinus surgery. These injuries are usually treated well endoscopically with a dacryocystorhinostomy and stenting if the rhinostomy from the sac does not lie open wide. Injury to the lacrimal apparatus most commonly occurs in anterior dissection involving the hard bone in front of the anterior lip of the maxillary sinus ostium. Conservative dissection in this area greatly reduces the likelihood of nasolacrimal injury.

CAROTID ARTERY INJURY

Management of injury to the internal carotid artery can be divided into two stages. Initial treatment involves stemming or stopping the bleeding and resuscitating the patient. Further treatment then involves more definitive management of the arterial injury. Control of bleeding by the surgeon and resuscitation by the anaesthetic team proceed simultaneously. Deep blind packing is likely to be required as are additional large bore intravenous access and blood transfusion.

Contemporary management of internal carotid artery injury, after resuscitation and stabilization of the patient most often involves the interventional radiologist as well as potential contributions from other specialties such as neurosurgery, intensive care and specialized anaesthesia. When these facilities are not available in the hospital where the injury occurred, consideration should be given to transferring the patient to a tertiary care facility, ensuring that the airway is secure at the time of transfer. Arteriography can be pursued in a dedicated radiological suite or in the operating room. Balloon technologies allow for bridging of the arterial breach. Temporary test balloon occlusion is carried out and this can be tolerated without

neurological sequelae. In addition, there is a low risk of stroke after permanent balloon occlusion and detachment. If there are neurological changes with temporary occlusion, a neurosurgical opinion can be obtained regarding the utility of an emergency internal carotid to external carotid bypass.

More recently, neuroradiologists have extended their experience obtained with stenting in, for example, the coronary circulation, to potentially using stents for internal carotid injuries. Endovascular placement of metal stents can be used to bridge the defect in the internal carotid wall[4] (Fig. 6.10). Such techniques are referred to as 'reconstructive techniques' in contrast to the 'deconstructive techniques' involved in balloon occlusion.

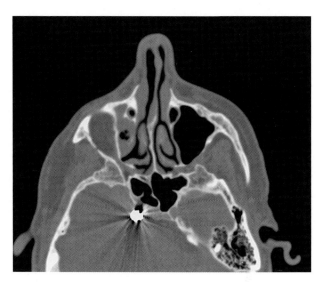

Figure 6.10 An expandable metal stent is seen in the sphenoidal course of the internal carotid artery on axial computed tomography (CT) scan.

CONCLUSION

Great strides have been made in the treatment of intracranial complications of sinus surgery. Technology has also provided advances for the treatment of carotid artery injuries. Orbital injuries, however, continue to be problematic. It goes without saying that the major thrust of surgical practice is careful planning and careful surgery to reduce the likelihood of occurrence of complications in the first place.

REFERENCES

1. Cumberworth VL, Sudderick RM, Mackay IS. Major complications of functional endoscopic sinus surgery. *Clin Otolaryngol* 1994; **19**: 248–53.
2. Tabaee A, Hsu AK, Shrime MG *et al.* Quality of life and complications following image-guided sinus surgery. *Otolaryngol Head Neck Surg* 2006; **135**: 76–80.

3. Graham SM. Complications in sinus surgery using powered instrumentation. *Oper Tech Otolaryngol* 2006; **17**: 73–7.

4. Graham SM, Carter KD. Major complications of endoscopic sinus surgery: a comment. *Br J Ophthalmol* 2003; **87**: 374.

5. Skedros DG, Cass SP, Hirsch BE *et al.* Sources of error in the use of beta-2-transferrin analysis for diagnosing perilymphatic and cerebral spinal fluid leaks. *Otolaryngol Head Neck Surg* 1993; **109**: 861–4.

6. Keerl R, Weber RK, Svaf W *et al.* Use of sodium fluorescein solution for detection of cerebrospinal fluid fistulas: an analysis of 420 administrations and reported complications in Europe and the United States. *Laryngoscope* 2004; **114**: 266–72.

7. Graham SM, Nerad JA. Orbital complications in endoscopic sinus surgery using powered instrumentation. *Laryngoscope* 2003; **113**: 874–8.

8. Graham SM, Carter KD. Combined approach orbital decompression for thyroid related orbitopathy. *Clin Otolaryngol* 1999; **24**: 109–13.

9. Graham SM, Thomas RD, Nerad JA. The transcaruncular approach to the medial orbital wall. *Laryngoscope* 2002; **112**: 986–9.

10. Hayreh SS. Central retinal artery occlusion. Retinal survival time. *Exp Eye Res* 2004; **78**: 723–36.

7

Orbital and lacrimal surgery

VIJAY R RAMAKRISHNAN, JAMES N PALMER

INTRODUCTION

The proximity of orbital structures to the paranasal sinuses allows for the logical extension of endonasal surgery to the treatment of orbital disease. Historical external approaches to the orbit are often considered the 'gold standard' with regards to safety, efficacy and extent of experience. Although both external and endonasal approaches continue to have a role in selected patients, the focus of this chapter will be the endoscopic approach to diseases of the orbit and lacrimal system. Advancements in technology, endoscopic skill and progressive understanding of surgical anatomy have paved the way for endonasal endoscopic management of sino-orbital and orbital disease. However, appropriate perioperative management and an excellent working relationship with a skilled ophthalmologist or oculoplastic surgeon are important for difficult cases and in the management of surgical complications.

This chapter will also review the minimally invasive approaches to the orbit and lacrimal system alongside their more traditional 'open' predecessors.

SURGICAL ANATOMY

Mastery of the intimate anatomical relationships of the paranasal sinuses to the orbital and lacrimal systems is essential prior to attempting endoscopic surgery in these regions. Anatomical knowledge of the orbital system should be correlated to the endoscopic view of the region for successful surgery, and intraoperative use of computed tomography (CT) image guidance can improve learning.

The anatomy of the orbital region can be conceptualized into bony, soft tissue, arterial and lacrimal.

Bony anatomy

The orbital cavity has four bony walls, with the medial wall and floor being notably thinner. The medial wall consists of contributions from the lacrimal, ethmoid and sphenoid bones from anterior to posterior, and along the anterosuperior aspect, the frontal bone. The anterior lacrimal crest is a continuation of the inferior orbital rim to the medial wall, whereas the posterior lacrimal crest is found on the lateral aspect of the lacrimal bone. Between the two crests is the lacrimal fossa, which contains the lacrimal sac (Fig. 7.1). The orbital floor is made of the orbital process of the maxilla, the zygomatic bone and the orbital plate of the palatine bone. The infraorbital nerve traverses the floor in an anterior direction from the infraorbital fissure. Travelling within the groove are the anterior superior alveolar nerve (V2) and the infraorbital nerve (V2) and artery. The anterior superior alveolar nerve gives off sensory branches and the infraorbital nerve and artery travel forwards to ultimately exit the groove through the infraorbital foramen in the maxilla. The orbital roof is comprised primarily of the orbital plate of the frontal bone, with a small posterior contribution from the lesser wing of the sphenoid. The lateral wall is formed by the orbital face of the zygomatic bone and the greater wing of the sphenoid. Whitnall's tubercle, the attachment site of the lateral canthal tendon, is found just inside the lateral orbital rim. The variably pneumatized sphenoid sinus provides medial access to the optic nerve and orbital apex (Fig. 7.2).

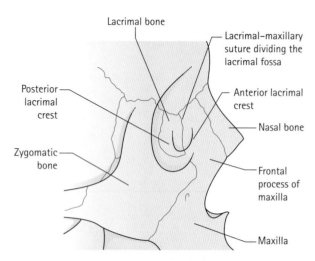

Figure 7.1   External bony relationships of the orbit.

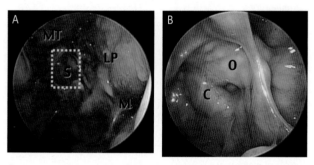

Figure 7.2   Endoscopic views along the medial wall of the orbit. (A) The yellow box is the opened face of the sphenoid sinus (S). (B) Note how superficial the optic nerve (O) and carotid artery are as they travel in the lateral wall of the sphenoid sinus, making them accessible for both surgery and complications. MT, middle turbinate; LP, lamina papyracea; M, maxillary sinus; C, carotid artery, and just above the optico-carotid recess.

Within the sphenoid, the bone overlying the optic nerve and carotid artery may be thin or dehiscent. The sphenoid bone permits passage of all neurovascular structures into the orbit.

Soft tissue anatomy and cranial nerves (CN)

The orbital soft tissues can be divided into intraconal and extraconal departments. The intraconal space lies within the fascial connections of the extraocular muscles and contains the extraocular muscles, retrobulbar fat, optic nerve and ophthalmic artery. The extraconal space contains orbital fat encased in the periorbita, which is the periosteal layer of the orbital walls. The medial rectus and superior oblique are the two muscles most at risk during endoscopic procedures as they traverse the thin lamina papyracea (Fig. 7.3).

The optic foramen lies at the superomedial aspect of the orbital apex, and transmits the optic nerve and the

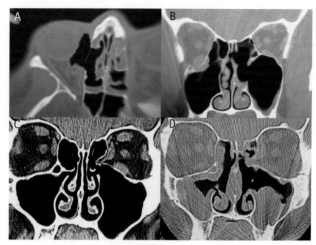

Figure 7.3   Damage to extraocular muscles during endoscopic sinus surgery. (A) Damage to the medial rectus muscle and optic nerve. (B) Damage to the inferior rectus muscle in the roof of the maxillary sinus. (C) Preoperative image of a well-functioning orbit prior to endoscopic sinus surgery and (D) postoperative image with new-onset medial rectus muscle palsy.

ophthalmic artery. The superior orbital fissure (SOF) is located lateral to the optic foramen. A common tendinous ring formed by the origin of the extraocular muscles, known as the annulus of Zinn, divides the superior orbital fissure and surrounds the optic foramen. Above the annulus within the SOF, the trochlear nerve (CN IV) and the frontal and lacrimal branches of CN V enter the orbit in the extraconal space. The portion of the SOF within the annulus of Zinn is known as the oculomotor foramen, and transmits CN III, nasociliary branch of CN V, CN VI, sympathetic fibres, the orbital branch of the middle meningeal artery, and ophthalmic veins. Posteriorly, the oculomotor foramen opens into the middle cranial fossa. The infraorbital fissure separates the greater wing of the sphenoid bone, which forms the lateral wall of the orbit, from the bone of the orbital floor. The infraorbital nerve and artery, along with branches of the sphenopalatine ganglion and inferior ophthalmic vein, travel through the infraorbital fissure.

Vascular anatomy

The arterial supply of the orbit and neighbouring ethmoid region comes from the internal carotid artery via the ophthalmic branch. The anterior and posterior ethmoid arteries arise from the ophthalmic artery. Because the anterior and posterior ethmoid arteries ultimately originate from the internal carotid artery, embolization of these arteries in the setting of epistaxis or oncological surgery is not recommended due to the risk of blindness, emboli and stroke.

The anterior ethmoid foramen lies in the medial orbital wall 24 mm back from the anterior orbital margin. The posterior ethmoid foramen is located another 12 mm posteriorly, and the optic foramen another 6 mm posteriorly. The optic foramen typically transmits the ophthalmic artery on the inferolateral aspect of the optic nerve, but it may enter on the inferomedial side in rare cases. The axial plane containing the anterior and posterior ethmoid arteries corresponds roughly to the level of the skull base.

Venous drainage lies within the connective tissue septa of the orbital fat, thus extensive fat manipulation at surgery carries a risk of haemorrhage.

Lacrimal anatomy

The lacrimal system is an excretory organ designed to transport tears from the lacrimal gland across the globe into the nose. The lacrimal system is frequently classified into an upper system and a lower system. The upper system consists of the lid margin, the upper and lower puncta, the upper and lower canaliculi, and the common canaliculus. The lower system is made of the lacrimal sac and the nasolacrimal duct, which empties into the inferior meatus at the membranous valve of Hasner (Fig. 7.4). The common internal punctum is the site of convergence between the upper and lower systems, and is important to identify endoscopically in procedures designed to open the lacrimal sac.

The lacrimal sac is located in a bony fossa bounded by the anterior and posterior lacrimal crests. The posterior portion of the lacrimal fossa consists of the thin lacrimal bone, whereas the anterior portion is made up of the thicker frontal process of the maxilla. The junction of these two bones, the lacrimal–maxillary suture, corresponds to the endoscopic landmark of the maxillary line. Fibres of the orbicularis oculi muscle around the lacrimal sac may contribute to function via a pumping

mechanism. Disorders of the nasolacrimal duct are much more common than diseases of the lacrimal sac, and this principle underpins the practice of dacryocystorhinostomy (DCR), or the marsupialization of the lacrimal sac into the nasal cavity.

PERIOPERATIVE ISSUES

Theatre set-up

Standard operating room set-up is employed during orbital and lacrimal cases. When present, the ophthalmological surgeon will usually stand at the head of the bed while the sinus surgeon sits or stands at the patient's right side. Image guidance may help, but is a matter of surgeon preference. There is no substitute for understanding the external and endoscopic anatomy. Standard instruments for sinus surgery are used, in addition to the use of a microdebrider and diamond drill. Although special instrument sets are available for DCR and orbital decompression, similar instruments may be borrowed from otological sets.

Lubricants and corneal protectors

The eyelids may be taped if direct access to the orbit is not required; lubricant and a corneal protector are placed when an open or combined approach is planned. The intermittent removal and replacement of the corneal protector is recommended during the case so that pupil reactivity may be checked, which is particularly important when globe retraction is necessary or if orbital haemorrhage occurs. Pupillary dilation may also be caused by injury to the branch of the oculomotor nerve that supplies the inferior oblique muscle and ciliary ganglion as it travels inferiorly within the intraconal space. Significant ocular pressure may lead to bradycardia or short periods of asystole. Intermittent relaxation of globe retraction will alleviate the vagally mediated physiological response. Communication with the anaesthetist is important in this scenario and intravenous atropine must be readily available.

Pre- and postoperative medication

Intravenous broad spectrum antibiotics are routinely used at the onset of endoscopic orbital and lacrimal surgery because sinonasal bacteria may be introduced into otherwise sterile environments. Intravenous steroids are routinely given for antiemetic benefit. In special circumstances, there may be an indication for higher doses of systemic steroids. Oral antibiotics, saline irrigation and topical eyedrops are continued postoperatively at the surgeon's discretion.

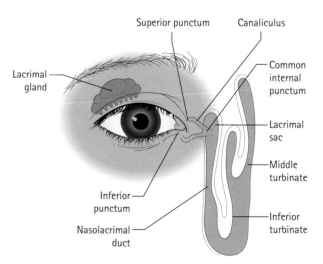

Figure 7.4 Anatomical relationships of the lacrimal system.

Postoperative concerns

In the recovery room, a visual acuity check is performed, and may be done serially if indicated. To minimize bruising and swelling, the head of the bed is kept elevated to at least 30° for 48 hours and ice packs are applied to the periorbital area for 10 minutes every hour while the patient is awake for the first 24 hours. Activity and nose-blowing limitations are implemented. Generally, the first postoperative clinic visit occurs 1 week later, but may be adjusted based on the surgery performed and surgeon or patient preference.

LATERAL CANTHOTOMY AND CANTHOLYSIS

All otorhinolaryngologists should understand the principles of lateral canthotomy and cantholysis. Normal intraorbital pressure is less than 20 mmHg. Increased intraorbital pressure can lead to optic nerve ischaemia and subsequent blindness. This most commonly occurs with orbital haemorrhage or haematoma, severe orbital emphysema, orbital cellulitis, orbital or subperiosteal abscess and Graves' exophthalmos. Signs and symptoms of acute intraocular hypertension include: pain, proptosis, vision loss, ophthalmoplegia, and development of a fixed, dilated pupil. Time is essential in the acute scenario because irreversible blindness may occur within 1 hour.

Canthotomy and cantholysis allow for pressure release by expansion of the orbital volume anteriorly. The orbit is confined by bony walls in all other directions, so anterior displacement of soft tissue is the best rapid intervention to decrease pressure. Immediate diagnosis and management of increased orbital pressure should be followed by identification and treatment of the underlying aetiology. Intravenous steroid and mannitol administration may be of additional benefit.

The procedure

The procedure is illustrated in Figure 7.5, and begins with infiltration of the lateral canthal region with 1 per cent lidocaine with 1:100 000 adrenaline (epinephrine). A horizontal incision is made from the lateral convergence of the upper and lower lids down to the orbital rim with a number 15 scalpel or sharp scissor as depicted in Figure 7.5B. The lower lid is then retracted anteriorly and inferiorly, and the inferior portion of the lateral canthal tendon is palpated with the tip of the instrument. Palpation of the taut, retracted tendon is often compared to the plucking of a guitar string. The inferior crus of the tendon is then cut and the orbital tissues should release anteriorly (Fig. 7.5C). The lower lid will freely swing and orbital fat may be visible. The inferior cantholysis is the crucial portion of this procedure. In one study, lateral canthotomy alone decreased intraocular pressure by 14 mmHg, whereas inferior cantholysis reduced pressure by 30 mm Hg.[1] The wound is left open until the

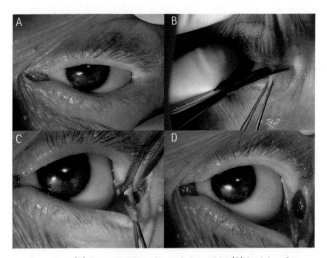

Figure 7.5   (A) Preoperative view of the orbit. (B) Incision for lateral canthotomy. (C) Identification and incision of the inferior canthal tendon, completing cantholysis. (D) View after lateral canthotomy and inferior cantholysis: by allowing the eyeball and orbital contents to come anteriorly, maximal immediate decompression is achieved.

primary disease is adequately controlled, and delayed repair may be carried out in the office using 5-0 monofilament suture, with an excellent cosmetic result.

APPROACHES TO THE MEDIAL ORBIT FOR LIGATION OF THE ETHMOID ARTERIES

Direct visualization and ligation are necessary for refractory epistaxis, transethmoid skull base approaches and surgical resection of highly vascular tumours. This is because, as mentioned earlier in the chapter, the ethmoid arteries, which provide the arterial supply to the ethmoid sinus and nasal cavity, ultimately arise from the internal carotid system and are therefore at high risk if they are embolized. Open approaches are reliable and successful, but are associated with scarring and potential disruption of the medial canthal anatomy and lacrimal system. A newer technique is the medial transconjunctival, or transcaruncular, approach. This approach avoids the external scar and disruption of the medial canthus and lacrimal sac. The medial transcaruncular approach may be combined with a lower lid transconjunctival dissection to expose the entire medial and inferior orbit. The endoscope is used to assist in either of the two open approaches described above as it enhances visualization of the posterior medial orbit with increased illumination and magnification. Both the approaches are discussed in detail below.

Traditional open approach

The Lynch incision and classical external ethmoidectomy approach can be used to reliably access the medial orbit. A corneal protector or tarsorrhaphy suture is initially placed. A 3 cm incision is marked halfway between the medial canthus and nasal dorsum, beginning at the inferior aspect of the medial brow and travelling inferiorly to the level of the medial canthus. The skin and subcutaneous tissues are divided sharply and the angular vessels cauterized. The periosteum is incised and subperiosteal dissection with a Freer elevator continues to the point of resistance at the medial canthal ligament. The ligament must be detached from its bony origin, which may be marked with a suture for reapproximation at the end of the procedure. The lacrimal sac is elevated from the lacrimal fossa and retracted with the lateral soft tissues. The lamina papyracea is then exposed.

The frontoethmoidal suture line is identifiable in most patients, and usually contains the ethmoid arteries. The anterior ethmoid artery is usually found 14–18 mm (range 9–27 mm) posterior to the lacrimal–maxillary suture.[2] The posterior ethmoid artery is found 10–11 mm posterior to the anterior ethmoid artery, but Kirchner *et al.* found it was absent in 22/70 patients.[2] Bipolar coagulation and division of the arteries may be carried out as they are identified.

Transcaruncular approach

The transconjunctival approach to the medial orbit is more often referred to as the transcaruncular approach, because the initial incision is placed over the caruncle. Thorough understanding of the anatomy is necessary for a simple and successful transcaruncular dissection. The pretarsal orbicularis oculi muscle sends fibres posteriorly to the posterior lacrimal crest, which maintains proper apposition of the lower lid to the globe. These fibres are known as Horner's muscle. The semilunar fold, or plica semilunaris, is the vascular fold of conjunctiva medial to the bulbar conjunctiva. Anterior to this is the caruncle, a mound of sebaceous tissue. Deep to the caruncle is an area of condensation of fascia of the medial canthal tendon, Horner's muscle, the medial orbital septum, the medial capsulopalpebral muscle, and Tenon's capsule.

The procedure begins with placement of a corneal protector. The medial orbit is infiltrated with 1 per cent lidocaine with 1:100 000 adrenaline. Infiltration of the conjunctival incision site may distort the anatomy, so this is done sparingly, or with enough time for adequate diffusion of the solution. The lids are retracted with Desmarres retractors, and the globe is gently retracted posterolaterally to flatten the caruncle and displace the orbital fat posteriorly. A 12–15 mm incision is made through the caruncle, or just posterior to the caruncle, with sharp scissors or a knife. This initial incision in the caruncle creates a natural plane that extends to the posterior lacrimal crest and medial orbital wall and which reflects the periorbita, orbital fat, and medial rectus laterally while protecting the lacrimal system and medial canthus anteromedially. Horner's muscle should

be identified and preserved; placement of a malleable retractor on the muscle will protect the medial soft tissues and lacrimal system. The tips of curved tenotomy scissors are used to palpate the posterior lacrimal crest and blunt dissection will identify the medial orbital wall. The periosteum is incised with a scalpel or needle-tip cautery, and subperiosteal dissection is carried out. The anterior and posterior ethmoid arteries can then be identified and cauterized or clipped prior to division. Dissection further posteriorly provides access to the orbital apex. Closure of the periorbita is difficult to achieve and unnecessary. The caruncle and conjunctiva are reapproximated with 6-0 fast absorbing gut suture and topical antibiotic/steroid drops are used for 1 week postoperatively.

Endoscopic transnasal ligation

Endoscopic transnasal ligation of the anterior ethmoid artery is possible in selected cases. Endoscopic transnasal ligation of the sphenopalatine artery is a popular procedure, and endoscopic transorbital ligation of the anterior ethmoid artery is also possible. The location of the artery in the anterior ethmoid cavity should be well known to the sinus surgeon. However, its location within the skull base or suspended in a bony mesentery precludes simple clipping or cauterization and division. Radiographically, its transition from the orbit into the ethmoid skull base occurs at the coronal plane of the posterior globe and can be identified as a pinch of soft tissue near the approximation of the superior oblique and medial rectus muscles (Fig. 7.6).

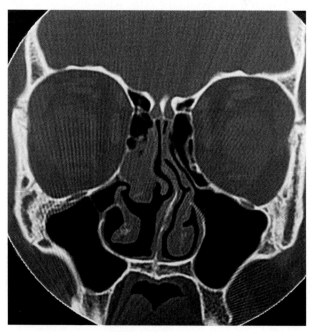

Figure 7.6 Coronal computed tomography (CT) scan demonstrating the anterior ethmoid artery exiting the orbit and crossing the ethmoid sinus at the point that the medial rectus and superior oblique muscles converge.

Surgery begins with routine maxillary antrostomy and complete anterior ethmoidectomy. With a 30° endoscope, the location of the anterior ethmoid artery is visualized, and may be confirmed with image guidance. A small opening in the medial orbital wall is created with a ball-tip probe or J curette and the lamina papyracea around the artery is removed. The periorbita is carefully preserved to prevent herniation of orbital fat into the operative field. A periosteal elevator is used to dissect in the subperiosteal plane anterior and posterior to the artery. An angled clip applier can then be used to clip the isolated vessel.

ORBITAL DECOMPRESSION

Indications

Decompression of the orbit may be indicated for:

- orbital haemorrhage
- orbital or subperiosteal abscess
- Graves' ophthalmopathy
- removal of orbital tumours
- biopsy of undiagnosed orbital lesions
- palliation of malignant tumours causing orbital symptoms.

Orbital haemorrhage may result from blunt or penetrating trauma, or as a complication of blepharoplasty or endoscopic sinus surgery. An injured vessel, often the anterior ethmoid artery, retracts into the orbit and continued bleeding increases intraorbital pressure. The pressure impairs blood flow to the retina and may stretch the optic nerve, leading to loss of colour vision or decreased visual acuity. Worrisome physical findings include elevated pressures, resistance to retropulsion, proptosis, relative afferent papillary defect and vision loss. As permanent vision loss may occur within 1 hour, the first surgical manoeuvre in the setting of acute increased intraocular pressure would be lateral canthotomy and cantholysis. Orbital decompression is an adjunctive measure, and may decrease intraorbital pressures by an additional 10 mmHg.

Orbital infections may occur as a complication of sinusitis. Common presenting symptoms and signs include periorbital oedema and erythema, nasal obstruction or congestion, purulent rhinorrhoea, facial pain and pressure, proptosis, ophthalmoplegia and loss of visual acuity. When evaluation suggests spread of infection into the post-septal space, CT scan with intravenous contrast is recommended. A subperiosteal abscess along the medial or superior orbital wall may be identified. Clinical judgement based on severity of disease, timing and response to medical management, and patient comorbidities, may suggest a role for surgical drainage of the abscess. Significant surgical expertise is required for using an endoscopic approach to a subperiosteal orbital access, given the vascularity and inflammation associated with the acute infection. It must

be stressed that open approaches to the orbit should be considered if there is any doubt as to the success of endoscopic drainage. General anaesthesia and topical vasoconstriction must be optimized in the endoscopic approach. Removal of the middle turbinate may be considered to optimize visualization and instrumentation. Depending on the location and extent of the disease, the frontal sinus may or may not need to be addressed. In severe infections or anatomically unfavourable cases, frontal sinus trephination may be of value if the frontal sinus is involved.

Oedema and fibrosis of orbital fat and extraocular muscles may occur in Graves' disease even with appropriate medical management. The orbitopathy may progress regardless of the clinical course of thyroid dysfunction. This results in exophthalmos, exposure keratitis, diplopia and loss of colour vision or visual acuity. Surgical decompression is offered when medical treatment fails, and may be considered for cosmesis. It must be acknowledged that even after successful decompression, fibrosis of the levator palpebrae muscle may contribute to a continued staring appearance, which may be addressed with a subsequent procedure. Nearly 30 per cent of patients with Graves' disease have preoperative diplopia, but new-onset diplopia in the postoperative patient can reach similar numbers depending on technical considerations.

The procedure

Decompression has historically been achieved through open approaches. However, endoscopic decompression of the medial and inferior orbit has certain advantages, including: lack of scar, preservation of medial canthal and lacrimal anatomy, decreased patient morbidity, better illumination and improved visualization. Open approaches to the orbital floor such as the transconjunctival and subciliary approach may also be added to endoscopic medial wall decompression. Open approaches to the medial orbit, as previously discussed, may also be used for medial decompression.

The procedure begins with standard uncinectomy, maxillary antrostomy, sphenoidotomy and frontal recess dissection. These sinuses are opened widely to provide adequate access to the orbit and to prevent postoperative obstruction and sinusitis after the orbital fat is ultimately released into the ethmoid cavity. The middle turbinate is routinely removed for decompression in Graves' cases. The skull base and medial orbital wall are thoroughly skeletonized. The lamina papyracea is palpated for its thinnest area, and this site is fractured and entered with an elevator or ball-tip probe. The surrounding thin bone of the lamina is then flaked away, but leaving the periorbita intact. Inadvertent entry into the periorbita at this point may spill orbital fat into the operative field prematurely and make subsequent dissection more difficult. The entirety of the medial orbital wall is removed, leaving the maxillary orbital strut, and perhaps 1–1.5 cm around the frontal recess to prevent subsequent frontal sinus obstruction from herniated orbital fat. For treatment of subperiosteal abscess, this is sufficient for drainage of the infection.

For treatment of Graves' ophthalmopathy or orbital haemorrhage, release of the orbital periosteum is necessary to achieve globe regression and alleviate pressure. The medial periorbita is incised serially from posterior to anterior, beginning superiorly and finishing inferiorly (Fig. 7.7). Alternatively, the periorbita may be resected, although some believe this may increase the risk of new-onset postoperative diplopia. When used for treatment of Graves' ophthalmopathy, approximately 2 mm of globe regression is expected from a medial orbital decompression. When combined with orbital floor decompression, approximately 5 mm of globe regression can be expected. When combined medial and floor decompression is planned, we prefer to preserve the maxillary strut and approach the orbital floor by a separate transconjunctival approach as this reduces the incidence of postoperative diplopia. Additional decompression of the lateral wall may add another 2 mm of globe regression, and may 'balance' the orbital decompression for prevention of diplopia. However, the addition of lateral decompression is substantially more involved, and the decreased risk of diplopia may not be as remarkable as many have reported.

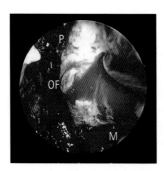

Figure 7.7   Endoscopic view of the lateral nasal wall as the periorbita (P) is pierced by a sickle knife and the orbital fat (OF) is allowed to prolapse into the ethmoid sinus as part of medial orbital wall decompression. M, maxillary sinus.

APPROACH TO ORBITAL APEX AND OPTIC NERVE DECOMPRESSION

The relative inaccessibility of the orbital apex has been an issue for surgeons for many years. Magnetic resonance imaging and CT are valuable in the evaluation of diseases of the orbital apex, but most lesions are diagnosed with tissue biopsy, which often ultimately defines treatment recommendations. The endoscopic transnasal approach to the orbital apex for biopsy or surgical resection has been a valuable development given the morbidity of traditional open approaches. Dissection in the crowded posterior orbit and apex has been historically difficult due to the presence of several important structures and lack of dead space for dissection. Transnasal approaches through the ethmoid and sphenoid sinuses have allowed for some degree of decompression, which may facilitate surgical dissection. The surgical approach must be individualized according to the location of the lesion and the surgical plan, whether

it be biopsy, subtotal resection and decompression, or complete resection. Use of the endoscope may also be beneficial in the open approaches.

Indications

Traumatic optic neuropathy, pseudotumour cerebri resulting in vision loss and severe dysthyroid orbitopathy are indications for decompression of the orbital apex. Traumatic optic neuropathy results from either direct or indirect trauma to the optic nerve. Direct injury to the nerve by projectiles or bone fragments is less common and is generally considered a contraindication to decompressive surgery due to its poor prognosis. Impingement of the nerve by fracture is considered to be an indication for surgical decompression, as improvement in vision may be achieved. Indirect injury to the optic nerve is thought to occur due to transmission of force from the injury or compression from haemorrhage or oedema within the nerve sheath. History and physical examination, along with maxillofacial and orbital CT, are necessary to make the diagnosis. Early therapy with high-dose intravenous corticosteroids is recommended based on studies performed for spinal cord injuries.

Studies on traumatic optic neuropathy have been unsatisfactory, given its rarity, lack of uniformity, and non-standardized steroid regimen. No randomized controlled trial has been carried out to compare outcomes from observation, systemic corticosteroids and surgery. Several case series have shown some benefit of surgery in the case of failed medical management, without any adverse events.[3,4] A multicentre study and a Cochrane review on traumatic optic neuropathy have concluded that there is no clear benefit for surgery in the management of this condition, but that it may be offered based on clinical judgement, surgical expertise and patient preference.[5,6] If vision does not improve with corticosteroid therapy, or if visual function deteriorates with tapering of corticosteroid dosage, surgical decompression may be offered with the understanding that prognosis is poor regardless of treatment strategy in these cases.

Surgical approaches

Open approaches to the medial orbit include the classical external ethmoidectomy approach and the medial transconjunctival approach, as previously described. The endoscope is helpful in either of these approaches in the posterior orbit, providing illumination and magnification. The inferior orbital apex may be accessed via a transconjunctival or transfacial approach to the orbital floor, or by an endoscopic transantral approach.

Conventional neurosurgical approaches to the orbital apex are tailored to the lesion. For small lesions, access may be obtained through a small frontal or frontotemporal craniotomy with removal of the orbital roof or lateral orbital wall. For larger lesions, the orbital rim is often included in the bone flap, such as in the orbitofrontal or orbitozygomatic approaches. These approaches are more useful for larger orbital lesions which extend into surrounding structures.

The endoscopic approach to the orbital apex begins with a complete sphenoethmoidectomy. The sphenoidotomy is enlarged in all directions with a Kerrison punch. It is helpful to enlarge the sphenoidotomy superiorly to the skull base, laterally to the orbit and inferiorly to the floor of the sphenoid sinus. The pituitary fossa, carotid artery, optic nerve and optico-carotid recess should be identified within the sphenoid sinus. Remember that the optic nerve lies within a few millimetres from the carotid artery within the sphenoid sinus, and either structure may be clinically dehiscent. Careful and complete skeletonization of the medial orbit and skull base is carried out before proceeding any further. In the setting of trauma, the lamina papyracea and skull base may be mobile, and blood may fill the sinuses. Otherwise, the lamina papyracea is left intact unless access to the orbit is required.

For optic nerve decompression, the medial wall of the orbital apex is identified and confirmed with image guidance, and the bony covering known as the optic tubercle is thinned with a diamond drill. The remaining eggshell bone is gently teased away with a thin probe or elevator. Fenestration of the nerve sheath is optional for traumatic optic neuropathy, and carries the risk of cerebrospinal fluid (CSF) leak. If it is carried out, an incision in the superomedial quadrant will minimize risk of injury to the ophthalmic artery.

In orbital tumours, thinning or erosion of the overlying bone may have occurred and the use of a punch or drill may not be necessary. After thorough bone removal, the underlying annulus of Zinn is incised with a sickle knife and the medial orbital apex is exposed. Lesions in this region are then accessible for biopsy. Blunt dissection can be achieved with a ball-tip probe or maxillary sinus seeker. Care must be taken not to place too much stretch or tension on this area if exposure is limited. A three-handed technique may be of benefit if traction is needed on the lesion for surgical dissection and removal. In the setting of severe dysthyroid orbitopathy (Graves'), this orbital apex decompression technique is combined with orbital decompression.

ENDOSCOPIC DACRYOCYSTORHINOSTOMY

External DCR has been considered a historical 'gold standard' in the treatment of nasolacrimal duct obstruction, with consistent reports of success rates around 90 per cent. This procedure is performed via a skin incision anterior to the medial canthus, osteotomy of the lacrimal bone at the anterior lacrimal crest, anastomosis of lacrimal mucosal flaps to nasal mucosa and stent placement. The advantages

of the endoscopic approach to DCR include: absence of scar, avoidance of disruption of medial canthal anatomy, preservation of the orbicularis oculi pump mechanism, less pain, less operative time, decreased blood loss, the ability to address concurrent nasal pathology, and the opportunity to perform surgery in the setting of acute dacryocystitis. Initial resistance to endoscopic approaches was warranted, as results were inconsistent and often less successful than the traditional open approach. However, with improved understanding of lacrimal anatomy and the use of powered instrumentation, endoscopic DCR has now achieved results comparable with traditional open approaches.[7–9] In addition, the endoscopic approach has been particularly useful in revision cases, where there is a need to address concurrent sinus pathology or ensure proper location and size of the osteotomy.

Procedural considerations

The location and extent of the lacrimal sac is the anatomical key to this procedure. In the endoscopic view, recall that the anterior half of the sac is covered by the thicker bone of the frontal process of the maxilla and the posterior half by the thinner lacrimal bone. The junction of these two bones is seen endoscopically as the maxillary line (Fig. 7.8). This location can be confirmed with image guidance, or passage of a lighted pipe from above.

The agger nasi region is injected with 1:100 000 adrenaline, and the maxillary line is identified. Septoplasty may be necessary to provide adequate exposure. The uncinate process is removed, and if needed the agger nasi cell may be opened. If encountered, concurrent ethmoid disease should be addressed at this point. An anterior vertical incision, and superior and inferior horizontal mucosal incisions are made over the location of the lacrimal sac on the lateral nasal wall. After elevation of the mucosal flap over the frontal process of the maxilla and lacrimal bone, the flap is trimmed or debulked with a microdebrider or through-cutting instrument. The thin lacrimal bone may be dissected and removed with an elevator, but the thicker bone of the frontal process of the

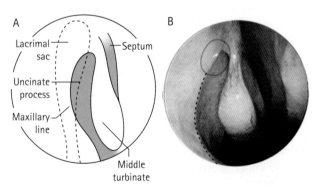

Figure 7.8 (A, B) Endoscopic anatomy useful for identification of the lacrimal sac.

maxilla is best removed with a 15° high-speed diamond bur. A lacrimal probe is inserted through the upper or lower punctum to confirm adequate bone removal for creation of a wide neo-ostium, and also to tent the lacrimal sac medially for incision with a sharp sickle or DCR spear knife. A vertical incision, and upper and lower horizontal incisions are made to create anterior and posteriorly based lacrimal mucosal flaps. These flaps are precisely resected with through-cutting instruments or a microdebrider. The edges of the nasal and lacrimal mucosa should closely approximate to minimize the amount of exposed bone. The final neo-ostium should be about 10–20 mm in height and 10–15 mm in width, with the common internal punctum easily visualized. Silicone lacrimal intubation stents are routinely placed and tied intranasally (Fig. 7.9). Additional nasal packing is generally not required.

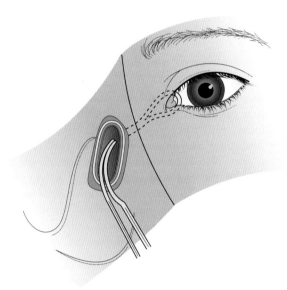

Figure 7.9 Schematic demonstrating the external and intranasal portions of silicone stent placement in dacryocystorhinostomy. Note both ends of the silicone stent are placed through the inferior and superior canaliculi and brought into the intranasal area and secured by either a knot on itself or a suture to the lateral nasal wall or vestibule.

Postoperative issues

The use of postoperative stents has been the subject of recent controversy. Stents have been used historically in both external and endoscopic DCR for many years. The duration of stenting has always been debated. Recently, a prospective randomized trial has shown improved outcomes at 6 months postoperatively without the use of silicone stents.[10] Currently, we keep silicone stents in place for 6 weeks postoperatively.

Safety of intranasal use of topical mitomycin C has been established, although efficacy or indications for its use remain unclear.[11] A prospective trial has demonstrated that topical application (0.4 mg/mL for 4 minutes followed by saline irrigation) results in larger ostial diameter at 6 months postoperatively.[12] However, the correlation of ostial size to successful outcome has not been thoroughly established. Currently, we reserve the use of topical mitomycin C application for revision DCR cases or in patients with sarcoidosis.

ORBITAL FRACTURES

Recently experience has been growing in the endoscopic management of orbital blowout fractures. Several publications have described a number of approaches for endoscopic repair of orbital floor and medial orbital fractures. The main advantages of the endoscopic technique over open approaches are the ability to visualize the posterior bony shelf and operate acutely in the presence of globe injury, elevated orbital pressures or periorbital oedema. It is important to remember that acceptable open techniques exist for both of these types of fracture and not all cases will be straightforward when using endoscopic approaches. Transcutaneous approaches, such as the subciliary approach to the orbital floor or Lynch approach to the medial orbit, should be familiar to the otolaryngologist. More recently, transconjunctival approaches to the inferior and medial orbit have been well described in the literature.

Orbital floor fractures may be accessed via a Caldwell–Luc-type approach or through a transnasal route. Fractures medial to the infraorbital nerve, and trap-door fractures are the best candidates for endoscopic fracture reduction. Lateral floor fractures may be difficult to manage endoscopically, and typically favour an open approach. Severely comminuted fractures or those with abundant orbital fat herniation may also be easier to manage with an open approach.

The endoscopic approach

The endoscope assisted open approach to the orbital floor begins with a sublabial approach and creation of a 1.0 × 2.0 cm maxillary osteotomy. A notch can be created along the inferior aspect of the osteotomy for stabilization of the endoscope. To determine the type of fracture and amount of fat herniation 0° and 30° endoscopes are utilized to thoroughly inspect the fracture site. Conservative elevation of the mucosa around the fracture site will reveal the bony edges as the orbital soft tissues are reduced. If a trap-door type fracture, or a large single bone fragment, is hinged on the medial orbital strut, simple reduction may be all that is necessary. More frequently, comminution of the fracture necessitates meticulous removal of individual fragments. The posterior bony shelf must be identified. An alloplastic implant, such as porous polyethylene, can then be trimmed to size and inserted through the osteotomy. The implant is stabilized on the posterior strut first, and then anteriorly and/or medially. Care is taken to prevent entrapment of any orbital soft tissue. Intermittent gentle force may be applied to the globe to confirm stability of the implant. Forced ductions must be carried out prior to completion of the procedure.

The transnasal route can be used to access the orbital floor and medial orbital wall. For orbital floor fractures, the uncinate process is removed and a wide maxillary antrostomy is created, with constant attention to visualization of the herniated orbital tissues. A microdebrider is not used in this dissection, and precise handling of suction instrumentation is necessary to minimize soft tissue herniation and bleeding. Bone fragments must be identified and removed to avoid reduction back into the orbital soft tissues. The orbital tissue is reduced with inflation of a saline balloon placed in the maxillary sinus, which may be stored intranasally or taped externally to the cheek for the duration of treatment. One group has had success with balloon inflation for a period of 7–10 days.[13]

Similarly, for medial orbital blowouts, the uncinate process, bulla ethmoidalis, basal lamina and ethmoid air cells are removed with through-cutting instruments and Blakesley forceps. Fractured bone chips from the lamina papyracea are removed. A microdebrider is not used, and care is taken to identify herniated orbital tissues and avoid unnecessary suction trauma. A thin Silastic sheet is cut to size and placed in the ethmoid cavity to facilitate reduction of orbital fat. Merocel sponges are placed between the Silastic sheet and the middle turbinate to reduce the herniated orbital soft tissue. Forced ductions are always carried out prior to the conclusion of the case. Merocel packing is kept in place for a period of 3–4 weeks. Oral antibiotics which cover sinonasal flora are administered for the duration of nasal packing. Postoperative CT scans are recommended for these treatments, as direct visualization of the reduction is not possible, and rigid reconstruction of the orbital wall is not performed (Fig. 7.10). If inadequate reconstruction is discovered, then revision surgery by a more traditional approach may be recommended.

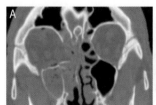 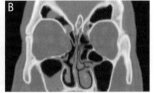

Figure 7.10 (A) Preoperative and (B) 5 months postoperative computed tomography (CT) scans in endoscopic medial orbital wall fracture repair.

COMPLICATIONS

Corneal abrasion

Corneal abrasion may occur inadvertently prior to, during, or after surgery. If a known abrasion has occurred, or there are symptoms of sharp pain, aggravated by opening and closing the eye accompanied by tearing and occasionally photophobia, diagnosis is confirmed with fluorescein staining. The eye should be examined to confirm the absence of a foreign body. Treatment usually consists of antibiotic eyedrops and abstaining from wearing contact lenses while healing. The eye may be patched for comfort, and healing can be expected to occur within 1–7 days depending on the size of the abrasion. Topical anaesthetic or steroid drops should not be administered. Large abrasions associated with considerable inflammation may require the use of cycloplegic medications to reduce pain associated with ciliary muscle spasm.

Oedema, emphysema and ecchymosis

Some degree of oedema, emphysema and ecchymosis may occur when orbital tissues are manipulated. This may be minimized with strict precautions against strenuous activity and nose blowing, avoidance of medications known to cause platelet or clotting dysfunction, elevation of the head of the bed and application of ice to the face postoperatively. However, these also may be signs of orbital haemorrhage or marked orbital emphysema (Figs 7.11 and 7.12). Worsening pain and vision loss are worrisome for increased orbital pressure as a result

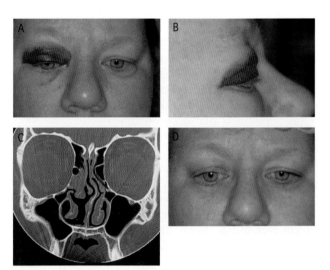

Figure 7.11 Inadvertent injury to the anterior ethmoid artery and resultant immediate orbital haematoma. (A, B) Orbital pressures were not elevated, and the patient was kept under observation. (C) Preoperative computed tomography (CT) scan demonstrating an exposed anterior ethmoid artery in the ethmoid. (D) Two weeks postoperatively.

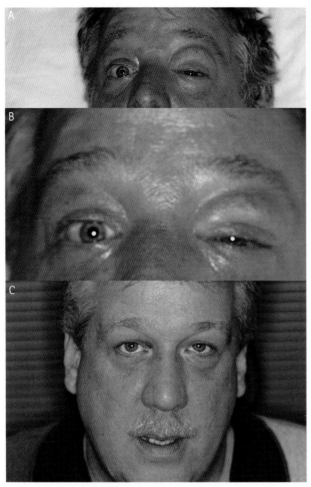

Figure 7.12 Immediate postoperative images of a patient with a coughing bout in recovery room. (A, B) The nasal packing was immediately removed and ocular pressures were checked and found to be normal; based on symptoms of crepitus, a diagnosis was made of preseptal emphysema, and the patient was kept under observation. (C) Patient at 2 weeks: no symptoms present.

of either circumstance. Immediate examination must be performed, including pupil size, symmetry and reactivity, visual acuity and measurement of intraocular pressure. If concerning, intravenous administration of steroids and mannitol is recommended. Lateral canthotomy and cantholysis may be necessary in the setting of elevated pressure and vision loss. Immediate consultation by an ophthalmologist or oculoplastic surgeon is mandatory.

Blindness

Blindness as a result of postoperative orbital haemorrhage or emphysema should not occur with appropriate patient awareness and availability of medical and surgical staff. Blindness and diplopia as a result of intraoperative injury to the optic nerve or rectus muscles are additional feared complications of sino-orbital surgery. These may result from direct trauma to the muscles, intraorbital portion

of the optic or ophthalmic nerves, or the intracanalicular segment of the optic nerve in the superolateral sphenoid sinus. Bone fragments in orbital fractures have the potential to cause injury to the optic nerve or recti muscles. Pupil examination with a swinging flashlight test may provide a clue to optic nerve or retinal injury. Examination of the extraocular movements may demonstrate a gross identifiable abnormality. A CT scan can be helpful to ascertain a site of injury or presence of haematoma or bone fragment. Incision of the annulus of Zinn may also contribute to postoperative diplopia, as this fascial ring forms the attachment of the rectus muscles. Often, diplopia of uncertain origin is managed expectantly, and treated in a delayed fashion with prism lenses or strabismus surgery.

Cerebrospinal fluid leak

A CSF leak may occur after surgery around the optic nerve. After leaving the chiasm, the intracranial segment of the nerve travels approximately 1.5 cm in the subarachnoid space. Within the optic canal, the dural–periosteal layer splits. The inner layer continues as a dural layer around the optic nerve, and the outer layer continues to form the periorbita. The subarachnoid space is maintained to the posterior aspect of the globe, so incisions of the nerve sheath anywhere along its course may lead to CSF leak. Fenestration of the nerve sheath in surgery for traumatic optic neuropathy theoretically should cause a CSF leak; however, this phenomenon is rarely encountered. This may be explained by associated nerve oedema or haemorrhage, which precludes drainage of CSF through the fenestration. If a CSF leak occurs, a free mucosal graft is placed and secured with fibrin glue without the use of additional packing.

CONCLUSION

The extension of endoscopic sinus surgical techniques into the treatment of orbital and lacrimal disease has become gradually accepted over time. Certain benefits are offered over traditional approaches; however, the following requirements must be met prior to the otolaryngologist undertaking endoscopic sino-orbital or lacrimal surgery:

- a thorough understanding of the surgical anatomy
- sufficient endoscopic skill and experience
- availability of appropriate instrumentation and image guidance if indicated
- established working relationship with a knowledgeable ophthalmologist or oculoplastic surgeon.

The early recognition and treatment of intraoperative and postoperative complications is crucial when working near the orbit. Finally, care of the patient does not end with surgery and meticulous postoperative monitoring and treatment are important.

REFERENCES

1. Yung CW, Moorthy RS, Lindley D et al. Efficacy of lateral canthotomy and cantholysis in orbital hemorrhage. *Ophthal Plast Reconstr Surg* 1994; **10**: 137–41.
2. Kirchner JA, Yanagisawa E, Crelin ES. Surgical anatomy of the ethmoid arteries. *Arch Otolaryngol* 1961; **74**: 382–6.
3. Li KK, Teknos TN, Lai A et al. Traumatic optic neuropathy: result in 45 consecutive surgically treated patients. *Otolaryngol Head Neck Surg* 1999; **120**: 5–11.
4. Wang BH, Robertson BC, Girotto JA et al. Traumatic optic neuropathy: a review of 61 patients. *Plast Reconstr Surg* 2001; **107**: 1655–64.
5. Yu Wai Man P, Griffiths PG. Surgery for traumatic optic neuropathy. *Cochrane Database Syst Rev* 2005; CD005024.
6. Levin LA, Beck RW, Joseph MP et al. The treatment of traumatic optic neuropathy: the International Optic Nerve Trauma Study. *Ophthalmology* 1999; **106**: 1268–77.
7. Ramakrishnan VR, Hink EM, Durairaj VD et al. Outcomes after endoscopic dacryocystorhinostomy without mucosal flap preservation. *Am J Rhinol* 2007; **21**: 753–7.
8. Wormald PJ. Powered endoscopic dacryocystorhinostomy. *Laryngoscope* 2002; **112**: 69–72.
9. Ben Simon GJ, Joseph J, Lee S et al. External versus endoscopic dacryocystorhinostomy for acquired nasolacrimal duct obstruction in a tertiary referral center. *Ophthalmology* 2005; **112**: 1463–8.
10. Smirnov G, Tuomilehto H, Teräsvirta M et al. Silicone tubing is not necessary after primary endoscopic dacryocystorhinostomy: a prospective randomized study. *Am J Rhinol* 2008; **22**: 214–17.
11. Selig YK, Biesman BS, Rebeiz EE. Topical application of mitomycin-C in endoscopic dacryocystorhinostomy. *Am J Rhinol* 2000; **14**: 205–7.
12. Deka A, Bhattacharjee K, Bhuyan SK et al. Effect of mitomycin C on ostium in dacryocystorhinostomy. *Clin Experiment Ophthalmol* 2006; **34**: 557–61.
13. Jeon SY, Kwon JH, Kim JP et al. Endoscopic intranasal reduction of the orbit in isolated blowout fractures. *Acta Otolaryngol* 2007; **558**: S102–9.

8

Endonasal surgery of the anterior skull base

DANIEL B SIMMEN

INTRODUCTION

There has been an impressive evolution in endoscopic skull base surgery over the past few years. The rhinologist has emerged as an important member of the interdisciplinary skull base team as experience has grown in the use of less invasive techniques to remove sinus tumours. Endonasal endoscopic approaches have become the standard for the surgical treatment of inflammatory sinus diseases and benign sinus tumours over the past few years. Although endoscopic resection of malignant tumours has been controversial, there is increasing evidence that there are many advantages to the endoscopic approach to remove many nasal and skull base tumours. The fundamental reasons behind this evolution are the new knowledge about the anatomy from the endoscopic perspective, and the development of instruments and image guidance that allow a more direct and magnified vision of what the surgeon can do (Fig. 8.1). A reduction in the mortality and morbidity – including less disruption of the brain and eye – of the surgery, being able to deal with most complications, a recognition that an 'en bloc' resection of most skull base tumours was a good concept but is rarely achievable, thus negating one of its main *raisons d'être*, and an accumulating volume of evidence add weight to the use of the endonasal approach in skull base surgery.[1,2]

The management of tumours of the skull base must be done as part of a multidisciplinary team and the surgeon should be able to undertake an external approach and know how to deal with the majority of possible complications (Fig. 8.2). This includes being able to change to an external approach if necessary at any time during procedure. The following principles apply to the planning of an endoscopic procedure of the skull base:

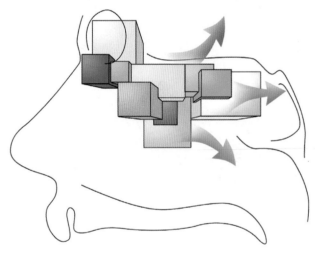

Figure 8.1 Evolution from endonasal sinus to skull base surgery – rhino-neurosurgery. The arrows illustrate the transcribriform, transsphenoidal–transclival and transpterygoid approaches.

- understanding the pathology of any lesion of the skull base is essential in its management
- involvement of other relevant disciplines in making a treatment plan
- extensive range of equipment is needed to do this type of surgery
- imaging should be done to define the extent of any tumour and when it is very vascular, angiography can contribute regardless of whether or not there is preoperative embolization
- preoperative counselling is important.

The gold standard for many tumours of the anterior skull base has been the craniofacial resection (Fig. 8.3). However, with this approach a craniotomy involves a

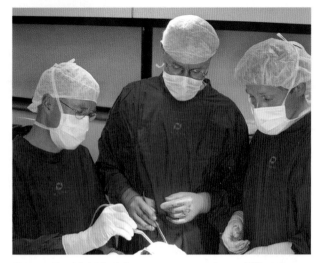

Figure 8.2 Multidisciplinary team approach – an ENT surgeon, a maxillofacial surgeon and a neurosurgeon carrying out a skull base procedure.

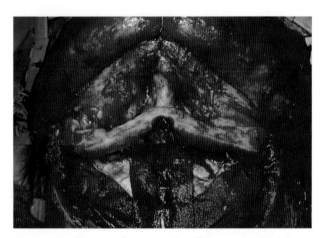

Figure 8.3 The craniofacial resection. This approach has been overtaken more and more by endonasal rhino-neurosurgical procedures.

great deal of bony work, with possible sequelae including the resorption of bone, osteomyelitis, a coronal flap that frequently causes some hair loss and a scar, being an inpatient for several days, some obtunded function (albeit temporary, due to retraction of the frontal lobes), epilepsy and intracranial complications. These tumours often cross the boundary between the nasal cavity and the brain and an approach through the nose provides a direct corridor for removal of these tumours and is often preferable to going via the intracranial cavity. The primary goal with these approaches is to address the pathology without displacing normal neural and vascular structures. Although the goal is to remove any tumour, whether *en bloc* or piecemeal with a margin, this is not always possible whether the approach is endoscopic or craniofacial. An example would be a tumour that invaded the basisphenoid. It may be possible to dissect it off its bony remains with a coarse diamond drill around much of the periphery of the tumour and

preserve the optic nerves and carotid arteries; however, a 'clear' margin may not be achievable. In these patients the pathology and its response to radiotherapy, with or without chemotherapy, need to be considered by a multidisciplinary team to determine the best treatment strategy (Fig. 8.4).

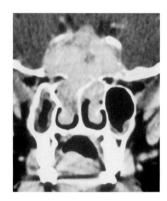

Figure 8.4 A malignant tumour in the sphenoid sinus illustrating an interdisciplinary team approach to determine the best treatment strategy.

FROM SINUS TO SKULL BASE SURGERY

Endoscopic sinus surgery for inflammatory diseases over the past decades has evolved hand in hand along with new perspectives as to what can be achieved surgically in the nasal cavity and skull base. For example, large mucocoeles, extensive benign tumours and fungal disease have expanded the scope of what the endoscopic surgeon can achieve. Surgery in this area has extended outside the normal remit of the rhinologist to encompass removal of the dura, the basisphenoid and periorbital tissue, as well as reconstruction of the skull base.

The extended applications around the anterior skull base surgery include:

- extended frontal sinus surgery – median drill out procedures
- dacryocystorhinostomy
- management of severe epistaxis – sphenopalatine artery, maxillary artery, anterior ethmoid artery
- management of cerebrospinal fluid (CSF) leaks, repair of dura
- orbital decompression, optic nerve decompression.

All surgeons wishing to be involved in skull base surgery have to learn these specific procedures. This usually involves gaining experience starting with endoscopic surgery for benign nasal disease before expanding their repertoire to deal with the removal of more invasive pathology. A surgeon must be able to carry out the extended applications listed above before addressing the resection of a skull base tumour. A team approach benefits from learning and using the bimanual technique, along with experience using the wider angled endoscopes, malleable instruments and powered drills.[3]

PLANNING THE SURGERY – AREAS AT RISK

Anterior skull base lesions pose a challenge because of the proximity of important structures. Surgeons require extensive knowledge and skills to be able to carry out precise and technically safe resections of these lesions. Planning the operation involves determining the best route of resection and this is based on individual experience and skills, and the site and extent of the lesion. Along with this the surgeon needs to have in mind the potential areas at risk and how to manage them (Fig. 8.5). The endonasal approach often provides a minimally invasive approach and has the potential to be as surgically thorough in the extent of the removal of the tumour compared with an external or craniofacial approach. However, because of the limited access and space available when using the endoscopic technique, dealing with complications is more difficult and therefore training is needed to manage these (see Chapter 4).

For anterior skull base surgery the key anatomical issues are as follows (Fig. 8.6).

- The frontal sinus – how far laterally its mucosa and, if necessary, the lateral and posterior walls can be removed. On one end of the spectrum is a hypoplastic or poorly pneumatized frontal sinus whose lining and contents can readily be removed, although this requires a lot of drilling as the 'beak' (see below) of the sinus is very thick.

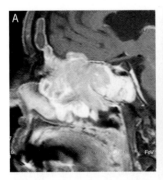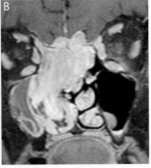

Figure 8.5 (A) Saggital and (B) coronal magnetic resonance images of an adenocarcinoma in the anterior skull base: these tumours pose a challenge to the surgeons because of the proximity of important structures involved. Planning and determining the best route of resection are crucial for successful removal.

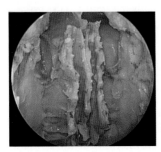

Figure 8.6 Endoscopic view to the anterior skull base in an injected specimen. The septum and middle turbinate have been partially removed with a fronto-sphenoethmoidectomy on both sides to expose the entire extent of the anterior skull base.

At the other end is a well-pneumatized frontal sinus that will need angled endoscopes and frontal sinus curettes to visualize and remove disease that lies lateral to the sagittal plane of the middle of the orbit. Both the angled endoscope and the malleable frontal sinus curettes may need to be placed through the contralateral nostril and across the space created by a large median drainage procedure to get to the lateral aspect of the frontal sinus.

- Lacrimal sac, orbit and optic nerve – any tumour that abuts or involves these structures often has to be removed without causing any serious visual sequelae. Much depends on the pathology and the site of the lesion.
- Cribriform plate and ethmoid bone – this area has become less of an issue as it is now known that it can readily be removed and reconstructed.
- Vascular anatomy of the anterior skull base – proximity to the carotid artery or cavernous sinus is of major importance. Removing disease that is next to these structures, let alone disease invading them, requires a lot of experience and careful planning.
- The pterygopalatine fossa – this area contains the maxillary artery anteriorly but otherwise it has few landmarks, being filled with fat and a plexus of veins.

SURGICAL ANATOMY OF THE ANTERIOR SKULL BASE

Frontal sinus

The precise anatomical knowledge of the frontal sinus is important as this sinus is a key landmark in anterior skull base surgery (see also Chapter 12). The frontal sinus is usually anterior to the lesion and by exposing the sinus with a frontal sinusotomy and median drainage procedure the posterior wall of the sinus defines the start of the cranial base resection (Fig. 8.7). The nasal process of the frontal bone is thick and forms a 'beak' that restricts both the anterior access and drainage of the frontal sinus. The anteroposterior distance between the beak and the cribriform plate determines the ease with which the frontal sinus can be reached and how much drilling of the beak will be required.

The frontal intersinus septum varies greatly in its position and has to be outlined carefully prior to the surgery as it helps to define the midline of the skull base and the position of the crista galli. Access to the lateral aspect of the frontal sinus is now possible using angled

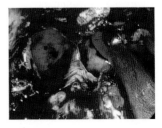

Figure 8.7 Endoscopic view of a median drainage procedure in a skull base tumour identifying the posterior wall of the sinus, which defines the start of the cranial base resection.

endoscopes through the contralateral side, having done a median drainage procedure, or through a septal window.

Lacrimal sac, orbit and optic nerve

Another important anatomical key landmark is the lacrimal sac, which helps the surgeon to find their way into the frontal sinus, especially if the anatomy is distorted by the lesion (Fig. 8.8). The fundus of the lacrimal sac in the lateral nasal wall and the periorbital tissue can usually be identified with ease. This is done by removing the anterior lacrimal crest with a Kerrison punch and diamond drill to reveal the magenta-coloured lacrimal sac.

Follow the periosteum of the orbit to reach the orbital apex where the optic nerve can be identified (Fig. 8.9). It is essential that the periorbita is kept intact as a breach in it will result in periorbital fat prolapsing into the nasal cavity and obscuring what lies behind it. The medial wall of the orbit is made up of the lamina papyracea of the ethmoid bone, the palatine bone and more posteriorly the thicker bone of the sphenoid that makes up the apex of the orbit (Figs 8.10 and 8.11). The degree of pneumatization of the sphenoid sinus determines whether the optic nerve indents, or is even dehiscent in, its lateral wall. The same applics to the posterior ethmoid sinuses, which can envelop the optic nerve before it reaches the sphenoid

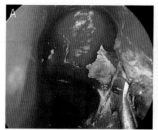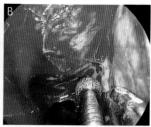

Figure 8.10   (A) Removing the lamina papyracea on the left side with the Cottle elevator and (B) more posterior towards the optic nerve, the thicker bone of the sphenoid sinus is removed with a diamond drill.

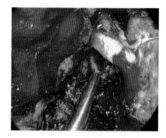

Figure 8.11   Endoscopic intraoperative view of a skull base tumour being removed to expose the orbit and optic nerve in the lateral wall of the left sphenoid sinus.

sinus if there is a sphenoethmoid cell (Onodi cell). The inferomedial strut of the maxillary bone is often thick but a portion is worth preserving as this reduces the possibility of developing diplopia. The bone in the floor of the orbit and lateral to the infraorbital nerve is also thick and more difficult to remove (Fig. 8.12).

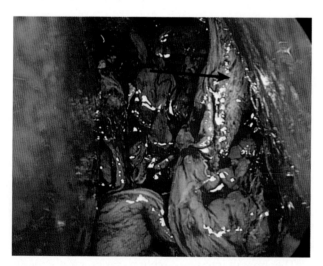

Figure 8.8   The lacrimal sac exposed on the left side (arrow) in a skull base tumour resection. With the help of the sac and its duct, the maxillary sinus can be identified, and the fundus of the sac guides the surgeon into the frontal sinus.

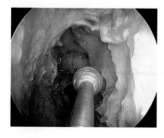

Figure 8.9   Exposing the periosteum of the orbit and optic nerve by removing the lamina papyracea of the ethmoid bone with a coarse diamond drill. The optic nerve can be seen above and distal to the head of the diamond bur.

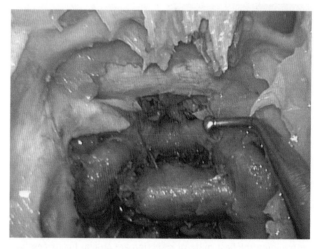

Figure 8.12   Anatomy of the posterior part of the anterior skull base. The ball probe indicates the optic chiasm, above the dura of the exposed planum sphenoidale, both carotid arteries beside the cavernous sinus with the pituitary gland in between.

Cribriform plate and ethmoid bone

The skull base is made up anteriorly of the posterior wall of the frontal sinus, which consists of thick frontal bone that extends posteriorly to form the roof of the ethmoid sinuses (fovea ethmoidalis) on either side of the cribriform plate that is part of the ethmoid bone. The cribriform plate joins the fovea through the lateral lamella and this can be almost non-existent when the cribriform plate and fovea ethmoidalis are on the same plane, or it can form the thin vertical bone connecting them, depending on how far the cribriform plate dips into the nose. Posteriorly, the sphenoid sinus and the posterior ethmoid air cells form the skull base. The dura is attached to the cribriform plate and the olfactory fibres penetrate into the nasal cavity along the septal mucosa and the medial surface of the superior and middle turbinate. The dura is very thin and very vulnerable in the cribriform plate area but it becomes thicker towards the planum sphenoidale and towards the orbital roof (see Fig. 8.6, p. 73).

Pterygopalatine fossa

The pterygopalatine fossa lies posterior to the posterior wall of the maxillary sinus. The maxillary artery is exposed as soon as the posterior wall of the maxillary sinus is removed. The space is filled with fat and a venous plexus as well as branches of the maxillary artery that supply the pterygoid muscles, and these are very tortuous and variable (Fig. 8.13).

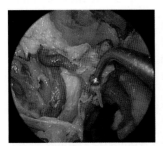

Figure 8.13 Endoscopic view into the right pterygopalatine fossa in an injected cadaver specimen. The maxillary artery is well exposed after removing the fat and after removing the bone at the level of the sphenopalatine foramen.

Vascular anatomy of the anterior skull base

In dealing with tumours along the anterior skull base, knowledge of the vascular anatomy is important as it helps to keep the operating field under control, promotes visibility and helps avoid complications. In many cases it also helps to control the feeding vessels to minimize bleeding and optimize visibility for the resection to be done safely (Fig. 8.14).

The sphenopalatine artery splits into three or more branches on exiting the foramen. The foramen becomes a slit whose anterior margin is a lateral 'knuckle' of bone called the crista ethmoidalis. The crista ethmoidalis comes off the lateral nasal wall near the root or posteroinferior base of the middle turbinate. The anterior branch of the sphenopalatine artery comes around the crista and can be found as it runs forwards in the lateral nasal wall over the posterior fontanelle (Fig. 8.15). The internal carotid artery can have pathological branches that supply the skull base lesion and other feeding vessels can come from the middle meningeal artery, the vidian artery or from the external carotid system, or from the ascending pharyngeal or maxillary artery (Figs 8.16 and 8.17).

The anterior ethmoid artery is a branch of the ophthalmic artery and therefore it originates within the orbit before

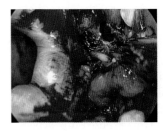

Figure 8.15 Exposure of the branches of the sphenopalatine artery on the right side in a skull base tumour case. The septal branch above the crista ethmoidalis has been coagulated while one conchal branch above and one conchal branch below the crista are still visible.

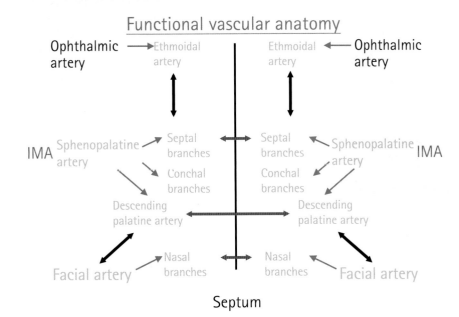

Figure 8.14 Vascular anatomy of the nose illustrating the ipsilateral and contralateral communication of the arteries. An important factor is the cross-talk between the ethmoid arteries and branches of the sphenopalatine artery ipsilaterally and contralaterally along the septum. IMA, maxillary artery.

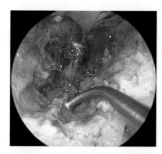

Figure 8.16 Vidian artery in the floor of the right sphenoid sinus in a injected specimen. Communication between the internal and the external carotid arteries is not uncommon through anastomosis.

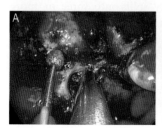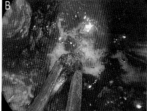

Figure 8.17 Intraoperative view of the bony crest in the sphenoid floor (A) containing the nerve and artery and (B) coagulation of the vidian artery coming off the internal carotid artery.

travelling medially through the bone of the anterior skull base – the fovea ethmoidalis (the part of the frontal bone that forms the roof of the ethmoid sinuses). The artery is normally enclosed to a large extent within a bony canal but often part of this is very thin or dehiscent. It can often be located just behind a supraorbital cell that is an extension of the suprabullar recess. It may travel in a coronal plane, but often it is oblique, travelling more anteriorly as it goes medially. It gives off branches to the septum (anterior nasal branch), lateral nasal wall and intracranially (anterior meningeal artery) (Fig. 8.18). How exposed it is depends in part on the degree of pneumatization of the sinuses and how 'deep' the cribriform plate 'dips' into the nasal airway (Fig. 8.19).

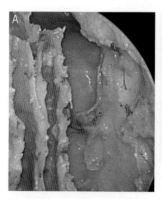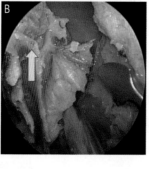

Figure 8.18 Endoscopic view of the skull base in an injected specimen showing (A) the anterior ethmoid artery leaving the orbit on the left side and (B) a close-up of the final branch into the septum – the anterior nasal branch of the ethmoid artery (arrow).

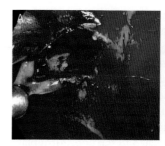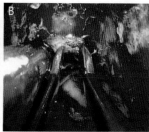

Figure 8.19 (A) Anterior ethmoid artery exposed in the left skull base. (B) Bipolar coagulation of the artery.

SURGICAL TECHNIQUE

The surgical strategy is individualized as no two tumours are exactly alike. The strategy depends on:

- localization and degree of expansion into the intracranial cavity or orbit (staging)
- tumour biology:
  - benign or malignant, invasiveness
  - soft, friable or hard, vascular content
- *en bloc* or piecemeal resection
- patient's health status
- repair of the defect.

Generally, the philosophy is to expose the tumour widely around its circumference before starting to mobilize and resect the lesion. An exception to this is when the tumour mass needs to be reduced at the beginning of the surgery in order to obtain access. This may lead to bleeding and a loss of visibility. There are several strategies to help the surgeon gain space around the tumour without debulking it. An ethmoidectomy around the lesion, including a large maxillary sinusotomy, and exposing the lacrimal system can help to expose important landmarks (fundus of the lacrimal sac, orbit) and create a cavity to gain space to work around the tumour. In very big lesions occupying the whole nasal cavity a medial maxillectomy should be performed as a first step. This is done by making an incision anterior to the inferior turbinate, removing the edge of the pyriform aperture along with the anterior and medial wall of the maxillary sinus and the anterior lacrimal crest. Very often a sphenoethmoidectomy on the opposite side can also help to clarify the anatomy and define the level of the skull base and the sphenoid sinus on the non-diseased side.

Mobilization of the cartilagenous and bony septa can help in skull base surgery as well and allows access for instruments and endoscopes from the contralateral side. Removal of the back of the vomer and the anterior wall of the sphenoid creates space posteriorly. Anterior access depends on doing a median drainage approach to the frontal sinus and a septal window helps in the bimanual approach with one surgeon being able to hold the endoscope and keep the site free of blood while the other can resect or drill with one hand and keep tension on the tissue with the other. The frontal sinus and the sphenoid provide the anterior and posterior landmarks for most anterior skull base tumours and exposing these are usually the initial steps from which the other tumour margins are defined. Wide exposure of the frontal sinus and the roof of the ethmoid sinuses starts to define the skull base. The bone can be resected or drilled away all around the tumour, starting with the posterior wall of the frontal sinus and then along the ethmoid roof on one or both sides according to the site of the lesion and the surgical plan (Fig. 8.20). Neurosurgical pattée or ribbon gauze soaked in 1 in 1000 adrenaline (epinephrine) can be used to retract the tumour, reduce bleeding and peel it away from surrounding structures.

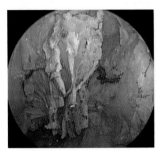

Figure 8.20 Diathermy of both anterior ethmoid arteries close to their exit from the orbit and thinning down the ethmoid roof to the level of the dura allows the cribriform plate to be mobilized and resected in one piece.

Depending on the morphology of the lesion the tumour can be dissected from the dura with cutting instruments or powered instruments such as drill or shaver systems (Fig. 8.21). A large coarse diamond drill is best as this is efficient and avoids skidding off pieces of bone and wrapping soft tissue around it. The shaver must be avoided if orbital fat or brain is exposed as the shaver efficiently removes these tissues. If the tumour is malignant and the dura has to be resected, the dura should be defined and opened all around the lesion. It is cut with microscissors starting anteriorly from the frontal sinus to the posterior aspect of the resection. With this manoeuvre the lesion can be mobilized and dropped down into the nasal cavity away from the intracranial space, and all the intracranial vessels can be preserved (Fig. 8.22).

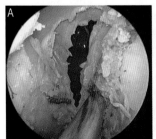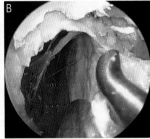

Figure 8.21 The posterior wall of the frontal sinus is opened and the dura incised with microscissors (A) and then the crista galli is dissected intracranially and the anterior meningeal artery is coagulated after coming off the anterior ethmoid artery before fully mobilizing the cribriform plate (B).

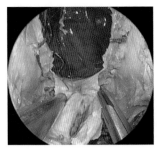

Figure 8.22 The dura has been cut all around the tumour mass with microscissors and is dropped down into the nasal cavity.

If there is extension into the brain, the neurosurgeon takes over and resects the lesion from the brain and manages the intracranial vessels. In specific pathology such as aesthesioneuroblastomas the olfactory bulb and tract are resected to the level of the planum sphenoidale and optic chiasm (Fig. 8.23). Finally frozen sections are taken around the lesion to check that the margins of resection are tumour free.

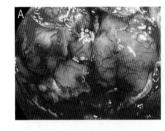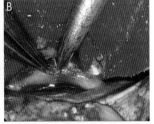

Figure 8.23 (A) Intraoperative view after dropping down the tumour into the nasal cavity with the exposed frontal lobes and (B) the view towards the optic chiasm and planum sphenoidale that still holds the tumour.

Closure of the defect

Large defects of the anterior skull base are challenging to close and require precise technical work. The prime graft materials needed to close large defects of the anterior skull base are free fascia grafts – mainly fascia lata and abdominal fat are needed along with glue. The fascia is first of all placed intracranially over the planum sphenoidale and then on both sides as an underlay along the orbital roof and finally over the posterior wall of the frontal sinus (Fig. 8.24). A second overlay is placed over the entire area

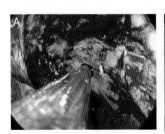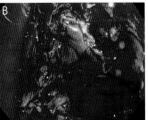

Figure 8.24 Closure of the defect using a free fascia graft (A) as a underlay intracranially and (B) then a second fascia graft in an overlay technique.

of the resection and secured with small fat grafts. The use of fibrin glue or similar products can further help to secure the graft (Fig. 8.25). We have found that bone or cartilage is rarely needed to close a defect in the anterior skull base. If a watertight closure cannot be obtained with this technique, a vascularized flap from the septal mucosa helps. This pedicle flap is based on the septal branch of the sphenopalatine artery and can further help support the fascia (Fig. 8.26).

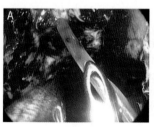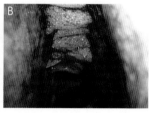

Figure 8.25 (A, B) Fibrin glue and small fat pads help to further secure the grafts.

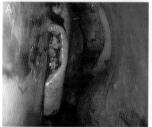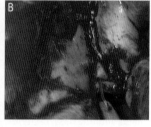

Figure 8.26 (A) Mobilization of a vascularized pedicled septal mucosal flap (Hadad flap) on the left side prior to the tumour resection and (B) close-up view showing the septal branch of the sphenopalatine artery that is the feeding vessel for the flap.

COMBINED ENDONASAL AND CRANIOFACIAL APPROACH

Most anterior skull base tumours that appear to approximate or involve the dura on imaging have not yet traversed it and can be resected endoscopically. The place of surgery is limited in poorly differentiated tumours that have traversed the dura and invaded the cerebrum as current evidence is that this rarely prolongs life expectancy and it usually adds to patient morbidity, reducing the patient's quality of life in their remaining months of life. Under these circumstances palliation is often the treatment of choice. In well-differentiated or moderately differentiated tumours that have traversed the dura but have not invaded the cerebrum, resection and radiotherapy with or without chemotherapy may have a role but these tumours usually require a craniofacial approach. The endoscope can still have a valuable role in defining and removing the intranasal part of the disease. Under these circumstances the intranasal component of

the disease is important to delineate to obtain surgically clear margins.

THE TIMING OF CHEMOTHERAPY OR RADIOTHERAPY

The timing of chemotherapy or radiotherapy is controversial. If radiotherapy is done postoperatively it should be started at least 6 weeks after any resection based on historical data on the treatment of squamous cell carcinomas of the head and neck. Preoperative radiotherapy affects healing, particularly when a free graft is used to close a skull base defect. Radiotherapy can reduce the vascularity of a tumour but it can make it more difficult to define the tissue plane between a tumour and the surrounding tissue. The number of skull base tumours is not large, even in big tertiary referral centres, and a prospective randomized multicentre study is needed to answer many of the questions related to the management of these tumours. If chemotherapy is indicated, and this usually applies to poorly differentiated tumours, neuroendocrine tumours or rhabdomyosarcoma, and particularly if there are metastases, then even if the tumour shrinks greatly, the current belief is that all the area that was originally involved with tumour should be removed. Should the tumour respond to the first few courses of chemotherapy it is usual practice for some further courses to be given after the resection of the tumour to kill any residual malignant cells although there is no hard evidence to substantiate this. Extra care needs to be taken with the preoperative work-up to ensure that the patient is fit for surgery in relation to their neutrophil and platelet counts.

COMPLICATIONS

It is important to extubate a patient without them coughing on a cuffed endotracheal tube in order to avoid a marked rise in intracranial and CSF pressure. Positive pressure on a face mask should be avoided as it might cause aerencephalus. It is also advisable to nurse the patient 30–45° head up in the hours after surgery to reduce the CSF pressure that might otherwise 'test' the seal of any reconstruction of the skull base. Antibiotics are not given preoperatively when there is an active CSF leak as they do not reduce the incidence of meningitis but make it more likely that the organism that causes it will be a more resistant strain. Antibiotic prophylaxis is used in skull base reconstruction in part because of the frequent use of a free graft and in part because the nasal vestibule, airway and nasopharynx (unlike healthy paranasal sinuses) are not sterile. Patients are advised not to strain or lift heavy weights for 2 weeks and that their diet avoids constipation to avoid episodes when their CSF pressure is markedly increased. Patients are advised not to blow their nose or stifle sneezes for 4 days after surgery. A variety of

nasal packs or dressings are used to support the graft or
vascularized pedicle that is used to reconstruct any skull
base defect. Dissolvable packs such as oxidized cellulose
can be left in position and kept clean by douching that
can be started after 4 days. Non-absorbable packs are
used less frequently but if they are used, they are usually
removed after 1 week and the layer between this and the
graft, one of resorbable material, is left in place.

POSTOPERATIVE MANAGEMENT

Postoperative imaging has little to offer initially as many
of the changes seen are non-specific. Even after several
months, there are non-specific changes on computed
tomography (CT) and magnetic resonance imaging
(MRI) that often cause more concern than being helpful.
Where mucosa has been removed and the underlying
bone has been drilled there is often an excessive amount
of granulation tissue for several months that can alarm
the endoscopist and cause concern that this represents
residual disease. Usually patience and douching pay off
and the florid amount of polypoidal granulation tissue
settles down. If this fails to show any sign of happening
after 4 months a biopsy is warranted, but frequently the
patient and the surgeon will be relieved to find that it is
due to non-specific inflammatory tissue.

Initial symptoms of diplopia may resolve but if not they
are very annoying. Horizontal diplopia may result from
scarring of the medial rectus if the medial wall of the orbit
and periorbital tissue has been removed. Little can be done
to correct this and often a frosted lens is required. Diplopia
looking straight ahead, such as when reading, is relatively
unusual but can result after a maxillectomy when the
whole of the medial wall and floor of the orbit as well as the
periorbital tissue has been removed. Preserving an inferior
medial strut of bone between the orbit and maxilla reduces
this complication, as has been advocated in endoscopic
orbital decompression.

Symptoms of crusting can persist for several months
until the cilia regenerate. It is important to explain to the
patient that until this time regular douching is required
otherwise mucus builds up and becomes locally infected
giving off toxins that delay the regeneration of cilia.
Regular douching is required until no crusts or 'casts'
have been produced for a month. If the patient has had
radiotherapy then regular douching may be required as
the mucus glands and cilia may never fully recover (Fig.
8.27).

Delayed haemorrhage is rare. One rare cause that
invokes concern is a pseudoaneurysm of the carotid artery.
If the carotid is uncovered in removing a tumour in
the sphenoid sinus, and in particular if the adventitia is
damaged in any way, a pseudoaneurysm can result. The
likelihood of this may be reduced by placing fascia or a
vascularized septal flap based on the sphenopalatine artery
over the site. In any event its development should be

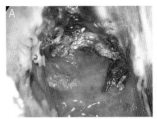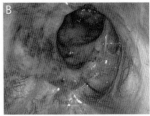

Figure 8.27   (A) Crusting and infected oedematous mucosa
several months after the operation and (B) the regenerated and
ciliated mucosa at 2 years after the surgery with ongoing local
treatment.

excluded by endoscopy and if necessary MRI angiography.
If a pseudoaneurysm develops it needs managing with
the help of an interventional neuroradiologist, who will
determine if there is enough cross-circulation from the
other carotid artery and vertebral arteries and find out if
occlusion is possible.

Postoperative monitoring to check for recurrent disease
is best done with nasal endoscopy, palpation of the neck
for cervical lymphadenopathy and depending on the
pathology on CT of the chest. Regular follow-up is needed
for a minimum of 5 years in these patients, ideally for 10
years.

CONCLUSION AND FUTURE DIRECTION

The role of the endoscope in removing skull base tumours is
expanding thanks to advances in endoscopes, instruments,

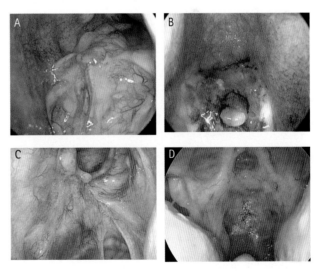

Figure 8.28   (A) A skull base tumour filling the entire nasal
cavity; therefore mobilizing the septum helps to gain space as
well as working anterior to the tumour into the frontal sinus.
(B) Creating a median drainage procedure is a key step in this
surgery. (C) Endoscopic view of the median drainage and anterior
skull base with fascia repair and (D) an endoscopic view of the
posterior skull base with the epipharynx and pituitary gland as
well as the optic chiasm above 7 years after the operation and
radiotherapy.

the four-handed technique and a better understanding of how to delineate the anatomy around tumours from an endoscopic perspective. Surgical experience, like other areas of medicine, comes by building up a repertoire whose building blocks include endoscopic medial maxillectomy and dacryocystorhinostomy, frontal sinus median drainage procedures, orbital decompression, pituitary surgery and the repair of CSF leaks and encephalocoeles, before embarking on the endoscopic resection of malignant skull base tumours (Fig. 8.28).

The pathology and staging of a tumour remain the primary determinants of prognosis and it is important to treat these tumours as part of a multidisciplinary skull base team. Resecting 'one or two' of these tumours 'every now and then' does not serve patients well.

REFERENCES

1. Eloy JA, Vivero RJ, Hoang K *et al.* Comparison of transnasal endoscopic and open craniofacial resection of malignant tumours of the anterior skull base. *Laryngoscope* 2009; **119**: 834–40.

2. Buchmann L, Larsen C, Pollack A *et al.* Endoscopic techniques in resection of anterior skull base/paranasal sinus malignancies. *Laryngoscope* 2006; **116**: 1749–54.

3. Robinson S, Wormald PJ. Endoscopic management of benign tumors extending into the infratemporal fossa. A two-surgeon transnasal approach. *Laryngoscope* 2009; **115**: 1818–22.

9

Pituitary and parasellar surgery

ALDO C STAMM, JOÃO F NOGUEIRA JR

INTRODUCTION

Endoscopic pituitary and parasellar surgery (EPPS) is a well-established technique for the treatment of sellar and parasellar tumours, especially pituitary adenomas, craniopharyngiomas and meningiomas.[1] The advantages it offers, compared with microscopic approaches, include a superior close-up view of the relevant anatomy and an enlarged working angle along with panoramic vision within the surgical area.[1,2] Several studies have shown that EPPS decreases postoperative discomfort and hospitalization time as well leading to faster recovery in comparison with the conventional microscopic technique. Compared with open transsphenoidal surgery, EPPS is associated with shorter operative times and less blood loss.[1–3]

Access to the pituitary gland through the nasal cavity and sphenoid sinus has been described since the past century, using several approaches including the sublabial microscopic to endoscopic transsphenoidal approach. The sellar region and planum sphenoidale can be approached endoscopically directly using the transnasal, transseptal, modified transseptal or transnasal/transseptal binostril method.[1,2,4,5]

It is often the otorhinolaryngologist who performs the surgical approach through the nasal cavity to the sphenoid sinus because they are more familiar with the anatomy and instrumentation, and have the requisite technical skills, and the neurosurgeon who removes the tumour.[1,5,6] This multidisciplinary team approach is not only important in this surgery but is vital in the preoperative assessment of these patients and their postoperative management. Radiologists, intensivists, endocrinologists, anaesthetists and paramedical staff also play a key role.[5]

In order to help the reader understand the place of EPPS, we have divided this chapter into sections on the different approaches that can be used, a description about surgical techniques in pituitary surgery and then about how to access the planum sphenoidale and cavernous sinus.

PITUITARY SURGERY

Traditionally surgery for pituitary adenomas has been done with microscopes using the transsphenoidal approach. Since the introduction of the rigid endoscope in sinonasal surgery, the pituitary can be visualized better and there is a lower risk of injuring the nasal structures.[5,6] A team approach with endocrinologists, radiologists, anaesthetists, neurosurgeons and otorhinolaryngologists minimizes the likelihood of endocrine problems, cerebrospinal leaks, anterior septal perforation and other functional nasal problems.[5]

Indications and contraindications

The indications for transnasal endoscopic pituitary surgery include pituitary adenomas whose volume causes neurological problems through a pressure effect or endocrine disorders such as prolactinomas, excessive growth hormone or adrenocorticotropic hormone (ACTH) production.

The contraindications for this surgery include patient comorbidities that preclude them from undergoing general anaesthesia.

Instrumentation

Good instrumentation is paramount for the endoscopic approach to the sellar and parasellar regions. The necessary equipment includes a high-quality 0° and 45° rigid endoscope, a camera and monitor, endoscopic bipolar forceps (preferably with a suction channel), long drills with a shaft that is housed to avoid abrading the alar margin, a variety of long dissection instruments and haemostatic materials. A 5 mm wide-angled 0° endoscope is ideal for these procedures, providing an improved field of view as well as illumination[5] (Fig. 9.1).

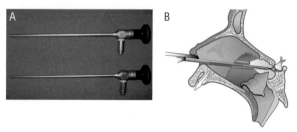

Figure 9.1 Instrumentation. (A) A novel 5 mm 0° endoscope (top) versus the traditional 4 mm 0° endoscope (bottom). (B) The long-shanked drill necessary for work on the sella.

Preoperative assessment

The preoperative evaluation must include a careful clinical history, physical examination and imaging studies. The physical examination will include an endoscopic assessment of the nasal cavity to visualize any nasal lesions, document septal integrity, deviation and other anatomical findings. An informed discussion is mandatory, with a clear explanation about the diagnosis, surgical plan, possible complications and the roles of both the physician and the patient in the anticipated postoperative care plan.

IMAGING

Coronal, axial, and parasagittal computed tomography (CT) of the paranasal sinuses and skull base is essential in the preoperative assessment. It is also necessary to evaluate the size of the sphenoid sinus, the position of the internal carotid artery, the intersinus septum, and the presence of a sphenoethmoidal (Onodi) cell (Fig. 9.2). Magnetic resonance imaging (MRI) is important to demonstrate the size and extension of the tumour and any involvement of the internal carotid artery or cavernous sinus (Fig. 9.2).

The approach

Several transnasal endoscopic approaches to the pituitary have been described, such as:

- transnasal – direct or modified with the removal of the posterior nasal septum
- transseptal – direct and modified, also with the removal of the posterior septum

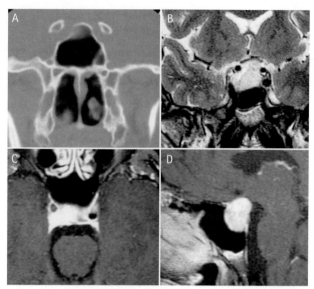

Figure 9.2 Imaging studies. (A) Coronal computed tomography (CT) image showing the sphenoid sinus. (B) Coronal magnetic resonance (MR) image showing the relationship between a pituitary tumour, the internal carotid arteries and the sphenoid sinus. (C) Axial MR image taken to evaluate the lateral extension of the tumour and any involvement of the cavernous sinus. (D) A sagittal MR image.

- transnasal combined with transethmoid and the removal of the middle turbinate
- transseptal/transnasal modified approach.

Each one of these approaches has its advantages and disadvantages.[5,6]

We are going to discuss the binostril approach (transseptal/transnasal), which has recently been described. This approach requires the creation of a nasal septal flap on one side, pedicled from the area of the sphenopalatine foramen, which can be used to close any dural defect and avoids the possibility of a large posterior nasal septal perforation.[6]

PREPARATION

Hypotensive general anaesthesia helps with the patient placed in a supine position on the operating table, the head elevated 30°, the neck slightly flexed and the head extended and turned towards the surgeon. Cottonoids soaked with adrenaline (epinephrine; 1:1000) are placed in the nasal cavity for 10 minutes before the surgical procedure begins. The nasal septum is infiltrated with 2 per cent lidocaine and 1:100 000 adrenaline. A Killian incision, as in septal surgery, is made, generally on the right side of the nose.

A mucoperichondrial/mucoperiosteal flap is raised on both sides. The posterior part of the nasal septum is removed, saving the inferior portion as a reliable landmark for the midline. A nasal septal flap, pedicled on the sphenopalatine bundle, is created on one side. The flap starts with incisions at the posterior choanal arch and is brought forward as far anteriorly as necessary. Multiple modifications regarding length and width are possible (Fig. 9.3).

This binostril approach has several advantages. It allows two surgeons to simultaneously manipulate surgical instruments using both the nostrils. This avoids instruments obstructing the surgical field when they are confined to one side of the nasal cavity. A robust pedicled septal flap helps to close any skull base defect and preserves the nasal septal mucosa on one side, thus avoiding a posterior septal perforation.[6]

At the creation of the nasal septal flap special attention should be given to the free borders of the septal flap as these can bleed and require cautery; occasionally, haemostatic absorbable material is also needed. The anterior wall of the sphenoid sinus must be exposed and opened, facilitating the identification of the principal anatomical structures of the sphenoid sinus, such as the prominences of the internal carotid arteries, optic nerve, clivus and planum sphenoidale. Any inter- and/or intrasinus septae are resected using strong through-cutting forceps. It is best not to grab and twist the septae, as an unpredictable segment of bone that overlies the carotid artery can be removed. The mucoperiosteum of the sphenoid sinus covering the floor of the sella is displaced laterally.

The next step consists of widely resecting the floor of the sellar bone, exposing the dura from one internal carotid artery (ICA) to the opposite ICA, and from the planum sphenoidale to the clivus. This is usually performed with a diamond bur or a micro-Kerrison punch[5,6] (Fig. 9.4).

DURAL QUADRANGULAR INCISION

Since the advent of microscopic approaches, surgeons conventionally have chosen to open the dura by making an 'X-like' or cruciate shaped incision (Fig. 9.5). These

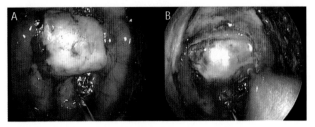

Figure 9.4   Wide resection is the key to this surgery. (A) Floor of the sellar bone exposed. (B) The dura exposed from one internal carotid artery (ICA) to the opposite ICA and from the planun sphenoidale to the clivus. This procedure is usually carried out with a diamond bur.

incisions are considered the 'gold standard' by many authors.[6] The traditional incision is usually made with a sickle knife or with a number 11 blade that allows the creation of a dural flap which can be repositioned after removal of the tumour. However, the dural flap created with the cruciate incision can occasionally get in the way of the surgeon, especially when using suction. The use of bipolar cautery with retraction of these flaps has been described.

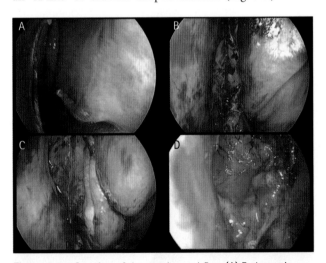

Figure 9.3   Creation of the nasal septal flap. (A) Endoscopic view (0° endoscope) of left nasal cavity. A vertical anterior septal incision was made with a surgical blade. (B) A horizontal incision. (C) Folding the nasal septal flap into the nasopharynx. (D) The final position of the nasal septal flap. Note the integrity of the nasal septum at the end of the procedure.

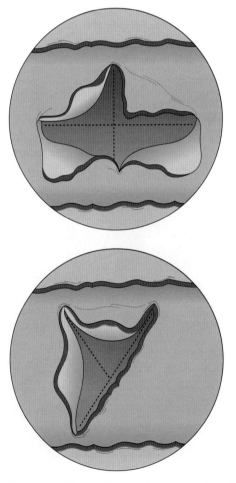

Figure 9.5   A traditional sellar dura incision, cruciate or 'X-like' shaped, as classically described in the literature.

We have described, and always carefully make, a quadrangular dural incision while trying to visualize the precise localization of the cavernous sinus, the superior and inferior intercavernous sinuses, and both ICAs through the exposed dura. These structures represent the anatomical limits of the dural opening. The limits of the quadrangular, or in some cases rectangular, incision are (Fig. 9.6):

- lateral: medial to both ICAs and cavernous sinus
- superior: inferior to the superior intercavernous sinus
- inferior: superior to the inferior intercavernous sinus.

RESECTION OF THE TUMOUR

The dura mater is removed along with any attached fragment of tumour, and sent for histopathological examination. Resection of the tumour begins laterally with a 45° endoscope and curved suction tube, first identifying the angle between the arachnoid and the ICA. The arachnoid is the limit of the superior and posterior dissection (classically known as the diaphragma sellae). When complete removal is accomplished, the arachnoid frequently descends to fill the space occupied by the tumour. This can partially obstruct the surgeon's view, and is one cause for incomplete tumour removal. In pituitary adenoma surgery, dissection is more important than use of the curette. Bleeding is carefully controlled with the use of warm saline irrigation, oxidized cellulose and bipolar cautery.

Reconstruction

At the end of the surgery, a piece of the nasal quadrangular cartilage can be positioned so as to protect the arachnoid membrane. If a cerebrospinal fluid (CSF) leak occurs then a piece of fat or fascia lata can be placed over the defect (Fig. 9.7). The previously created nasal septal flap is placed back in its original position if there is no CSF leak or it can be placed at the floor of the sella if there is a perioperative CSF leak.[5,6] After this the sphenoid sinus cavity is filled with Spongostan and the nasal cavity is also packed (Fig. 9.7).

NASAL PACKING

The nasal pack is removed the day after the surgery if there has been no perioperative CSF leak. If there was a perioperative CSF leak the pack is removed between the third and fifth postoperative day. All patients routinely receive wide-spectrum antibiotics during the operation and for 7 days postoperatively.

Postoperative care

Patients are asked to avoid moderate or intense physical activities, straining, nose blowing and sneezing for approximately 30 days, especially when there has been a perioperative CSF leak. To prevent constipation a high-fibre, soft diet is recommended. Patients are also asked to frequently irrigate their nose with 0.9 per cent or 3 per cent saline solution.

At the first postoperative visit, between the seventh and tenth day after the operation, we usually look for signs of infection, bleeding, crusting and adhesions, as well as any signs of a CSF leak. Patients often complain of some nasal obstruction in the first few days and they are warned that this is normal. The urine output is checked to exclude diabetes insipidus.

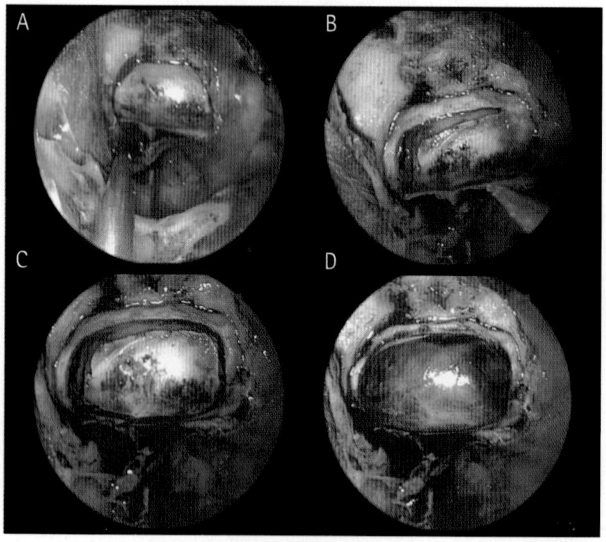

Figure 9.6 Quadrangular incision. (A) Exposure of sellar dura. (B) Incisions for a quadrangular or rectangular area in sellar dura. (C) Completed incisions. (D) Exposure.

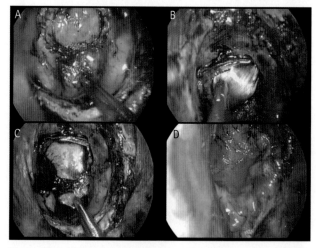

Figure 9.7 Reconstruction. In cases of cerebrospinal fluid (CSF) leaks (A) a piece of fat or (B) fascia lata is placed over the defect. (C) A piece of the nasal quadrangular cartilage can be placed so as to protect the arachnoid membrane. (D) The nasal septal flap has been repositioned to cover the dural defect.

PLANUM SPHENOIDALE AND CAVERNOUS SINUS ENDOSCOPIC SURGERY

The endoscopic management of lesions involving the planum sphenoidale is a relatively novel concept, but it offers some advantages over traditional craniotomies as it optimizes the exposure, helps to minimize the risk of complications and also avoids nerve damage and excessive brain retraction.

Indications and contraindications

The indications for an endoscopic approach include lesions involving the planum sphenoidale and tuberculum sella. The most common pathology in this area is a meningioma, but it can also be useful for lesions that compromise the suprasellar cistern and pre- and postoptic chiasmal lesions such as pituitary microadenomas, craniopharyngiomas, Rathke's pouch cysts and even optic nerve gliomas.

The contraindications include patient comorbidities that preclude prolonged general anaesthesia, unfavourable anatomy such as a small sphenoid sinus, when there is a small space between the ICAs or between the optic chiasma and the pituitary gland, and a lack of specialized equipment/instruments.

Planum sphenoidale approach

An uncinectomy with a total ethmoidectomy is performed. The superior turbinate is resected to allow access to the entire front wall of the sphenoid. In some cases, the middle turbinates also need to be resected. Commencing at the sphenoid ostium, the maximum amount of the front wall of the sphenoid sinus is removed. At this stage, a posterior pedicled mucoperiosteal flap, based on the septal branch of the sphenopalatine artery, is usually developed.[7-9]

A posterior septectomy is performed and the mucosa of the posterior sphenoid wall removed. The thick bone of the tuberculum sellae and the sella is then removed. An area the width of the entire intercarotid roof is thinned down to 'egg shell' thickness with a high-speed diamond drill and then removed. We are especially careful not to damage the optic nerves by excessive heat generated by the use of the drill, with short periods of drilling and copious irrigation.

A Kerrison rongeur (Karl Storz, Tuttlingen, Germany) may be used for additional bone removal. The area exposed is much wider and higher than the area exposed in standard pituitary surgery, and bone removal continues along the sphenoid planum (Fig. 9.8). The posterior ethmoid arteries are coagulated and divided. The dura mater is carefully opened above and below the intercavernous sinus, exposing the suprasellar region and optic chiasm, avoiding any damage to the attached vessels. The intercavernous sinus is coagulated or packed with haemostatic material. Dural dissection is critical and it is

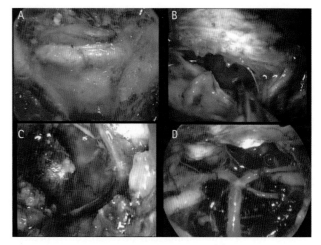

Figure 9.8   Planum sphenoidale approach. (A) Bone is removed from a much wider and higher area than in standard pituitary surgery and continues along the sphenoid planum. (B) Opening of the dura. (C) Visualization and dissection of the tumour. (D) Visualization of the basilar artery, its branches and the third cranial nerve.

imperative to identify the internal carotid arteries in the paraclinoid region, the anterior cerebral arteries (A1 and A2), the anterior communicating artery, and the recurrent artery of Heubner. The optic nerve and chiasm must be identified more superiorly and also the pituitary stalk.

Sharp extra-arachnoid dissection of the tumour proceeds using the two-surgeon binostril technique. One surgeon handles the endoscope and sharp dissection whilst the co-surgeon performs suction and uses forceps to retract. Dissection in the arachnoidal plane is highly recommended whenever possible, and also the avoidance of excessive coagulation and traction, as this reduces the possibility of minor surgical trauma to neurovascular structures.[7-9]

Reconstruction

A pedicled rotation flap forms the foundation to repair any defect. Free fat grafts are used to fill any dead space as well as forming a buttress for a subdural (or extradural intracranial) fascial graft. This is then covered with both pedicled mucoperiosteal/perichondrial flaps. Fibrin tissue glue is used to secure the repair. Gelfoam is placed on the area followed by conventional nasal packs, which are supported by an inflated Foley balloon catheter.

Postoperative care

Antibiotics are given perioperatively and continued postoperatively while the nasal packing remains in place for 7–14 days. The onset of diabetes insipidus is monitored by measuring serum and urine sodium/osmolality. Patients are confined to bed for 48 hours with 30° head elevation, and told to avoid straining, Valsalva manoeuvres, and nose blowing. Lumbar drains are not routinely used unless there is an additional comorbidity, such as intracranial hypertension or prior radiotherapy. Discharge usually occurs 3–5 days after surgery.

CAVERNOUS SINUS

The endoscopic transnasal approach permits the exploration not only of the whole cavernous sinus, but of those areas adjacent to the sphenoid sinus. For this reason, at this time, only the parasellar and middle cranial fossa areas of the cavernous sinus can be explored. At present pituitary adenomas that extend inside the cavernous sinus are the main indication for this approach (Fig. 9.9).

Surgical approach

After a traditional approach, as described for obtaining access in pituitary surgery, a 45° endoscope is introduced in order to inspect the most lateral parts of the tumour. Then gentle suction is used with curved forceps that contain a suction channel. The completeness of the removal of the parasellar portion of the lesion is usually confirmed when venous bleeding starts and this can be controlled with gentle irrigation followed by packing with haemostatic material. When the lesion involves the entire cavernous sinus, a lateral compartment approach

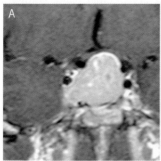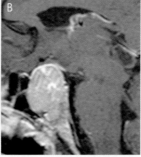

Figure 9.9 Magnetic resonance image of a pituitary adenoma with cavernous sinus invasion. (A) Coronal image. Note the position of the internal carotid arteries. (B) Sagittal image.

is indicated. Pituitary adenomas, because of their soft consistency, currently are the simplest lesion to remove through this approach.[5,6]

The corridor lateral to the ICA is delineated by the intracavernous tract of the ICA posteriorly, by the vidian nerve inferiorly and by the medial pterygoid process anteriorly. It is possible to expose the neurovascular structures inside the anterior part of the cavernous sinus. In this region, the oculomotor nerve (cranial nerve III), the abducens nerve (VI) and the maxillary branch of the trigeminal nerve (V2) form a layer on the inner wall, as opposed to the trochlear (IV) and the ophthalmic branch of the trigeminal nerve (V1), which are lateral.

REFERENCES

1. Cappabianca P, Alfieri A, de Devitiis E. Endoscopic endonasal transsphenoidal approach to the sella: towards functional endoscopic pituitary surgery. *Minim Invasive Neurosurg* 1998; **41**: 66–73.
2. Har-El G. Endoscopic transnasal transsphenoidal pituitary surgery – comparison with the traditional sublabial transseptal approach. *Otolaryngol Clin North Am* 2005; **38**: 723–35.
3. Cappabianca P, de Devitiis E. Endoscopy and transsphenoidal surgery. *Neurosurgery* 2004; **54**: 1043–50.
4. Nguyen-Huynh A, Blevins NH, Jackler RK. The challenges of revision skull base surgery. *Otolaryngol Clin North Am* 2006; **39**: 783–99.
5. Stamm AC. Transnasal endoscopic-assisted skull base surgery. *Ann Otol Rhinol Laryngol* 2006; **196** Suppl: 45–53.
6. Stamm AC, Pignatari SSN, Vellutini E *et al.* A novel approach allowing binostril work to the sphenoid sinus. *Otolaryngol Head Neck Surg* 2008; **138**: 531–2.
7. Stamm AC, Pignatari SNP. Transnasal endoscopic surgical approaches to the posterior fossa. In: Anand VK, Schwartz TH, eds. *Practical endoscopic skull base surgery*. San Diego: Plural Publishing, 2007.
8. Stamm A, Pignatari SSN. Transnasal endoscopic-assisted surgery of the skull base. In: Cummings C, Flint P, Harker L, eds. *Otolaryngology head neck surgery*, 4th edn. Philadelphia: Elsevier, 2005:3855–76.
9. Stamm AC, Vellutini E, Harvey RJ *et al.* Endoscopic trans-nasal craniotomy and the resection of craniopharyngioma. *Laryngoscope* 2008; **118**: 3675–82.

10

Endoscopic management of nasal tumours

ALDO C STAMM, JOÃO F NOGUEIRA JR, MARIA L S SILVA

INTRODUCTION

Nasal tumours account for 0.2–0.8 per cent of all tumours. They are two or three times more frequent in males, are rare in infants and increase in incidence after 35 years, reaching their peak between the fifth and seventh decades.[1] Over the past decade, the role of the endoscopic sinus surgeon, as well as the concept of a multidisciplinary team,[2] has expanded what can be achieved in the management of diseases in the nose, paranasal sinuses and skull base. Advances in endoscopic instrumentation, along with imaging and surgical experience in the endoscopic repair of large skull base defects, have all opened up new and exciting possibilities.[3]

Initially advocated for inflammatory disease, nasal endoscopic approaches are now being used increasingly for the treatment of nasal and paranasal sinus tumours, previously resected through more traditional (transfacial or craniofacial) approaches.[1,3] Some of these lesions, such as inverted papillomas, juvenile nasopharyngeal angiofibromas (JNAs) and aesthesioneuroblastomas (ENBs) have received particular attention in the recent literature. The endoscopic management of other benign lesions such as osteomas, other fibro-osseous tumours, and schwannomas, reflects a fundamental change from the more traditional therapeutic concepts and modalities.[3] This chapter will discuss the current and future endoscopic management of benign and malignant nasal tumours including inverted papilloma, JNA and ENB.

INDICATIONS AND CONTRAINDICATIONS

The endoscope is a tool to help access and visibility but its use should not compromise tumour resection.

The excellent magnification and access that the endoscope provides mean that an external approach is only warranted when the tumour invades the orbit, infratemporal fossa or traverses the dura. The current evidence supports the endoscopic management of nasal tumours including inverted papillomas, JNAs, ENBs, and most benign tumours, such as fibrous dysplasia and schwannomas.[3,4]

The main practical contraindications are a lack of adequate instrumentation or the absence of a multidisciplinary team, and the location and pathology of the tumour. It is important that a multidisciplinary team take into consideration the pathology, staging and evidence base that is available before arriving at a treatment plan. For example a poorly differentiated squamous cell carcinoma that has involved the cerebrum may best be managed by palliative treatment alone, which could include radiotherapy, steroids, antiemetics and analgesics but not surgery.

Historically, *en bloc* resection of skull base tumours has been advocated although in reality their removal is often done piecemeal if the tumour involves the periorbita or basisphenoid. Tumours located adjacent to, or involving, large important blood vessels such as internal carotid artery or the cavernous sinus pose a management challenge, whether by endoscopic or traditional open approaches (Table 10.1). It is increasingly recognized that malignant tumours that involve the basisphenoid cannot be removed with an adequate margin by any technique but that many of these tumours can be removed to a large extent endoscopically and, in conjunction with chemo- and/or radiotherapy, may produce better results with less morbidity. The scarcity of these tumours means that much of the literature relates to case series and not to controlled trials.

Table 10.1 Indications, endoscopic approach and possible contraindications for the endoscopic management of inverted papilloma (IP), juvenile nasopharyngeal angiofibroma (JNA) and aesthesioneuroblastoma (ENB)

	Endoscopic approach	Indications	Possible contraindications*
IP	Medial maxillectomy, complete sphenoethmoidectomy with or without turbinate removal	Tumours located at the maxillary, ethmoid and sphenoid sinus	Tumours located laterally in the frontal sinus
JNA	Medial maxillectomy, complete sphenoethmoidectomy if necessary, pterygoid approach	Tumours located in the nasal cavity and paranasal sinus	Giant tumours with cranial or cavernous sinus extension
ENB	Endoscopic assisted transnasal craniectomy	Tumours confined to the nasal cavity, paranasal sinus, dural and intradural invasion at the midline	Tumours with orbital involvement or lateral brain involvement

*Possible contraindications at this time.

INSTRUMENTATION

Before addressing the endoscopic management of these nasal and paranasal sinus tumours, it is paramount to focus on instrumentation. In our opinion, good instrumentation is essential to carrying out the safe and effective endoscopic resection of malignant tumours and to obtain an adequate margin.

The necessary equipment includes high-quality endoscopes (0°, 45° and 70°); video equipment (camera and monitor); long endoscopic bipolar forceps, preferably suction bipolar; long and delicate drills; long dissection instruments, and haemostatic materials (Fig. 10.1). Image guidance systems, when available, are also helpful for evaluating the tumour resection margins.

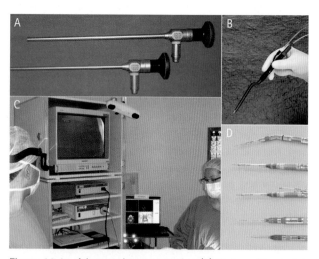

Figure 10.1 Adequate instrumentation. (A) High-quality crystal clear endoscopes, straight and angled. (B) Long bipolar forceps. (C) High-quality video equipment, light source and, if available, image guidance system. We use a portable laptop-based optic image guidance system. (D) Long handpiece drills with diamond and cutting burs.

MULTIDISCIPLINARY TEAM

The introduction of multidisciplinary teams has resulted in improved survival and a reduction in complication rates.[2] For the endoscopic management of nasal tumours, a team approach is needed in the preoperative assessment and in planning the treatment. Ideally, a multidisciplinary team will include otolaryngologists, head and neck surgeons, neurosurgeons, radiologists, intensive care doctors, endocrinologists, anaesthetists, oncologists, pathologists and skilled paramedical staff.

INVERTED PAPILLOMAS

Inverted papillomas are benign neoplasms that may be locally invasive; 5–15 per cent are malignant at presentation and 3 per cent undergo malignant change from an initially benign pathology.[5] They comprise between 0.5 per cent and 4 per cent of primary nasal tumours, and the peak age of presentation is between the fifth and sixth decades. There is a strong male preponderance.[3,4]

Histological, clinical and imaging features

Histologically, inverted papillomas are characterized by an invagination of neoplastic epithelium into the underlying stroma, without transgression of the basement membrane. The most common sites of occurrence are along the lateral nasal wall, particularly in the middle meatus. The aetiology of inverted papillomas remains unclear but a considerable body of evidence suggests a role for human papillomavirus (HPV) in the pathogenesis.[3,4,6] The classical presenting symptoms are unilateral nasal obstruction and intermittent epistaxis, and inverted papillomas must be always part of the differential diagnosis of a unilateral nasal mass, particularly when it originates from the lateral nasal wall.[3,4] Although the clinical appearance of an inverted papilloma is often highly suggestive, the presence of surrounding polyps and inflammation can mask the process.

On computed tomography (CT), inverted papillomas appear to have soft-tissue density, which enhances heterogeneously with contrast (Fig. 10.2). Changes to the bony sinus walls are common, with hyperdense areas or remodelled bone within the tumour. These radiographic features are indistinguishable from those of inflammatory polyps with entrapped debris, so CT is not a sensitive method of diagnosis.[3,4] Magnetic resonance imaging (MRI) is, however, more capable of separating soft tissue from secretions, and can further characterize the features of the lesion. Thus it is an important preoperative investigation to determine whether an opaque CT of the frontal or maxillary sinus indicates the presence of secretions or inverted papilloma as well as to assess whether there is any intracranial or orbital extension of the tumour, which would influence treatment decisions.[3]

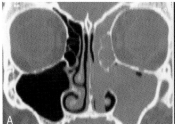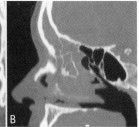

Figure 10.2   Computer tomography of an inverted papilloma. (A) Coronal view with unilateral involvement of the left maxillary, ethmoid and frontal sinuses. (B) Sagittal reconstruction showing the anteroposterior extension. Note that the posterior ethmoid and sphenoid sinuses are clear of the disease.

Inverted papillomas have been reported to have a high propensity for recurrence, with a recurrence rate of 5–30 per cent, regardless of whether they have been treated with the traditional open surgical approach of lateral rhinotomy or midfacial degloving with medial maxillectomy.[5] Early studies of less invasive endoscopic techniques have generally demonstrated a greater incidence of recurrence,[3,4,6] and the advances in endoscopic techniques mean that it is usually not only possible, but preferable to remove the papilloma endoscopically.[7–11] Another advantage of endoscopic techniques described in recent studies is a significantly reduced length of admission compared with traditional methods.[6–11] Because of the association of the inverted papilloma with squamous cell carcinoma it is important to remove all diseased mucosa and submit it for histological examination.[3,4,6]

The endoscopic surgical approach

Various endoscopic surgical techniques have been described, ranging from an endoscopic spheno-ethmoidectomy and wide middle meatal antrostomy to an endoscopic medial maxillectomy and dacryocystorhinostomy. The surgeon must gain as much visibility and access as is necessary to achieve complete removal of the tumour, and this should also enable the patient to be followed up by endoscopic examination. Endoscopic medial maxillectomy is our approach of choice in cases of inverted papillomas that involve the anterior wall and floor of the maxillary sinus and for the removal of malignant sinonasal neoplasms restricted to the lateral wall of the nasal cavity or the medial maxillary sinus (Fig. 10.3).

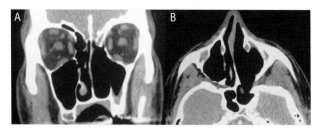

Figure 10.3   Postoperative computer tomography scans following medial maxillectomy for an inverted papilloma. (A) Coronal view. (B) Axial view. Note the limits of the resection.

The procedure begins with resection of the anterior third of the middle turbinate and radical ethmoidectomy. The lamina papyracea and the fovea ethmoidalis are exposed and also the sphenoid sinus rostrum. If necessary, the ethmoid arteries are cauterized with bipolar cautery. The uncinate process, lacrimal bone and the anterior lacrimal crest are removed along with the nasolacrimal duct, the inferior turbinate and the rim of the pyriform aperture. A Hajek–Kofler or Kerrison punch efficiently removes the anterior lacrimal crest and a coarse diamond bur helps when the bone becomes too thick for the jaws of the punch. After elevation of the nasal mucosa, the bone of the pyriform aperture and the medial wall of the maxillary sinus are removed with a drill or osteotome. The large middle meatal antrostomy is extended to the nasal floor and to the posterior wall of the maxillary sinus.

The mucosa of the nasal wall and the tumour are both dissected off the lateral surface of the maxillary sinus. When the lining is dissected off the posterior wall of the maxillary sinus and the crista ethmoidalis, cauterization of the sphenopalatine artery is usually required. The posterior attachment of the inferior turbinate is cut and the lateral wall along with the tumour is removed. Generally, the nasolacrimal duct is transected obliquely to avoid stenosis of the duct and epiphora. Stenting of the lacrimal sac during surgery is not necessary. Currently, extended endoscopic medial maxillectomy, which includes the removal of the posterior wall of the maxillary sinus, also permits access to the pterygomaxillary area and pterygopalatine fossa. The sphenoid and frontal sinus are opened if the tumour extends into them and the diseased mucosa removed.

The extent of the endoscopic surgical procedure is tailored based on the extent of disease.[7–10] Inverted papillomas involving the inferomedial wall of frontal sinus (which is typically the case in the vast majority in whom there is frontal sinus involvement) can be removed by carrying out a modified Lothrop or Draf III procedure. In cases where there is lateral or more superior involvement of the frontal sinus the disease may be removed but these require an array of curved instruments. However, where an inverted papilloma involves most of the frontal sinus, particularly when it is well pneumatized, an osteoplastic flap may be needed to gain adequate exposure.[4,6,7] Nowadays, endoscopic transnasal piecemeal resection is done more often than an *en bloc* resection.[8–11] In some cases, inverted papillomas are intimately associated with bone. Here, bone removal or thinning with a diamond bur is prudent. This is typically performed over the lamina papyracea and fovea ethmoidalis.

The skill and experience of the endoscopic surgeon are key factors in the success of the procedure.[4,6–11] In addition, strict attention must be paid to identifying the site of attachment of the tumour and aggressive resection of a margin of mucosa and bone at this location. Because of the propensity of inverted papilloma to reoccur and to harbour malignancy, frozen sections are desirable at the margins to ensure complete removal of the tumour. The same endoscopic techniques can be performed in revision cases, when recurrence occurs.[4,6,7]

JUVENILE NASOPHARYNGEAL ANGIOFIBROMAS

General considerations

Juvenile nasopharyngeal angiofibromas are histologically benign, highly vascular tumours found in male teenagers and young adults (Fig. 10.4). Recurrent epistaxis and nasal obstruction are the two most common presenting symptoms.[12–14] These tumours have the potential to cause life-threatening complications secondary to bleeding and intracranial extension. However, they can be cured by complete excision,[12–14] via the traditional open or endoscopic approaches. A number of open surgical approaches have been advocated, including transfacial (through lateral rhinotomy or midfacial degloving incisions), transmaxillary and infratemporal procedures.[12] Recently, endoscopic resection of these tumours is gaining increasing acceptance. This method of management provides several advantages over more traditional open surgical techniques, including lower costs and lower morbidity and improved outcomes, such as the avoidance of facial incisions and deformity, and preservation of a greater amount of the anterior surface of the maxilla.[12,15]

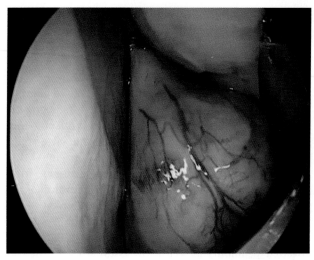

Figure 10.4   Endoscopic view (0° 4 mm endoscope) of a juvenile nasopharyngeal angiofibroma in the left nasal cavity of a 14-year-old boy.

The endoscopic surgical approach

Endoscopic removal of JNAs in the nasal cavity, with extension into the sinuses and pterygopalatine fossa and with limited extension into the infratemporal fossa, has a good success rate. As the size of the JNA increases, for example when the tumour spreads laterally into the infratemporal fossa, novel adaptations to the endoscopic approach have been developed to allow safe removal. A bimanual technique using a transseptal/transnasal binostril approach, with the nasal septum being preserved, allows better leverage and traction of the tumour. With two surgeons holding several instruments at the same time, this has meant that more laterally placed tumours can be removed. This bimanual technique means that a drier surgical field can be achieved due to constant suction.[14,16]

A large number of case reports and case series of the endoscopic removal of JNAs with early intracranial or intracavernous infiltration have been published.[14,17] Large tumours can be delivered through the mouth or reduced in size *in situ* using a laser or harmonic scalpel. To maximize the possibility of complete endoscopic resection, the tumour must be adequately exposed and bleeding controlled. The general consensus is that preoperative embolization reduces intraoperative blood loss.[14] Usually the tumour is located in the posterior half of the nasal cavity and is often seen between the middle turbinate and septum.[14]

In large tumours (Figs 10.5–10.7) the first surgical step is generally the creation of a transseptal/transnasal binostril approach.[14,16] This is achieved by making an anterior septoplasty incision in one nostril and a posterior nasal septal cartilage incision on the other side. Once the approach is prepared, an uncinectomy and a large middle meatal antrostomy are carried out to expose the posterior

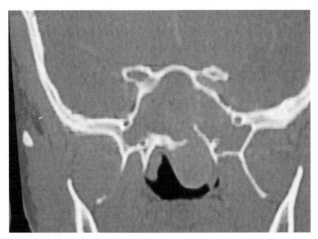

Figure 10.5   Coronal bony window computed tomography scan demonstrating a mass that is completely obstructing the left posterior nasal space with erosion through the floor of the sphenoid.

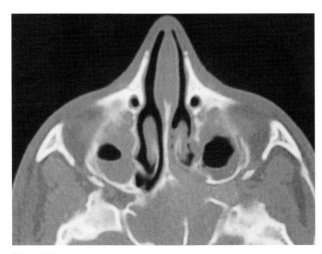

Figure 10.6   Axial bony window computed tomography scan demonstrating widening of the sphenopalatine fossa and extension into the sphenoid.

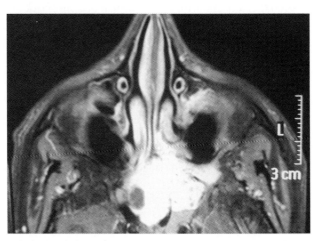

Figure 10.7   T1-weighted magnetic resonance image with gadolinium enhancement demonstrating a vascularized mass extending into the pterygopalatine fossa.

wall of the maxillary sinus. The tumour must never be touched as it will lead to bleeding that will compromise the surgical field. A complete ethmoidectomy is also carried out to expose the anterior wall of the sphenoid sinus. The lower third of the superior turbinate can be removed, the natural ostium of the sphenoid identified and a large sphenoidotomy created. Often the tumour will extend through the floor of the sphenoid sinus, or even occupy the entire sinus.

To achieve complete exposure of the tumour and to facilitate removal of its lateral (infratemporal fossa) extension, if present, an endoscopic medial maxillectomy should be performed. This allows the entire posterior and lateral wall of the maxillary sinus to be accessed and removed. Angled through-cutting Blakesley forceps, Kerrison punches and coarse diamond burs are used to remove the posterior wall of the maxillary sinus and expose the tumour within the pterygopalatine fossa and any infratemporal extension. The maxillary artery is visualized (Fig. 10.8) and it is important to clip it or cauterize it laterally and thoroughly as otherwise there will be severe bleeding. Other visible vessels are also cauterized with bipolar or monopolar diathermy. A Freer suction is used to free the tumour from its attachments. This dissection leaves the tumour attached to a pedicle that protrudes through the enlarged sphenopalatine foramen. This region is then explored to make sure no tumour is left. One of the major causes of JNA recurrence are tumour remnants in the region of the sphenopalatine foramen or the vidian canal.[14,16,17] After the removal of the bulk of the tumour, it is important to carefully scrutinize the area, particularly around the pterygoid plates, to ensure that it has been completely removed (Fig. 10.8).

Tumours extending into difficult anatomical areas such as the orbital apex, cavernous sinus and parasellar region present considerable challenges, whether they are approached endoscopically or by an open procedure.[14,16,17]

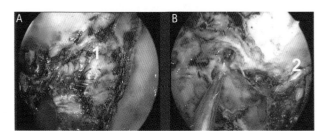

Figure 10.8   Endoscopic view (0° 4 mm endoscope) of juvenile nasopharyngeal angiofibroma surgery. (A) Removal of the posterior wall of the maxillary sinus, exposing the pterygoid fossa, the fat within it and the maxillary artery (1). (B) End of the surgery: note the internal carotid artery (at the end of the suction tube), infraorbital nerve (2) and the wide surgical field following tumour removal.

Vascular considerations

Revision surgery can also be done by an endoscopic approach, but it is important to be aware of the vascular supply and the tumour's relationship with major vessels in order to remove it completely and minimize the risk of life-threatening haemorrhage. Some tumours have a collateral supply from the internal carotid artery and it may be necessary to occlude that. Branches of the external carotid artery are best approached via superselective embolization with variable embolic agents. This is because the branches adjacent to the affected artery should be preserved to reduce the potential risk of ischaemia involving the face and neck and of impairment of cranial nerve function.[18] There is a 15–20 per cent rate of delayed cerebral ischaemic complications, resulting from the presence of an incomplete circle of Willis, thromboembolism arising from an acutely occluded carotid artery, and delayed collateral failure. The presence of complex vascular anatomy and rich anastomosis means that intracranial complications can occur due to backflow of embolic materials into the internal carotid or vertebral artery.[18]

When a considerable portion of a skull base tumour is supplied directly by the internal carotid artery, particle embolization from within the carotid artery may be performed safely under systemic heparin anticoagulation either by use of a balloon to temporarily occlude the carotid distal to the tumour supply, or by use of a balloon-guiding catheter proximal to the tumour vessels. The latter technique requires greater operator attention to avoid spilling particles into the cavernous segment where antegrade flow from the inferolateral trunk may carry the particles to the brain. Major complications include cerebrovascular accidents (CVAs), blindness, ophthalmoplegia, facial nerve palsy and necrosis of the soft tissues.[19] The most serious risk is inadvertent embolization of the internal carotid artery leading to a CVA. In high-flow lesions, there is rapid shunting of blood into the venous circulation and small emboli can pass through the lesion and into the pulmonary bed leading to an infarction.[20,21] General complications, such as sensitivity to the embolic or contrast material, are rare.

Bent and Wood stated that the complication rates for embolization in epistaxis resemble those of arterial ligation at around 13–48 per cent.[20,21] Central neurological deficits may occur if polyvinyl alcohol (PVA) circulates intracranially via the external and internal carotid anastomoses, or from dislodgement of embolic plaques during catheterization of the artery.

AESTHESIONEUROBLASTOMAS

Aesthesioneuroblastomas are rare, malignant neuro-ectodermal tumours that arise in the olfactory vault of the nasal cavity and can metastasize to cervical lymph nodes,

bone and lung. Although there is no consensus about their treatment, many believe they are best treated by combining surgery with adjuvant therapy such as radiotherapy and chemotherapy.[22,23]

Craniofacial resection with or without a bifrontal craniotomy has been considered as the conventional surgical approach for resecting ENBs, and is considered the gold standard against which all other treatments are compared. Craniofacial resection has the advantage of providing excellent intradural and extradural exposure of the structures of the anterior cranial fossa, and facilitates multilayer reconstruction using a pericranial flap to reduce the likelihood of a cerebrospinal fluid (CSF) leak. The associated morbidity is usually related to retraction of the frontal lobes, the loss of olfactory function, epilepsy and resorption of the anterior wall of the frontal sinus.[1,24]

Staging classifications

Currently, the visualization provided by the use of endoscopes during tumour resection is unsurpassed, resulting in their use becoming more and more popular. However, it is also critical that the important principles of oncological resection are not overlooked. The Kadish staging system, although widely utilized and frequently modified, has recognized limitations.[25] One acknowledged problem with the Kadish is its lack of recognition of metastases. In our experience, an additional shortcoming of the Kadish system is its inability to provide remarkable guidance about which surgical approach works best as the stages cannot readily be applied to the concepts of endoscopic transnasal resection.

Whereas the Kadish system differentiates between tumours confined to the nose and those involving the sinuses, with endoscopically assisted transnasal craniectomy (EATNC) this differentiation becomes of limited importance in terms of surgical approach, and is of limited prognostic importance. On the other hand, for tumours that extend beyond the nose and paranasal sinuses, it becomes critically important to differentiate whether the tumour involves the dura or the orbit, because the appropriate surgical approach differs markedly, and this differentiation is not achieved with the Kadish staging system.

In terms of dural involvement we, like many surgical oncological centres, believe that it is also important to know whether the tumour involves just the dura or extends intracranially. If it extends into the cerebrum or orbit it is often best managed by a craniofacial approach.[26,27] We utilize the Stamm–Kennedy staging system shown in Table 10.2 and Figure 10.9.

Endoscopically assisted transnasal craniectomy

A problem with the earlier endoscopic approaches to skull base tumours was that the surgery was often performed

Table 10.2   Novel Stamm–Kennedy aesthesioneuroblastoma staging system

Staging	Location	Recommended treatment
I	Nasal cavity and/or paranasal sinuses	Endoscopically assisted transnasal resection*
II	I + dural involvement	Endoscopically assisted transnasal craniectomy (EATC)*
III	Orbital invasion	EATC ± orbital exenteration + radiation therapy ± chemotherapy
IVa	Intradural involvement and tumour located medial to the medial orbital wall	EATC + radiation therapy ± chemotherapy
IVb	Intradural involvement and tumour located lateral to the medial orbital wall	Craniofacial resection + radiation therapy ± chemotherapy
V	Metastasis (regional or distant)	Individualized approach (craniofacial resection + radiation therapy + chemotherapeutic options)

* Radiotherapy if poorly differentiated

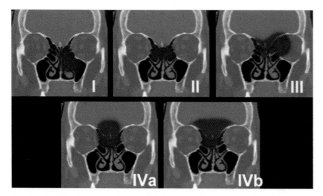

Figure 10.9   A normal coronal computed tomography (CT) scan edited to illustrate the novel Stamm–Kennedy aesthesioneuroblastoma staging system. See Table 10.2 for details of the stages.

with only one hand. This disadvantage has been overcome with the development of the binostril technique that allows two surgeons to work together.[15] In cases where septal resection is not required for oncological resection, the second surgeon can access the tumour with a transseptal approach and use a vascular nasoseptal Hadad flap.[28]

Stammberger and colleagues published a series of three patients in which a 100 per cent success rate was achieved with a combination of transnasal endoscopic surgery and radiosurgery (gamma knife). The patients were selected on the basis of no tumour infiltration of the dura, no intracranial extension, no deep infiltration of the orbit and no remarkable extension into the pterygopalatine fossa. In addition, any involvement of the posterior wall of the frontal sinus would have excluded the endoscopic approach. All three patients remained free of disease with excellent quality of life at follow-up (71, 50 and 39 months).[29,30]

There are some clear attractions of the EATNC approach over traditional craniofacial surgery with lower hospitalization times and costs. When the tumour is confined to a single side of the nasal cavity, it is possible to preserve olfactory function and the procedure causes no deformity or external incisions. Patients undergoing EATNC have a lower rate of morbidity compared with those submitted to a craniofacial approach, with or without bifrontal craniotomy.[1] However, the appropriate selection of patient for this surgical approach is essential, and the Kadish staging system does not provide guidance in this regard. Although the proposed revised staging system is, in our opinion, more appropriate for EATNC, it still does not take into account the histological characteristics of the tumour. The importance of following sound oncological principles in endoscopic resection of skull base tumours cannot be overemphasized. The oncological surgical resection should never be compromised for the sake of an endoscopic resection.

We perform EATNC under controlled hypotensive general anaesthesia. The patients are positioned supine on the operating table (reverse Trendelenburg position of up to 30°) and the head slightly extended and turned toward the surgeon. Cottonoids containing 1:1000 adrenaline (epinephrine), are placed in the nasal cavity, especially over the areas of surgical access, and left in place for approximately 10 minutes. This surgical approach generally includes the resection of all involved structures of the skull base, including the nasal mucosa, bone and the underlying dura. For large tumours and those with involvement of the dura or near the midline, surgery is performed through both sides of the nasal cavity. The extent of bone removal depends on the relationship of the tumour to the crista galli.

In unilateral tumour cases the surgery is begun with a wide middle meatal antrostomy. The tumour may be debulked sufficiently to allow identification of the relevant anatomy and any sites of attachment are carefully identified for subsequent wide resection. The middle and superior turbinates are removed to the level of the skull base and a complete sphenoethmoidectomy is performed, including removal of the lateral wall of the orbit, exposing the periorbita. Next, the frontal recess and then the frontal sinus are exposed. The anterior and posterior ethmoid arteries are identified, coagulated and divided. The bone of the roof of the ethmoid sinus is removed, completely exposing the dura. The medial dissection is accomplished by removing the posterior and superior portions of the ipsilateral nasal septum. The perichondrium and periosteum of the contralateral side are preserved for use in the reconstruction. After skeletonization of the skull base, the roof of the ethmoid sinus is removed, including the ipsilateral cribriform plate, using either a diamond bur or a micro-Kerrison punch. The dura of the olfactory region including the ipsilateral olfactory nerve filaments is resected so that the tumour attachment can be removed *en bloc* if possible. The olfactory bulb is also resected on the affected side. Frozen sections are obtained of the margins to validate the oncological resection.

Following tumour removal, the dural defect is reconstructed with two layers of fascia lata harvested from the quadriceps muscle (one placed intradurally and the other extradurally), covered with a contralateral nasal septal mucoperiosteal graft or flap. The latter, pedicled at the sphenopalatine artery, is currently the method of choice for closure of the defect. Fibrin glue and nasal packing secures these grafts in place (Fig. 10.10).

In cases in which the tumour crosses the crista galli, we use a modified Lothrop or Draf III technique to widely expose the frontal sinus in addition to the exposure described above. As previously, the craniotomy is initiated with a diamond drill and completed with micro-Kerrison forceps, preserving the underlying dura and creating an osteotomy limited by the sphenoid plane posteriorly, the medial wall of orbits laterally and the posterior wall of frontal sinus anteriorly (Fig. 10.11). The dura is opened with an incision at the margin of the craniotomy window. During the identification of the falx cerebri at the most anterior region of the skull base, bleeding from the sagittal sinus can be controlled with pieces of oxidized cellulose. The falx is then detached from the crista galli, and the tumour removed *en bloc* along with the underlying dura. Freeing the tumour from the frontal lobe requires meticulous dissection. The dural defect is reconstructed in the same way as described above with two layers of fascia lata (one placed intradurally and the other

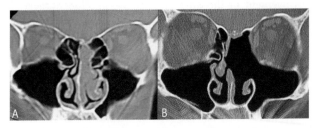

Figure 10.10 Coronal computed tomography scans in a patient with a unilateral tumour (A) before and (B) after an endoscopically assisted transnasal craniotomy approach.

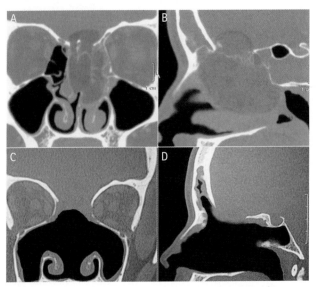

Figure 10.11 Endoscopically assisted transnasal craniotomy approach in a 26-year-old woman with recurrent epistaxes and nasal obstruction. A bilateral approach was performed. (A) Coronal computer tomography (CT) scan showing the bilateral tumour arising from the olfactory vault. (B) Sagittal reconstruction. (C) Postoperative coronal CT scan showing complete endoscopic removal of the tumour. (D) Sagittal reconstruction.

extradurally), and a vascular pedicle nasal flap including mucoperiosteum/mucoperichondrium is used to cover the grafts. If a vascular pedicle flap is not available because of involvement of the nasal septum, a mucoperiosteal flap from the floor of the nasal cavity may be used.

POSTOPERATIVE CARE

All patients undergoing endoscopic resection of nasal tumours are discharged in under 5 days. Nasal packing is performed routinely and it stays *in situ* for at least 3 days or longer if necessary. Intravenous antibiotics are given while the patient is in hospital followed by oral antibiotics up to 10 days. Saline solutions and vasoconstrictors are used for nasal cleaning after the discharge.

Patients return weekly for the first month for removal of crust and granulation tissue. After the first month, they are seen every 2 weeks or monthly depending on the healing progress. Investigations including MRI and CT, and endoscopic examination, are performed at 6 months and 1 year following surgery.

CONCLUSION

The endoscopic management of nasal tumours is an effective alternative approach for the removal of these lesions, with reduced morbidity and mortality. However, the selection of the approach must be based on the individual patient's pathology and extent of disease. There remain some limitations to the use of endoscopes in removing nasal tumours, for example ENBs with orbital involvement or extensive JNAs or inverted papillomas. Basic surgical oncological principles must be borne in mind during the endoscopic approach although an *en bloc* resection is not essential. The tumour may be resected in a piecemeal fashion, as long as there are free margins.

In the future, it is possible that novel chemotherapy drugs, instruments and surgical techniques will allow even safer resection of more extensive tumours with minimally invasive approaches.

REFERENCES

1. Howard DJ, Lund VJ, Wei WI. Craniofacial resection for tumors of the nasal cavity and paranasal sinuses: a 25-year experience. *Head Neck* 2006; **28**: 867–73.

2. Stamm AC, Vellutini E, Harvey RJ *et al.* Endoscopic transnasal craniotomy and the resection of craniopharyngioma. *Laryngoscope* 2008; **118**: 1142–8.

3. Banhiran W, Casiano RR. Endoscopic sinus surgery for benign and malignant nasal and sinus neoplasm. *Curr Opin Otolaryngol Head Neck Surg* 2005; **13**: 50–4.

4. Lawson W, Patel ZM. The evolution of management for inverted papilloma: an analysis of 200 cases. *Otolaryngol Head Neck Surg* 2009; **140**: 330–5.

5. Mirza S, Bradley PJ, Acharya A *et al.* Sinonasal inverted papillomas: Recurrence, synchronous and metachronous malignancy. *J Laryngol Otol* 2007; **121**: 857–64.

6. Lane AP, Bolger WE. Endoscopic management of inverted papilloma. *Curr Opin Otolaryngol Head Neck Surg* 2006; **14**: 14–18.

7. Pasquini E, Sciarretta V, Farneti G *et al.* Inverted papilloma: Report of 89 cases. *Am J Otolaryngol* 2004; **25**: 178–85.

8. Tomenzoli D, Castelnuovo P, Pagella F *et al.* Different endoscopic surgical strategies in the management of inverted papilloma of the sinonasal tract: Experience with 47 patients. *Laryngoscope* 2004; **114**: 193–200.

9. Kaza S, Capasso R, Casiano RR. Endoscopic resection of inverted papilloma: University of Miami experience. *Am J Rhinol* 2003; **17**: 185–90.

10. Kraft M, Simmen D, Kaufmann T *et al.* Long-term results of endonasal sinus surgery in sinonasal papillomas. *Laryngoscope* 2003; **113**: 1541–7.

11. Lawson W, Kaufman MR, Biller HF. Treatment outcomes in the management of inverted papilloma: an analysis of 160 cases. *Laryngoscope* 2003; **113**: 1548–56.

12. Douglas R, Wormald PJ. Endoscopic surgery for juvenile nasopharyngeal angiofibroma: where are the limits? *Curr Opin Otolaryngol Head Neck Surg* 2006; **14**: 1–5.

13. Wormald PJ, Van Hasselt A. Endoscopic removal of juvenile angiofibromas. *Otolaryngol Head Neck Surg* 2003; **129**: 684–91.

14. Robinson S, Patel N, Wormald PJ. Endoscopic management of benign tumors extending into the infratemporal fossa: a two-surgeon transnasal approach. *Laryngoscope* 2005; **115**: 1818–22.

15. Andrade NA, Pinto JA, Nobrega Mde O *et al.* Exclusively endoscopic surgery for juvenile nasopharyngeal angiofibroma. *Otolaryngol Head Neck Surg* 2007; **137**: 492–6.

16. Stamm AC, Pignatari S, Vellutini E *et al.* A novel approach allowing binostril work to the sphenoid sinus. *Otolaryngol Head Neck Surg* 2008; **138**: 531–2.

17. Onerci TM, Yucel OT, Ogretmenoglu O. Endoscopic surgery in treatment of juvenile nasopharyngeal angiofibroma. *Int J Pediatr Otorhinolaryngol* 2003; **67**: 1219–25.

18. Luo CB, Teng MM, Chang FC *et al.* Transarterial embolization of acute external carotid blowout syndrome with profuse oronasal bleeding by N-butyl-cyanoacrylate. *Am J Emerg Med* 2006; **24**: 702–8.

19. Kingsley D, O'Connor F. Embolization in otolaryngology. *J Laryngol Otol* 1982; **96**: 439–50.

20. Tseng YE, Narducci AC, Willirig JS *et al.* Angiographic embolisation for epistaxis: A review of 114 cases. *Laryngoscope* 1988; **8**: 615–19.

21. Bent J, Wood BP. Complications resulting from treatment of severe posterior epistaxis. *J Laryngol Otol* 1999; **113**: 252–4.

22. Dulguerov P, Calcaterra T. Esthesioneuroblastoma: the UCLA experience 1970–1990. *Laryngoscope* 1992; **102**: 843–9.

23. Liu JK, O'Neill B, Orlandi RR *et al.* Endoscopic-assisted craniofacial resection of esthesioneuroblastoma: minimizing facial incisions – technical note and report of 3 cases. *Minim Invasive Neurosurg* 2003; **46**: 310–15.

24. Lund VJ, Howard D, Wei W *et al.* Olfactory neuroblastoma: past, present, and future? *Laryngoscope* 2003; **113**: 502–7.

25. Kadish S, Goodman M, Wang CC. Olfactory neuroblastoma: a clinical analysis of 17 cases. *Cancer* 1976; **37**: 1571–6.

26. Zumegen C, Michel O. Classification and prognosis of esthesioneuroblastoma based on 7 treated cases. *Laryngorhinootologie* 2000; **79**: 736–42.

27. Vrionis FD, Kienstra MA, Rivera M *et al.* Malignant tumors of the anterior skull base. *Cancer Control* 2004; **11**: 144–51.

28. Hadad G, Bassagasteguy L, Carrau RL *et al.* A novel reconstructive technique after endoscopic expanded endonasal approaches: vascular pedicle nasoseptal flap. *Laryngoscope* 2006; **116**: 1–5.

29. Stammberger H, Walch C, Feichtinger K. The minimal approach to olfactory neuroblastoma: combined endoscopic and steriotactic surgery. *Laryngoscope* 2000; **110**: 635–40.

30. Stammberger H, Anderhuber W, Walch CH *et al.* Possibilities and limitations of endoscopic management of nasal and paranasal sinus malignancies. *Acta Oto-Rhino-Laryngologica Belg* 1999; **53**: 199–205.

11

Cerebrospinal fluid leaks

SCOTT M GRAHAM

INTRODUCTION

Few procedures reflect the tremendous benefits of endoscopic techniques in quite the same way as the endoscopic closure of cerebrospinal fluid (CSF) leaks. Although the ultimate chance of success may in some measure depend on the aetiology of the leak,[1] remarkable results of 90 per cent success rates at the initial attempt with success rates up to 97 per cent with revision have been published.[1,2] Despite these impressive figures, there continues to be isolated enthusiasm for open approaches in some neurosurgical centres. Some published neurosurgical series have success rates as low as 60 per cent with predictable sequelae from brain retraction and sacrifice of the olfactory nerves, to say nothing of the coronal flap and frontal craniotomy. Recent neurosurgical publications have recommended open approaches in the face of adverse prognostic factors such as prior radiation or elevated intracranial pressure.

Although rhinorrhoea can be a socially troubling symptom, the principal motivation for repair of CSF leaks is to reduce the risk of meningitis or other intracranial complications. The incidence of meningitis in patients with an active CSF leak has been quoted as 10 per cent year on year,[3,4] although a more recent study has suggested that the incidence may be as low as 0.3 per cent per year per active leak per person.[5] Daudia et al. found that in 111 patients with 190 years of active leaks, 21 developed meningitis resulting in an overall risk of 19 per cent although most occurred in the first year of the leak.

The repair of a newly diagnosed CSF leak is not an absolute surgical emergency and time can be taken to properly examine and investigate the patient. During this time the simple advice of telling the patient not to blow their nose or to sneeze 'with their mouth open' and not to use continuous positive airway pressure (CPAP) needs to be reinforced. Nonetheless, because of the risk of meningitis, surgical repair should be performed at the earliest reasonable opportunity. Even today meningitis is associated with a definite mortality rate. Few studies have followed patients with repaired leaks over the long term. A publication from the Mayo Clinic[6] identified recurrence of leaks in a group of 21 patients at an average of 50.8 months after corrective surgery. The longest interval to recurrence in this group of patients was 28 years.

In patients with a history of a CSF leak, it is worth checking the pneumococcal antibody titre, and if it is low, vaccination with a 23-valent polysaccharide Pnc vaccine or a 7-valent conjugate Pnc vaccine is recommended.[7] In recent years the spectrum of leaks seen in major centres has changed considerably. Most of the leaks seen today are either 'spontaneous', following trauma, or what might be termed a recognized complication after anterior skull base, sellar or parasellar tumour resection or after intranasal surgery. In many of these patients the bony defect is often substantial and this has required a reappraisal of reconstructive techniques.

Although there are a variety of classification systems of CSF leaks, perhaps the most useful is the time honoured system of classification by aetiology: congenital, spontaneous or post-traumatic. Post-traumatic CSF leaks can be further divided into those associated with head trauma, those seen as a complication of sinus surgery and those seen as a part of skull base surgery. A small number of patients with tumours also present with CSF leaks.

HEAD TRAUMA

Cerebrospinal fluid leaks are quoted to occur in perhaps 2 per cent of head injuries and 12–30 per cent of skull base fractures[8] (Figs 11.1 and 11.2). Most CSF leaks occur as a result of blunt trauma. They may present as CSF otorrhoea, CSF oto-rhinorrhoea or CSF rhinorrhoea. The conventional viewpoint is that most traumatic CSF leaks will heal with conservative treatment including bed rest. Insertion of a lumbar drain may sometimes be required. It is possible that only the sinus mucosal aspect of the defect closes as the dura does not regenerate. This produces a relatively fragile closure and work by Bernal-Sprekelsen et al.[9] has suggested a substantial continuing risk of meningitis in these patients. The authors suggest that this 'monolayer of protection' may be eroded by either the pulsatile effect of the brain or by inflammation within the nose.[9] With the widespread availability of endoscopic closure, performed with statistically small risks, this conservative management paradigm might be challenged, changing towards a more active interventionist policy.

Massive head trauma with complex comminuted and displaced fractures of the skull base can be incredibly difficult to treat. Open approaches may be of value for these patients. The decision to proceed with an open approach is sometimes made easier by the presence of intracranial injuries requiring attention or fractures of the posterior wall of the frontal sinus (Fig. 11.1). Free tissue transfer has been reported as being helpful in carefully selected groups.[10] In massive 'egg-shell' fractures of the sphenoid sinuses, fat obliteration can be considered, leaving the treatment of possible subsequent mucocoeles that may develop to a secondary procedure.

CONGENITAL CEREBROSPINAL FLUID LEAKS

Congenital CSF leaks in association with an encephalocoele or meningoencephalocoeles are uncommon. These are

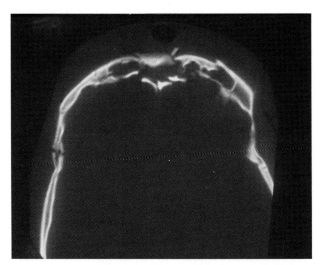

Figure 11.1   Fracture of the posterior table of the frontal sinus with associated cerebrospinal fluid leak.

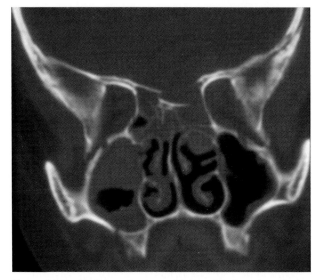

Figure 11.2   Skull base fracture with associated cerebrospinal fluid leak.

well diagnosed on magnetic resonance imaging (MRI) and this investigation is recommended when sinus opacity is demonstrated adjacent to a skull base defect (Figs 11.3 and 11.4). Brain tissue contained within the encephalocoele is invariably non-functioning and can be removed as part of the surgical procedure. Congenital abnormalities

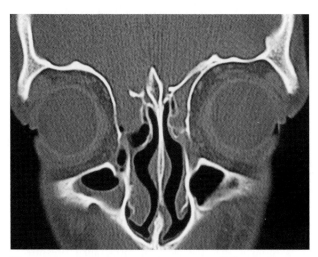

Figure 11.3   Coronal computed tomography (CT) scan showing a bony defect in the right fovea ethmoidalis.

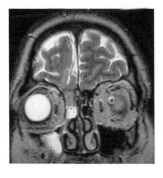

Figure 11.4   Magnetic resonance image showing a right encephalocoele.

of the inner ear such as Mondini dysplasia may present with substantial CSF leaks where the CSF has only briefly traversed the perilymphatic space. Such leaks, in addition to presenting as hearing loss or recurrent meningitis, may also present with CSF otorrhoea or CSF oto-rhinorrhoea.

CEREBROSPINAL FLUID LEAKS ASSOCIATED WITH TUMOURS

Tumours causing substantial erosion of the skull base may present with CSF rhinorrhoea. Occasionally where tumour shrinkage occurs, for example during induction chemotherapy, CSF leaks may also occur. The closure of the CSF leak is part of the surgical treatment of the tumour and for the closure to be successful it is important for the margins of the CSF leak to be clear of tumour, particularly in malignant disease. Persisting CSF leaks in the face of residual untreated tumour may present a considerable challenge. A study by Boudreaux and Zins,[11] described open treatment of CSF leaks in 14 high risk patients. Nine of these patients had malignant brain tumours. A success rate of 85 per cent was reported.

SPONTANEOUS LEAKS

A good deal of recent interest has centred on 'spontaneous CSF leaks' sometimes described as 'idiopathic'. The association of spontaneous leaks with middle-aged women with a raised body mass index is now well known. These leaks are thought to represent a variant of benign intracranial hypertension.[12] These patients have a generally elevated intracranial pressure, this diagnosis being made on lumbar puncture after surgical repair. It is not possible to measure this preoperatively as the persistent leak reduces the pressure although there may be radiological features of increased intracranial pressure such as an empty sella, enlarged ventricles or diffuse erosion of the skull base.[1] When the CSF is actively draining, for example, perhaps at the time of lumbar puncture for fluorescein installation prior to repair, the intracranial pressure is often reduced. It is thought that the elevated intracranial pressure is due to poor CSF resorption by the arachnoid villi.[12] This increased intracranial pressure with associated pulsatile forces produces thinning of bone that is most evident in the weakest areas of the skull base. Herniation of the meninges and brain, often with CSF leakage, most often occurs in the lateral recess of a well-pneumatized sphenoid (Fig. 11.5), or in the area of the lateral lamella of the cribriform plate and in the ethmoid roof. There may be multiple sites of weakness of the skull base.

Imaging and diagnosis are similar to other varieties of CSF leaks. In cases of multiple cranial base defects, intrathecal fluorescein can be helpful in localizing the exact location of active leakage (Fig. 11.6). Identification

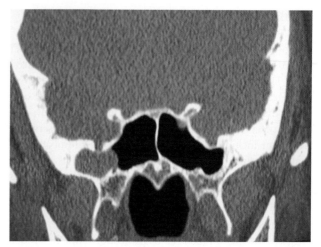

Figure 11.5   Defect in the lateral recess of the right sphenoid sinus.

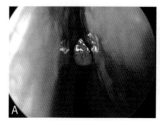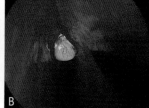

Figure 11.6   (A) Endoscopic appearance of a small meningocoele. (B) Endoscopic appearance of a small meningocoele after intrathecal fluorescein administration.

of 'spontaneous' as the likely aetiology of the leak preoperatively is helpful in counselling the patient.[1] Spontaneous leaks are most likely to recur and the success rates for endoscopic closure are worse than for other aetiologies.[1] In one study 21 per cent of spontaneous leaks recurred, going up to 46 per cent if there were radiological signs of a raised intracranial pressure, compared with 2 per cent if the leak was not spontaneous.[1] With spontaneous leaks there can be re-leakage at the site of repair, but there can be multiple areas of weakness of the skull base and with untreated underlying elevated intracranial pressure other areas may break down and leak.

Areas of substantial skull base dehiscence may benefit from additional reinforcement with a bone or cartilage graft. This is sometimes easier said than done with a thin bony skull base and difficulty in finding a reliable 'edge'. Cerebrospinal fluid leaks in the lateral recess of well-pneumatized sphenoid sinuses (Fig. 11.5) may be best approached by the transantral transpterygoid approach described by Bolger and Osenbach.[13] Postoperatively the elevated intracranial pressure may be helped by oral acetazolamide. Selected patients may benefit from shunting. Success with a gastric bypass for morbid obesity has also been described.[12]

CEREBROSPINAL FLUID LEAKS COMPLICATING SINUS SURGERY

A rate of serious complications in the order of 0.5 per cent is generally quoted for endoscopic sinus surgery. This category of serious complications would include CSF leaks diagnosed intraoperatively or postoperatively. Bachmann et al.[14] looked at the incidence of occult CSF fistulae during sinus surgery. They found a 3 per cent incidence of occult leaks utilizing the β-trace protein assay. They had reviewed 69 consecutive patients, 'all-comers', receiving surgery at the hands of an experienced surgeon in a tertiary referral centre. None of the patients with occult leaks displayed any symptoms or sequelae in the follow-up period of 6 months. The authors speculated that occult leaks may be more common than previously thought and that small leaks may self-heal. The important caveat to be included with this study is that these patients do need to be followed long term to determine the incidence of delayed meningitis.

Some of the details of CSF leaks complicating sinus surgery are covered in Chapter 6. Image-guided surgery, while indisputably helpful in individual cases, has not reduced the likelihood of complications in large case series. Powered instrumentation, the other great technical advance in sinus surgery in recent times, has changed the scale of complications, making brain parenchymal injury more likely than imminently treatable CSF leaks. With brain parenchymal injuries has come the need to exclude significant intracranial adverse vascular events using MR angiography.

As a general rule, CSF leaks complicating sinus surgery, diagnosed intraoperatively, should be repaired in the same anaesthetic session. Local intranasal tissue can be used for the repair with generally good results. The most likely anatomical sites for CSF leaks complicating sinus surgery are the very thin bone of the lateral lamella of the cribriform plate, the area of the anterior skull base where it is weakened by the anterior ethmoid neurovascular bundle and posteriorly where there may be confusion as to the exact anatomical relationship between the last posterior ethmoid cell and the sphenoid sinus. In unusual circumstances, a decision can be made not to repair the CSF leak in the same anaesthetic session. Where the degree of surgical disorientation is such that attempts at repair might result in further damage such as an orbital or brain parenchymal injury, an argument can be made for referring these patients to specialist centres for closure. The wound can be carefully packed with particular care being exercised during the 'wake-up' from anaesthesia. It is crucial that the patient does not receive positive pressure mask ventilation after extubation for fear of substantial pneumocephalus developing.

Cerebrospinal fluid leaks complicating sinus surgery may also become evident in the postoperative period. Any complaint of clear rhinorrhoea postoperatively needs to be taken seriously and investigated vigorously. The appropriate investigation of such leaks is dealt with later in the chapter.

REPAIR OF SURGICALLY INDUCED SKULL BASE DEFECTS

Endoscopic approaches to the anterior skull base and sellar and parasellar regions are increasingly employed for the treatment of a variety of pathological processes. Small defects can be repaired in the same way as defects of other aetiologies. For larger defects, free fat grafts can be successfully employed. More recently interest has focused on the use of vascularized tissue flaps. The idea of CSF leak repair utilizing vascularized septal or turbinate flaps is not new. Yessenow and McCabe reported excellent success rates more than 20 years ago with this tissue in transnasal, extracranial, non-endoscopic repair of CSF leaks.[15]

Most reports have focused on posterior septal flaps. The so-called, 'Hadad–Bassagastequy' flap utilizes septal mucoperiosteum and mucoperichondrium based on the nasoseptal artery. Kassam et al.[16] reported its general utility in 75 patients undergoing endonasal endoscopic cranial base surgery. Harvey et al.[17] reported on the experience of two skull base centres over a 12-month period in 30 patients. They reported using a variety of flaps, including the posterior septal flap as well as inferior turbinate and nasal floor flaps, and emphasized technical aspects relating to the flap including avoiding injudicious initial posterior septectomy, decisions regarding a concomitant hemi-transfixion or Killian septal incision and careful preservation of the flap during surgery. They also emphasized the use of multilayer skull base reconstruction initially supported by an inflated Foley catheter balloon.

INVESTIGATION OF CEREBROSPINAL FLUID LEAKS

A story of clear rhinorrhoea, sometimes tasting salty and often posturally provoked, with an appropriate antecedent history, is clinically suspicious for a CSF leak. Such patients must be investigated vigorously. As compelling as such a history appears, these patients do not always end up having CSF leaks as shown by Bateman and Jones in nine patients presenting with highly suggestive histories (Fig. 11.7).[18] Further investigation is therefore required. Endoscopic examination of the nose may be unrevealing but is part of the initial work-up.

The next goal is to obtain fluid for testing. Ideally this can be obtained at the office visit, sometimes with postural provocation. When this is unsuccessful we will sometimes ask the patient to run up the stairs in an effort to increase intracranial pressure and produce drainage or strain on a closed glottis. If this fails, patients are given vials to take home to catch fluid for testing. In the USA, the β_2-transferrin test is widely available and most

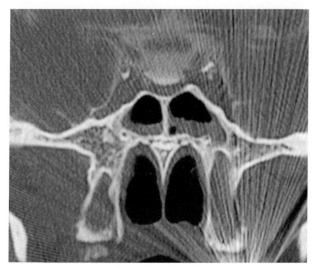

Figure 11.7   Fluid levels in both sphenoid sinuses wrongly interpreted as being due to cerebrospinal fluid. The patient was advised to have a craniotomy but declined. Their rhinorrhoea was found to be negative for immunofixation of β_2-transferrin and their secretions were due to allergic rhinitis.

commonly used. A downside of the test is that it may only be performed in certain major centres and thus it may take a few days to get a result. The β_2-transferrin test provides excellent sensitivity, specificity and positive and negative predictability in the diagnosis of CSF leaks.[19] A concomitant serum value enhances its utility. Occasional false positives have been reported in certain liver diseases or hereditary disorders of protein metabolism. It has been suggested in some European studies that β-trace protein is an even better test than β_2-transferin in detecting CSF leaks.[19]

IMAGING FOR DIAGNOSIS OF CEREBROSPINAL FLUID LEAKS

The clear majority of CSF leaks can be diagnosed using β_2-transferrin testing and reformatting of ultra fine cut CT scans of the sinuses. The coronal scan is most helpful in examining the ethmoid roof (see Fig. 11.3) but other views are useful in diagnosing leaks at other anatomical sites (Fig. 11.8). These images are most often obtained as

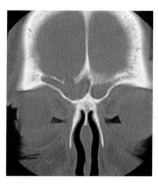

Figure 11.8   A spontaneous defect in the posterior wall of the frontal sinus. The patient was found to have a high pressure system after the defect was repaired and a shunt was inserted.

part of planning for image-guided surgery. Details of a bony defect may be seen or an area of opacification or an air–fluid level in an adjacent sinus. In the situation where there is an opaque sinus adjacent to a skull base defect, MRI should be performed to help diagnose a possible encephalocoele or meningocoele. Where a defect is not visualized in the sinuses, CT of the temporal bones should be performed to exclude CSF oto-rhinorrhoea.

In some centres, MRI cisternography is performed if fine cut CT and β_2-transferrin testing do not provide a diagnosis. A variety of technical modifications of the MRI enhance its ability to detect the area of the leak.[20] More commonly in cases where the diagnosis is unclear, CSF contrast studies are considered. This may utilize radiographic contrast such as iohexol or alternatively a radioactive tracer. These investigations require the patient to be actively leaking at the time of the study. As they need an intrathecal contrast agent of one sort or another, these tests are associated with a slightly greater risk than non-invasive studies. Radionuclide cisternography involves intrathecal administration of a tracer via a lumbar puncture followed by imaging once the tracer has had an opportunity to make its way to the skull base. Strategically placed nasal pledgets are also used. It is our practice to cut these pledgets into different shapes as this helps to identify their position in the nose after they come out. Radioactive tracers of different half lives can be considered. Localization of CSF leaks by gadolinium-enhanced MRI cisternography has also been described. Gadolinium is injected into the subarachnoid space. This is an 'off-label' use of gadolinium in the USA and requires separate consent. Aydin *et al.*[21] found this technique useful in 43 of 51 patients. No neurological sequelae were seen from the injection.

CONTROVERSIES IN REPAIR

Intrathecal fluorescein

It is my practice to use intrathecal fluorescein as part of the repair of all CSF leaks planned as a discrete procedure. Separate consent is obtained for the intrathecal use of fluorescein as its use via this route is not approved by the US Food and Drug Administration. There is at least a theoretical advantage to giving this while the patient is awake and a German publication describes employing intrathecal fluorescein the afternoon before surgery.[22] In this publication fluorescein is administered without CSF withdrawal to minimize CSF displacement.[22]

As a practical matter in the USA, fluorescein is mostly administered in the operating room after induction of general anaesthesia. Our neurosurgical colleagues perform a lumbar puncture and insert a lumbar drain, and 10 mL of the patient's CSF is withdrawn and mixed with 0.1 mL of 10 per cent fluorescein suitable for injection. The mixture is then reinjected slowly over 10 minutes timed by the clock. The patient is placed slightly head down and sufficient time is allowed for the fluorescein to equilibrate throughout the subarachnoid space. The nose is closely examined with 0° and angled telescopes and sites of leakage are disclosed by the bright green colour of the fluorescein (see Fig. 11.6). Usually the light of the telescope is sufficiently broad spectrum to achieve this – occasionally a blue light filter is helpful. The intrathecal fluorescein is of use, first, in diagnosing a CSF leak, second, in disclosing its exact location, and third, by its absence, providing evidence of success of the repair.

Complications of intrathecal use of fluorescein have been reported.[22] The most common complication cited has been seizures, but in general this has been associated with use of the wrong formulation of fluorescein, occipital application, a higher than recommended dose or rapid bolus injection. Other complications have been attributed to the simultaneous use of intrathecal radiographic contrast material. Citing these concerns, Zuckerman and Del Gaudio[23] described excellent success rates in 42 CSF leaks repaired without using intrathecal fluorescein or indeed lumbar drains. They relied on high-resolution CT and intraoperative image guidance for leak identification. The use of topical 5 per cent fluorescein applied intraoperatively to the surgical site has also been described.[24] This can also be used as an office-based diagnostic test. The authors recommend skin testing the patient with fluorescein eye drops to rule out allergy the day prior to the procedure.[24]

Lumbar drains

The routine use of lumbar drains in elective CSF leak repair is controversial. Our practice is to use one when intrathecal fluorescein has been employed. The drain is placed at the time of initial lumbar puncture and then 'closed' and reopened immediately prior to repair. Lumbar drains can be associated with important complications and their use requires specialist nursing management. In our hospital, patients with lumbar drains are managed on the neurosurgical floor.

We feel that the reduction in intracranial pressure afforded by the lumbar drain offers an extra measure of insurance for the repair. Certainly, however, series of successful repair without lumbar drains in selected patients with CSF leaks have been described.[1,23]

Technical aspects of the repair

The good news is that whatever preferences and prejudices a surgeon might have regarding specific aspects of the surgical repair, evidence can be found in the literature to support that view. Successful repair of CSF leaks must include identification of the exact site of leakage. This may require considerable dissection in difficult cases to find the site of the leak. In contrast to routine endoscopic sinus surgery where mucosal preservation and avoidance of scarring is of paramount importance, in cases of CSF leak repair, scarring incited by mucosal stripping helps form a dense repair. There is no literature favouring one graft material over another and therefore the choice is largely based on surgeon preference, ease of manipulation, cost, etc. Likewise, there is no literature on the use of onlay versus underlay grafts. In general free grafts have been preferred to vascularized flaps for smaller defects because of technical ease of manipulation and obviation of the potential for contraction with healing. Recent interest in closing large defects associated with skull base surgery has favoured pedicled flaps.[16,17] Although bone or cartilage grafts are helpful in medium-sized defects they have not been used for large repairs or generally in small defects. There is some evidence to support the use of fibrin glue to reinforce the closure. In a pig model, de Almeida et al.[25] showed that fibrin glue enhanced closures had superior graft adherence and higher 'burst pressures'. Neurosurgical authors[26] have recommended dural sealants as an adjuvant to surgical repair in high-risk patients. A concern is that these 'sealant' materials may add to the cost of the surgery without appreciably improving success rates.

We place a 'break-layer' of Gelfoam under the area of repair and then place a Merocel pack. The Gelfoam isolates the repair from shearing forces when the pack is removed. As mentioned earlier in the chapter, inflated catheter balloons[17] may provide temporary structural support after major skull base repairs.

CONCLUSION

Remarkable progress has been made in the endoscopic treatment of CSF leaks. Advances have occurred both in preoperative imaging and diagnosis as well as in technical refinements of the surgical closure. Areas of interest in the future might include a better understanding of how to manage patients with spontaneous leaks and improvements in the reconstruction of major skull base defects from endonasal craniotomies.

REFERENCES

1. Mirza S, Thaper A, McLelland L et al. Sinonasal cerebrospinal fluid leaks: Management of 97 patients over 10 years. *Laryngoscope* 2005; **115**: 1774–7.
2. Banks CA, Palmer JN, Chiu AG et al. Endoscopic closure of CSF rhinorrhea: 193 cases over 21 years. *Otolaryngol Head Neck Surg* 2009; **140**: 826–33.
3. Eljamel MS, Foy PM. Non-traumatic CSF fistulae: clinical history and management. *Br J Neurosurg* 1991; **5**: 275–9.
4. Eljamel MSM. The role of surgery and beta-2-transferrin in the management of cerebrospinal fluid fistula. MD thesis. Liverpool: University of Liverpool, 1993.

5. Daudia A, Biswas D, Jones NS. The relative risk of meningitis with cerebrospinal fluid rhinorrhoea. *Ann Otol Rhinol Laryngol* 2007; **116**: 902–5.

6. Gassner HG, Ponikau JU, Sherris DA *et al*. CSF rhinorrhea: 95 consecutive surgical cases with long term follow-up at the Mayo Clinic. *Am J Rhinol* 1999; **13**: 439–47.

7. Peabody RG, Leino T, Nohynek H *et al*. Pneumococcal vaccination policy in Europe. *Euro Surveill* 2005; **10**: 174–8.

8. Dalgic A, Okay HO, Gezici AR *et al*. An effective and less invasive treatment of post-traumatic cerebrospinal fluid fistula: closed lumbar drainage system. *Minim Invas Neurosurg* 2008; **51**: 154–7.

9. Bernal-Sprekelsen M, Bleda-Vazquez C, Carrau RL. Ascending meningitis secondary to traumatic cerebrospinal fluid leaks. *Am J Rhinol* 2000; **14**: 257–9.

10. Weber SM, Kim J, Delashaw JB *et al*. Radial forearm free tissue transfer in the management of persistent cerebrospinal fluid leaks. *Laryngoscope* 2005; **115**: 968–72.

11. Boudreaux B, Zins JE. Treatment of cerebrospinal fluid leaks in high risk patients. *J Craniofac Surg* 2009; **20**: 743–7.

12. Wise SK, Schlosser RJ. Evaluation of spontaneous nasal cerebrospinal fluid leaks. *Curr Opin Otolaryngol Head Neck Surg* 2007; **15**: 28–34.

13. Bolger WE, Osenbach R. Endoscopic transpterygoid approach to the lateral sphenoid recess. *Ear Nose Throat J* 1999; **78**: 36–46.

14. Bachmann G, Djenabi V, Jungehülsing M *et al*. Incidence of occult cerebrospinal fluid fistula during paranasal sinus surgery. *Arch Otolaryngol Head Neck Surg* 2002; **128**: 1299–302.

15. Yessenow RS, McCabe BF. The osteomucoperiosteal flap in repair of cerebrospinal fluid rhinorrhea: a 20 year experience. *Otolaryngol Head Neck Surg* 1989; **101**: 555–8.

16. Kassam AB, Carrau RL, Snyderman CH *et al*. Endoscopic reconstruction of the cranial base using a pedicled nasoseptal flap. *Neurosurgery* 2008; **63** (1 Suppl 1): ONS44–53.

17. Harvey RJ, Nogueira JF, Schlosser RJ *et al*. Closure of large skull base defects after endoscopic transnasal craniotomy. *J Neurosurg* 2009; **111**: 371–9.

18. Bateman N, Jones NS. Rhinorrhoea feigning cerebrospinal fluid leak: nine illustrative cases. *J Laryngol Otol* 2000; **114**: 462–4.

19. Michel O, Bamborschke S, Nekic M *et al*. Beta-trace protein (prostaglandin D synthase) – a stable and reliable protein in perilymph. *Ger Med Sci* 2005; **3**: Doc04.

20. Lloyd KM, Del Gaudio JM, Hudgins PA. Imaging of skull base cerebrospinal fluid leaks in adults. *Radiology* 2008; **248**: 725–36.

21. Aydin K, Terzibasioglu E, Sencer S *et al*. Localization of cerebrospinal fluid leaks by gaddolinium-enhanced magnetic resonance cisternography: a 5-year single center experience. *Neurosurgery* 2008; **62**: 584–9.

22. Keerl R, Weber RK, Draf W *et al*. Use of sodium fluorescein solution for detection of CSF fistulas: an analysis of 420 administrations and reported complications in Europe and the United States. *Laryngoscope* 2004; **114**: 266–72.

23. Zuckerman JD, Del Gaudio JM. Utility of pre-operative high resolution CT and intraoperative image guidance in identification of cerebrospinal fluid leaks for endoscopic repair. *Am J Rhinol* 2008; **22**: 151–4.

24. Saafan ME, Ragab SM, Albirmawy OA. Topical intranasal fluorescein: the missing partner in algorithms of cerebrospinal fluid fistula dissection. *Laryngoscope* 2006; **116**: 1158–61.

25. de Almeida JR, Ghotme K, Leong L *et al*. A new porcine skull base model: fibrin glue improves strength of cerebrospinal fluid leak repairs. *Otolaryngol Head Neck Surg* 2009; **141**: 184–9.

26. Weinstein JS, Liu KC, Delashaw JB *et al*. The safety and effectiveness of a dural sealant system for use with non-autologous duraplasty materials. *J Neurosurg* 2010; **112**: 428–33.

12

The frontal sinus

PETER-JOHN WORMALD

SURGICAL PHILOSOPHY

In the past the frontal sinus has been regarded as the most difficult area of endoscopic sinus surgery.[1-3] The frontal sinus is situated behind the frontal beak and the anatomy in this region can be quite variable. In addition the thin bone of the lamina papyracea (orbit) and lateral wall of the cribriform plate form the lateral and medial boundaries that are at risk during surgery in this region. The frontal recess may also vary considerably in size, and in patients with a narrow frontal recess, adhesion formation and postoperative fibrosis may occur after minimal surgical trauma.[4,5] Cells in the frontal recess may be positioned to a variable extent around the frontal recess, further narrowing or obstructing the recess. In the past these factors have led surgeons to suggest that surgery in this region should not be performed and that surgically treating the maxillary sinus ostium and bulla ethmoidalis may result in resolution of disease in this area;[5] however, the so-called minimally invasive sinus treatment (MIST) has not been shown to achieve this goal.[6] Another suggestion that has been made is that the frontal sinus should only be operated on if there were symptoms that could be related directly to the frontal sinus. However, this argument is also flawed as we know that frontal pain or headaches are only one symptom of chronic frontal sinusitis and that the diseased frontal sinuses also contribute substantially to the symptoms of nasal obstruction, rhinorrhoea and postnasal drip.

The aforementioned philosophy is also not consistent with the philosophy generally applied to all the other nasal sinuses. An accepted philosophy is that disease in a maxillary, ethmoid or sphenoid sinus that has not responded to maximal medical treatment should be surgically removed and the ostium of maxillary and sphenoid sinus opened to improve ventilation and drainage of those sinuses. It does not make sense that the frontal sinuses should be treated any differently. The philosophy in this chapter is that patients who have undergone maximal medical treatment and who have continuing symptoms of chronic sinusitis and in whom a sinus or sinuses remain diseased, should have the diseased sinuses surgically addressed irrespective of which sinus this is.[4,5]

THE PATIENT WITH POOR PROGNOSIS

It is important to realize that a number of factors influence the outcome of surgery in the frontal recess and sinus. The most important of these are the size of the frontal recess, the presence of obstructive cells around the frontal recess, the overall severity of disease as reflected by the Lund and Mackay score, presence of new bone formation, lateralization of the middle turbinate and the presence of eosinophilic mucus and polyps.[5] Patients with small frontal sinus recesses have a greater likelihood of developing postoperative oedema and obstruction of the recess than patients with large frontal recesses. This is also seen in patients with eosinophilic mucus and polyps. It remains unclear why the size of the frontal recess appears to be related to surgical outcome. In some patients where all factors are controlled and disease is quiescent in the sinuses with large ostia such as the maxillary and the sphenoid, why do these patients develop oedema and progressive obstruction of their narrow frontal recess? Is it purely related to the ventilation of the sinus or are there other factors at play? It is not uncommon to see healthy mucosa in a widely opened maxillary and sphenoid sinus but to have polypoid mucosa or polyps obstructing a narrow frontal recess. Is this due to poor ventilation and does this result in initial mild oedema of the mucosa with accumulation of eosinophilic mucus within the sinus followed by increasing mucosal oedema and finally polyp recurrence?

Other factors too play a role, such as the presence of obstructive cells around the frontal recess requiring surgery through the recess and in the frontal sinus. This may traumatize the recess, resulting in loss of mucosa, and this may in turn predispose the patient to postoperative fibrosis, adhesion formation and retention of secretions. Patients with a high Lund and MacKay score will often have associated eosinophilic mucus and nasal polyps. Even though all the polyps and eosinophilic mucus are removed during surgery, the patient has a predisposition to react very strongly (overactively) to inhaled environmental stimulants that may initiate mucosal oedema and formation of eosinophilic mucus. It is still unclear as to whether this is due to fungus, superantigen stimulation, biofilm or chronic infection, or a combination of these.

The other important prognostic factor is new bone formation in the frontal recess and frontal recess region indicating chronic osteitis. After removal of this chronically infected bone the remaining bone will usually show ongoing osteitis that results in the formation of thick layers of fibrous tissue, which will often partially or completely block the frontal recess with recurrence of frontal sinus disease. Finally frontal stenosis can occur in some patients in whom the middle turbinate has lateralized or who have had a previous middle turbinectomy with subsequent lateralization of the stump; this can result in frontal sinus disease.

THREE-DIMENSIONAL RECONSTRUCTION OF THE ANATOMY

It is beyond the scope of this chapter to explain in detail all the variations of the anatomy that occur in the frontal recess. There are excellent reference texts where this can be found.[4,5,7–9] Understanding the anatomy of the frontal recess includes knowledge of the agger nasi cell and its

relationship with the various cells that occur around the frontal recess. These variations consist of the four types of frontoethmoidal cell, intersinus septal cell and frontal bullar cell.[5,10] Brief definitions of these are provided in Table 12.1.[5,10] Frontoethmoidal cells are ethmoid cells that contact the frontal process of the maxilla. Cells that occur in the frontal recess but do not have contact with the frontal process of the maxilla are suprabullar or frontal bullar cells.

In order to illustrate the need to fully understand these variations an example of a three-dimensional (3D) reconstruction is provided. It would also be of value to review the preoperative assessment in Chapter 5 where an additional example is provided. The principle in 3D reconstruction is for the surgeon to fully understand the way the cells interact and how these cells alter and affect the drainage pathway of the frontal sinus. This understanding in turn allows for detailed surgical planning to be done by the surgeon before surgery is performed. This process can be likened to an elite skier doing the slalom course in his/her mind with each bend and jump pictured and the approach to each of these obstacles detailed. One will sometimes see the skier with their eyes closed mentally going through each step of the course before the run is started. In the frontal recess each cell is pictured and entry into each cell planned. In order to prevent placement of instruments through the roof of a cell, the drainage pathway that the instrument will be inserted into should be identified on computed tomography (CT) scans. This principle of not placing an instrument through the roof of a cell needs to be reinforced. Fracturing a cell by pushing an instrument through a solid bony structure such as the roof of a cell is an unsafe practice. If the surgeon is mistaken and the anatomy is different from what was thought, then pushing an instrument through a bony wall may result in the instrument been pushed into either the intracranial cavity with subsequent CSF leak or into the orbit with possible damage to the eye muscles, nerves or eyeball.

In the present example, the intersinus septal cell (ISSC) on the left side can be seen in all the coronal scans (Fig. 12.1). The process is to identify the first visible cell then follow it posteriorly before proceeding to the parasagittal

Table 12.1   Common variations seen in the frontal recess and frontal sinus

Agger nasi cell		A single cell seen directly adjacent to the 'axilla' (insertion) of the middle turbinate on the lateral wall
Frontoethmoidal cells	Type 1	A single cell above the agger nasi cell
	Type 2	Two or more cells above the agger nasi cell
	Type 3	A cell that pushes through the frontal recess into the frontal sinus
	Type 4	A type 3 cell that pushes into the frontal sinus and occupies more than 50 per cent of the vertical height of the sinus
Intersinus septal cell		A cell associated with the frontal sinus septum usually pushing and narrowing the frontal sinus drainage pathway laterally
Frontal bullar cell		A cell that enters the frontal sinus along the skull base pushing the drainage pathway anteriorly

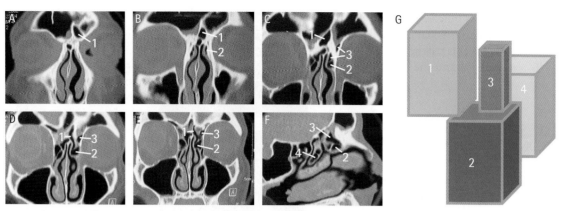

Figure 12.1   (A–E) Coronal computed tomography (CT) scans show the intersinus septal cell (1), agger nasi cell (2) and T1 cell (3). Cells 2 and 3 can also be seen on the parasagittal CT (F). In addition the bulla ethmoidalis can be seen on this scan (4). (G) A building block is placed for each cell.

scan and identifying the cell on this scan. In this example the ISSC is not seen on the parasagittal views as the cell sits medial to where the parasagittal slice has been taken. However, the agger nasi and T1 cells can be clearly seen on the parasagital scan, as well as the bulla ethmoidalis. Placing building blocks for each of these cells allows a 3D picture of the anatomy of the frontal recess to be developed. Once this is done, the axial scans are viewed to determine the frontal sinus drainage pathway (Fig. 12.2). This can then be drawn into the 3D picture and a surgical plan can be formulated.

SURGICAL PLAN

The surgical plan for the left side presented in Figures 12.1 and 12.2 would be to do an axillary flap, which will allow exposure of the anterior face of the agger nasi cell and accurate identification of this cell. The suction curette can then be placed in the drainage pathway behind this cell and the posterior wall and roof of the cell fractured away to reveal the T1 cell laterally and the drainage pathway

medially. This pathway proceeds medial to the T1 before turning lateral to the ISSC. The drainage pathway is sought with either the suction curette or, if the pathway is very narrow, a malleable frontal sinus probe. The probe is very gently slid up the region directly medial and posterior to the T1 cell but lateral to the medial wall of the ISSC. No pressure is placed on the probe and it should slide relatively easily up into the frontal sinus.

Once the pathway is confirmed the probe then curette is used to fracture the T1 cell laterally and anteriorly until the cell can be removed and the frontal sinus drainage pathway is clear of obstructing cells. If the medial wall of the ISSC is thin, it may be fractured and removed to further widen the frontal recess but in many patients, and in the example in this chapter, this wall is thick and cannot be removed by fracture. In *no* circumstances should a drill be used to remove these septations. We have found that using a drill in a narrow frontal recess such as this causes extensive loss of mucosa and will almost certainly result in a stenosed or fibrosed frontal recess postoperatively. It is much better to only remove the obstructing cells that can be fractured and removed with a giraffe forceps with

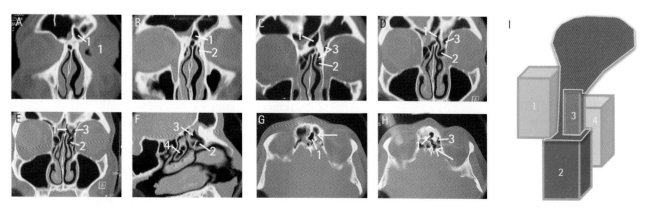

Figure 12.2   (A–H) The axial computed tomography (CT) scans (G–H) allow the frontal sinus drainage pathway to be identified (arrows) and followed from the frontal sinus into the ethmoids. (I) This pathway can then be drawn into the 3D drawing giving a full understanding of the frontal recess anatomy.

preservation of the frontal recess mucosa. The only time a drill is used in the frontal recess is when a frontal sinus drill-out is performed. Most patients will heal well if only the obstructing cells are removed and the frontal recess exposed.

SURGICAL ACCESS TO THE FRONTAL RECESS AND FRONTAL SINUS

One of the reasons surgery in the frontal recess and frontal sinus is thought to be difficult is due to the fact that both these regions are located above the 'axilla' of the middle turbinate and behind the 'beak' of the frontal process of the maxilla.[4,5] The axillary flap[11] was developed for two reasons.

- Removal of the bone that forms the axilla results in the surgeon entering the agger nasi cell: such an entry allows the surgeon to be certain as to where he or she is, as the agger nasi cell is easily identified on coronal and parasagittal CT scans and on the patient. This allows the surgical plan to be executed with high certainty and precision as the starting point is defined. Trying to identify the cells during a frontal recess dissection, when moving along the skull base from posterior ethmoids into the frontal recess, can be challenging for even the most experienced surgeon. Often surgery that is conducted in this manner is done by experience and feel rather than with certain identification of each cell and location of the frontal sinus drainage pathway. This posterior to anterior technique is valuable but is only recommended when prior surgery has been performed and there are few anatomical landmarks, or in patients with massive polyposis and few landmarks.
- The axillary flap is preferred for entry into the frontal recess and frontal sinus because it allows the 0° and 30° endoscopes to be utilized for the dissection rather than the 70° endoscope: it is well documented that using a 70° endoscope is technically more demanding and time consuming than using the less angled scopes. In all branches of surgery improving exposure of the surgical site aids the completeness and precision of the dissection. This is the advantage that the axillary flap gives to surgery of the frontal recess.

THE AXILLARY FLAP[5,11]

The incisions for the axillary flap are 8–10 mm above the axilla of the middle turbinate (Fig. 12.3). This incision is brought forward for 8–10 mm and then turns vertically and a parallel incision made under the axilla and over the insertion of the middle turbinate. The suction Freer is used to elevate the mucosa and tuck it between the middle turbinate and septum (Fig. 12.4). The mucosa must be dissected clear of the middle turbinate insertion as

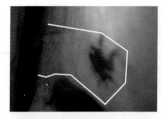

Figure 12.3   The incisions for the axillary flap in a left nasal cavity are outlined above the axilla of the middle turbinate.

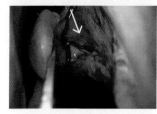

Figure 12.4   The mucosal flap is elevated off the anterior face of the agger nasi cell (arrow) and tucked between the middle turbinate and septum.

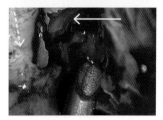

Figure 12.5   The anterior face of the agger nasi cell has been removed and the roof of the agger cell is seen (continuous arrow). The axillary flap can be seen tucked between the middle turbinate and septum (broken arrow).

leaving mucosa over this region will result in the flap being pulled into the surgical field every time a suction or other instrument is passed under the new axilla. Exposure of the insertion of the middle turbinate will allow the flap to remain undisturbed for the entire duration of the surgery until the flap is fetched and draped over the new axilla. Once the anterior face of the axilla has been removed with a Hajek–Koeffler punch the agger nasi cell can be clearly identified (Fig. 12.5). The surgeon now knows exactly where they are and can safely proceed with the surgical plan.

FRONTAL SINUS MINI-TREPHINE[5,8]

This technique is useful in patients in whom the frontal sinus drainage pathway cannot be found. This may occur in patients with very complex frontal anatomy, in patients with extensive or severe disease or in patients in whom severe bleeding obscures the drainage pathway. This technique may often 'save the day' when all else has been tried without success. The technique requires the 'frontal sinus mini-trephine kit' (from Medtronic ENT).

The landmarks for placing the trephine are the inferior medial aspects of the eyebrows. A line is drawn between the eyebrows and the midpoint identified, and the trephine placed 1 cm lateral to this midpoint along the line (Fig. 12.6). Although this should be the position of the trephine, the skin incision can be placed further laterally. I usually place the skin incision in the hairs of the medial end of the eyebrow. The hairs camouflage the incision very well once the trephine is removed. The skin over this area is mobile

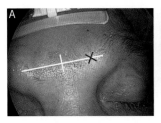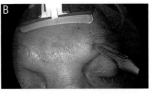

Figure 12.6   (A) A line is drawn from the inferior medial aspect of each eyebrow and the red X marks the position of the mini-trephine. (B) Note the scalpel incision is placed further laterally in the hairs of the eyebrow. Once the guide is placed the skin is pulled medially until it is correctly positioned.

so that once the incision has been performed and the guide placed through the incision, the guide can drag the skin medially until the trephine is correctly placed as previously stated. The trephine drill is 1 mm and is placed through the guide (Fig. 12.7). There is no built-in bur tip irrigation during drilling and the tip heats up very quickly so it needs to be removed from the guide and irrigated and cooled within 2–3 seconds of contacting the bone. This process is repeated until penetration of the frontal table is achieved. The bur only extends 11 mm beyond the guide so contact with the posterior wall of the frontal sinus should not be possible. The irrigation washes the bone bits away and cools the tip of the bur. If this is not done, the bur will heat up and cause a thermal injury to both the bone and surrounding skin, which can result in an ugly scar from the incision and may predispose the bone to infection.

Once the trephine has penetrated the anterior wall of the frontal sinus, it is withdrawn and the guidewire placed through the guide into the newly created bony trephine. The guide is withdrawn leaving the guidewire in place. The cannula is placed over the guidewire into the trephine and fixed in the bone of the frontal sinus (Fig. 12.8). The cannula can be removed at the end of surgery or left in place for a few days to irrigate the frontal sinus and frontal recess if this is

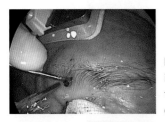

Figure 12.7   The bur is irrigated as it is placed through the guide onto the anterior face of the frontal sinus.

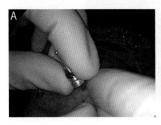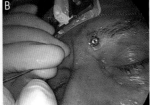

Figure 12.8   (A) The cannula is placed over the guidewire and into the frontal sinus. (B) The cannula is seen positioned in the frontal sinus.

thought to be necessary. Current indications for leaving the cannula in the frontal sinus for a few days postoperatively include a small frontal recess that has required excessive instrumentation to remove debris or cells from within the frontal sinus and may have lost considerable mucosa around the recess during this process, or marked inflammation or oedema of the mucosa of the frontal sinus and frontal recess that may benefit from topical steroid drops applied though the cannula for some days after surgery. After removal of the cannula a Steri-Strip is placed over the incision. The wound is not sutured. Cosmetically it heals very quickly and the 2 mm scar is well hidden in the hairs of the eyebrow.

FRONTAL SINUS DRILL-OUT, ENDOSCOPIC MODIFIED LOTHROP OR DRAF TYPE III PROCEDURE[3,5,12]

A number of patients will fail standard endoscopic sinus surgery either due to having poor prognostic factors such as narrow frontal recess, new bone formation or due to scar tissue formation and obstruction. In addition, in some patients with severe disease usually associated with asthma, nasal polyps and eosinophilic mucus, polyps will start to form, first in and around the frontal recess and second, this may slowly evolve to include the ethmoid cavity. The frontal drill-out procedure has been shown to be of considerable benefit in all these patient groups.[5,12,13] The frontal drill-out is always performed after complete clearance of the maxillary sinus, sphenoid and ethmoids, and in patients with severe disease and nasal polyps; the horizontal portion of the ground lamella is also removed. This opens up the posterior ethmoid/sphenoid complex and improves the aeration in this area. The frontal sinuses are then joined and widely opened into the nose. The average neo-frontal ostium should be 22 × 20 mm. This extended surgery with frontal sinus drill-out widely marsupializes all of the sinuses into the nasal cavity. This is no longer functional surgery as the functional surgery had previously failed.

This surgery is, however, effective in managing these patients, who are very difficult to treat, and will allow control of the nasal polyp regrowth and the reduction or elimination of recurrent sinus infections in most cases. We have found in our studies on this technique in patients who had previously had an average of six sinus operations that we were able to cure 75 per cent and in those remaining only 10 per cent required further revision surgery during a follow-up within 2 years.[12] Most of the 25 per cent that remained symptomatic after this surgery were in the poor prognostic fungal sinus group or had Samter's triad or an immune deficiency.

SURGICAL STEPS[5,12]

The first step is to completely clear the maxillary, ethmoid and sphenoid sinuses of all polyps and mucus. Once this has been done the mucosa is removed from above the axilla of the middle turbinate, exposing the underlying bone. This removal of mucosa is continued across the roof of the nose onto the septum. Next the mucosa overlying the septum is removed from the point adjacent to the middle turbinate for about 2 cm anteriorly (Fig. 12.9). The septal bone is removed and the opposite nasal cavity visualized. The septal window is lowered inferiorly until an instrument can be passed from one side of the nose under the axilla of the opposite side (Fig. 12.10). The window is brought anteriorly until an instrument can be passed from one side of the nose onto the frontal process of the maxilla for about 1 cm anterior to the axilla of the middle turbinate. The window should be taken right up the roof of the nose.

Next, bilateral frontal mini-trephines are placed through the eyebrows into the frontal sinuses. Aspiration is performed with syringes containing fluorescein-coloured saline to ensure the trephines are in the frontal sinuses and are not intracranial. The sinuses are irrigated allowing the frontal ostium to be identified. This also allows the posterior extent of the drill-out to be accurately identified, as the drill should never be posterior to the fluorescein-stained saline, which should allow some protection for the skull base as the frontal processes of the maxilla are drilled out.

Next the 3.2 mm straight round bur and a 0° endoscope are placed through one side of the nose across the septal window and drilling is begun on the opposite frontal process of the maxilla, anterior and just inferior to the axilla of the middle turbinate. The drilling is continued laterally and superiorly until the skin is exposed (Fig. 12.10). This skin exposure allows the lateral limit of the dissection to be identified. Drilling is then continued superiorly and laterally into the floor of the frontal sinus

without any drilling being performed medial to the frontal recess. This is repeated on the opposite side (Fig. 12.11). Once the floor of the frontal sinus has been entered, drilling can then proceed medially until the intersinus septum is identified and removed.

The next step is to identify the anterior projections of the olfactory fossa by looking for the first olfactory neurones, as this indicates the position of the forward projection of the skull base. This should be confirmed by using computer-aided navigation. The 0° endoscope is now placed through the right nostril and the drill through the left, and the 'frontal T' is drilled down onto the first olfactory neurone (Fig. 12.12). Drilling past the first olfactory neurone may cause a CSF leak so this landmark needs to be respected. Then the endoscope is changed to 30° and the bur changed to a 40° frontal finesse bur. The 70° reverse cut diamond bur may also be used if preferred. The lateral and anterior aspects of the neo-frontal ostium are now drilled away until the anterior face of the frontal sinus runs smoothly out into the nose (Fig. 12.13). There should be no lip between

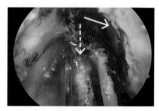

Figure 12.11   The microdebrider has now been placed from the left nostril across the septum (broken arrow) and under the axilla of the right middle turbinate. The opened left frontal sinus is indicated with the continuous arrow.

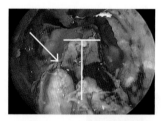

Figure 12.12   The two frontal sinuses have been joined by removal of the intersinus septum. This creates a frontal 'T' as indicated by the black lines. To make out the anterior projection of the olfactory fossae the olfactory nerve is identified (arrow).

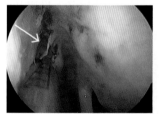

Figure 12.9   The septal window (arrow) is created with a microdebrider in the left nasal cavity.

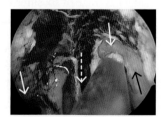

Figure 12.10   The microdebrider is placed from the right nostril across the septum (broken arrow) and under the axilla of the left middle turbinate. The axillae on both sides are marked with white arrows. A small area of skin has been exposed on the left side (black arrow).

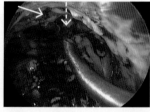

Figure 12.13   Using the 30° endoscope the anterior table of the frontal sinus is viewed (continuous arrow). Note how this runs smoothly out into the nasal cavity. The frontal sinus septum has been removed to the roof of the frontal sinus (broken arrow).

the frontal sinus and nasal cavity. Once this is achieved the ostium should be in the region of 20 × 22 mm depending on the individual patient's anatomy and available space. The ostium should also be oval and not crescent shaped (Fig. 12.14). Crescent shaped ostia have a much greater tendency to stenose, as the anteroposterior diameter is much smaller than the larger oval-shaped ostium. On average the frontal ostium will circumferentially stenose by about 30 per cent and if the anteroposterior diameter of the neo-ostium is small this may lead to obstruction and recurrence of frontal symptoms.[13]

The frontal sinus mini-trephines may be left *in situ* for 2 to 3 days postoperatively and irrigations of the frontal sinus done through these trephines. This helps keep the neo-ostium clear of blood clots. Before these trephines are removed a steroid-based cream (not ointment as petroleum base causes irritation) may be injected through the trephines into the frontal sinus. This helps lessen the crusting that can occur on the raw bone of the new ostium. The first postoperative visit is at 2 weeks where all blood clot and crust is removed and the cream suctioned from the frontal sinuses. Healing can take up to 8 weeks as the bone mucosalizes and regular toilet is usually required to keep the ostium clean and healing well.

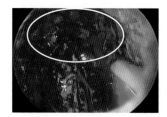

Figure 12.14 Using a 0° endoscope the frontal ostium is viewed and it can be seen that by lowering the frontal 'T' and smoothing the anterior wall of the frontal sinus, an oval shaped neo-ostium is created.

REFERENCES

1. Kennedy DW, Senior BA. Endoscopic sinus surgery – a review. *Otolaryngol Clin North Am* 1997; **30**: 313–30.
2. Thawley SE, Deddens AE. Transfrontal endoscopic management of frontal recess disease. *Am J Rhinol* 1995; **9**: 307–11.
3. Ramadan HH. Surgical causes of failure in endoscopic sinus surgery. *Laryngoscope* 1999; **109**: 27–9.
4. Wormald PJ. Surgery of the frontal recess and frontal sinus. *Rhinology* 2005; **43**: 83–5.
5. Wormald PJ. *Endoscopic sinus surgery, anatomy, 3-D reconstruction and surgery*, 2nd edn. New York: Thieme Medical Publishers, 2007.
6. Catalano PJ, Roffman E. Outcome of patients with chronic sinusitis after minimally invasive sinus technique. *Am J Rhinol* 2003; **17**: 17–22.
7. Wormald PJ. Three dimensional building block approach to understanding the anatomy of the frontal recess and frontal sinus. *Oper Tech Otolaryngol* 2006; **17**: 2–5.
8. Wormald PJ, Chan SZX. Surgical techniques for the removal of frontal recess cells obstructing the frontal ostium. *Am J Rhinol* 2003; **17**: 221–6.
9. Wormald PJ. The agger nasi cell. The key to understanding the anatomy of the frontal recess. *Otolaryngol Head Neck Surg* 2003; **129**: 497–507.
10. Kuhn FA. Chronic frontal sinusitis: the endoscopic frontal recess approach. *Otolaryngol Head Neck Surg* 1996; **7**: 222–9.
11. Wormald PJ. The axillary flap approach to the frontal recess. *Laryngoscope* 2002; **112**: 494–9.
12. Wormald PJ. Salvage frontal sinus surgery: the modified Lothrop procedure. *Laryngoscope* 2003; **113**: 276–83.
13. Tran K, Beule A, Singhal D *et al*. Frontal ostium restenosis and function after modified endoscopic Lothrop procedure. *Laryngoscope* 2007; **117**: 1457–62.

The posterior ethmoid cells and sphenoid sinus

DHARMBIR S SETHI, BOAZ FORER

INTRODUCTION

The paranasal sinuses are divided into two anatomical groups. The maxillary sinus, the frontal sinus and the anterior ethmoid cells form the anterior group. The posterior group includes the posterior ethmoid cells (PEC) and the sphenoid sinus. The posterior group is closely related to the orbital apex, optic nerve and the cavernous sinus. Although pathology in the posterior group is not as common as in the anterior group, disease in this cell complex may cause serious complications including impairment of vision, blindness, cranial nerve palsies and thrombophlebitis of the cavernous sinus.

The spectrum of pathology that affects the posterior group is similar to that of the anterior group and commonly results as an extension from the anterior group. However, isolated pathology may occur in the PEC or the sphenoid sinus. Because of the proximity of the posterior group of paranasal sinuses to the orbital apex, optic nerve, cavernous sinus, sella turcica, petrous apex, middle and posterior cranial fossa, pathology may often extend to the sphenoid sinus and the PEC directly or along the paths of least resistance. The sphenoid sinus has remained a neglected sinus for most of the past century. However, it is likely that owing to the lack of diagnostic modalities such as computed tomography (CT) and magnetic resonance imaging (MRI), and nasal endoscopy, in the past pathology affecting this cell complex may have been under-reported. In the past two decades, since the popularity of endoscopic sinus surgery, the emergence of current imaging technology and availability of image-guided systems, the sphenoid sinus has become the gateway for endoscopic surgery of the skull base, providing minimally invasive access to the middle and posterior cranial fossa.

The objective of this chapter is to review and discuss the:

- gross and endoscopic anatomy of the posterior group of paranasal sinuses
- pathology affecting these sinuses
- endoscopic approaches to the PEC and the sphenoid sinus
- complications.

SURGICAL ANATOMY

Located posterior to the basal lamella the PEC are larger in size and fewer in number than the anterior ethmoid cells. The boundaries of the PEC are: the basal lamella anteriorly, lamina papyracea laterally, skull base superiorly, the superior turbinate medially, and the medial turbinate lamella inferiorly. The size of this cell complex depends on the degree of encroachment by the anterior ethmoid cells anteriorly and the sphenoid posteriorly. Their relationship with the sphenoid sinus depends on the presence or absence of a sphenoethmoid cell (also known as Onodi cell), which is a posterior ethmoid cell that pneumatizes posterolaterally and posterosuperiorly in relation to the anterior wall of the sphenoid. In the presence of the Onodi cell, the sphenoid sinus is located inferiorly and medially, and not posteriorly, in relation to the most posterior cell of the PEC. The PEC drain into the superior meatus.

The sphenoid sinus is subject to considerable variation in size and shape and to variation in the degree of pneumatization.[1] Based on the extent of pneumatization, the sphenoid sinus has been classified into three types:

- conchal – in this type the area below the sella is a solid block of bone without an air cavity. The conchal type is common in children under the age of 12 years, after which pneumatization begins within the sphenoid sinus
- presellar – in this type, the air cavity does not penetrate beyond a plane perpendicular to the sellar wall (Fig. 13.1A)
- sellar – this type is the most common, occurring in 76 per cent of individuals. The air cavity extends into the body of the sphenoid below the sella and may extend as far posteriorly as the clivus (Fig. 13.1B).

A sellar-type pneumatized sphenoid sinus can be compared with a pyramid-shaped six-sided box, the larger side of which is facing forward and forms the anterior wall, which is shaped like the keel of a ship and is termed the sphenoid rostrum. The medial third of the anterior sphenoid sinus wall is a free surface in the nasal cavity. This area is called the sphenoethmoidal recess (SER) and the sphenoid sinus ostium opens into it. The roof of the sphenoid sinus is flat and termed the planum sphenoidale. It is limited posteriorly by the sellar floor, laterally by the optic nerve prominences and anteriorly by the anterior wall of the sphenoid sinus. The width of the planum sphenoidale anteriorly, between the lamina papyracea on either side, has been measured in cadaver studies at 26 ± 4 mm and narrows to 16 ± 3 mm posteriorly at the posterior aspect of the tuberculum sella.[2]

The posterior wall of the sphenoid sinus is made up of the sellar floor in the upper part and by the clivus in the lower part (Fig. 13.1A). It is limited laterally by the carotid prominences, superiorly by the roof or the planum sphenoidale and inferiorly by the floor of the sphenoid sinus. The lateral wall of the sphenoid sinus shows the prominence of the optic nerve anterosuperiorly and the cavernous carotid artery posteroinferiorly (Fig. 13.1B).

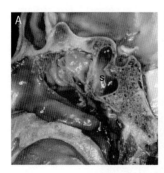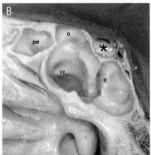

Figure 13.1   (A) Sagittal section of a cadaver head showing the right lateral wall of the sphenoid sinus. Note the presellar type of pneumatization of the sphenoid sinus (S). The posterior extent of pneumatization does not extend posterior to the anterior wall of the sella (asterisk). (B) The sphenoid sinus in this specimen extends posterior to the anterior wall of the sella (asterisk) as far back as the clivus. The structures identified on the lateral wall of the sphenoid sinus are the cavernous carotid artery (c), optic nerve (o) and the second branch of the trigeminal (V2). Note the relation of the posterior ethmoid cell (pe) to the sphenoid sinus.

The floor of the sphenoid sinus is formed by the clivus posteriorly and the sphenoid rostrum anteriorly. The extent to which the clivus participates in formation of the posterior wall or the floor of the sphenoid sinus depends on the pneumatization of the sphenoid sinus. The ostium of the sphenoid sinus is located in the SER and varies in size from 1 mm to 4 mm. In most cases it can be identified lateral to the nasal septum and medial to the superior turbinate about 1.5 cm superior to the posterior choana. The septae within the sphenoid sinus vary greatly in size, shape, thickness, location and completeness. The cavities within the sinus are seldom symmetrical and are often subdivided by irregular minor septae.

A sphenoid sinus with presellar type pneumatization on one side and sellar type on the other side is not uncommon. A single major septum separating the sinus into two large cavities has been reported in only 68 per cent of specimens and may be off the midline by as far as 8 mm.[3] The most common type of sphenoid sinus has multiple small cavities in the large paired sinuses. The smaller cavities are separated by septae oriented in all directions. These intersinus sinus septae or the accessory septae may terminate onto the carotid canal in 40 per cent, and onto the optic nerves in 4 per cent.[4]

The lateral wall of the sphenoid sinus is related to the cavernous sinus, which extends from the orbital apex to the posterior clinoid process. The cavernous sinus contains delicate venous channels, the cavernous part of the internal carotid artery, the third, fourth and the sixth cranial nerves, and fibro-fatty tissue. The internal carotid artery is the most medial structure within the cavernous sinus and forms a discernible prominence on the posterolateral aspect of the lateral wall of the sphenoid sinus. This prominence is clearly identified in a well-pneumatized sphenoid sinus, forming a serpiginous bulge marking the course of the carotid artery. The bone separating the artery and the sphenoid sinus is thinner over the anterior than the posterior parts of the carotid prominence and is thinnest over the part of the artery just below the tuberculum sellae. A layer of bone less than 0.5 mm thick separates the artery and sinus in nearly 90 per cent of sinuses and areas with no bone between the artery and the sinus may be present in nearly 10 per cent.[4] On the anterosuperior aspect of the lateral wall of the sphenoid sinus is another bulge formed by the optic nerve as it traverses the optic canal from the optic chiasma to the orbital apex. There are areas where no bone separates the optic sheath and sinus mucosa. In nearly 80 per cent of the optic nerves, less than 0.5 mm of bone separates the optic nerve and sheath from the sinus mucosa. In more than half of cases, both the optic nerve and the cavernous carotid artery are separated from the sphenoid sinus mucosa by bone of 0.5 mm or less in thickness. The incidence of dehiscence of these structures has been noted to be 4 per cent and 8 per cent, respectively.[4]

The prominence of the internal carotid artery is separated from the prominence of the optic nerve by a pneumatized diverticulum on the lateral wall of the sphenoid sinus called the optico-carotid recess. The extent of pneumatization varies, and in some cases it extends through the optic strut into the anterior clinoid process. In a well-pneumatized sphenoid sinus, the pterygoid canal and a segment of the maxillary division of the trigeminal nerve may be identified in the lateral recess of the sphenoid sinus (Fig. 13.1B). The trigeminal ganglion and the first and third trigeminal divisions are separated from the lateral wall of the sphenoid sinus by the carotid artery.

The roof of the sphenoid, the planum sphenoidale, extends anteriorly in continuation with the roof of the ethmoid sinus. At the junction of the planum sphenoidale and the posterior wall of the sphenoid, the sphenoid bone is thickened to form the tuberculum sella. Inferior to the tuberculum sella, on the posterior wall, is the sella floor, which forms a midline bulge. Often the dura may be visible through this thin bone, imparting a bluish hue to the sellar floor that aids in its recognition. Removal of the sellar floor provides access to the sella turcica.

POSTERIOR ETHMOID AND SPHENOID PATHOLOGY

Pathology may occur concomitantly in the PEC and the sphenoid sinus or result as an extension of pathology in the anterior group. Though uncommon, it may be isolated, arising within the PEC or the sphenoid sinus. Occasionally, pathology may extend into these sinuses from the surrounding region such as the orbit, skull base, middle cranial or the posterior cranial fossa. In 1999, the senior author of this chapter reported a series of 21 isolated sphenoid lesions treated in a 4-year period.[5] This experience has broadened to more than 250 cases of isolated sphenoid lesions in the past 15 years. Most posterior sinus lesions can be categorized into either inflammatory or neoplastic disease. The majority of the lesions seen in clinical practice are due to inflammation. Primary neoplastic diseases are rare but sinus invasion from an adjacent malignant neoplasm is relatively more common.

INFECTIOUS PROCESSES

Chronic bacterial sinusitis

Chronic sinusitis most commonly involves the anterior group of the sinuses but may often involve the PEC and the sphenoid sinus (Fig. 13.2). Isolated sphenoid sinusitis, on the other hand, is even less commonly observed. Both the sphenoid and PEC drain into the SER and subsequently into the superior meatus. Hence inflammatory disease usually affects these sinuses together.

Presenting symptoms include a deep-seated headache over the vertex, temporal or retro-orbital area. As the maxillary division of the trigeminal nerve is intimately related to the sphenoid sinus some patients may present clinically with pain in the maxillary nerve (Fig. 13.3A). Involvement of the third, fourth and sixth cranial nerves or periorbital oedema should alert the physician to possible ophthalmic vein or cavernous sinus involvement (Fig. 13.2C). Endoscopic findings in inflammation of the PEC and sphenoid sinus include mucosal oedema, polypoid hypertrophic mucosa and or mucopus in the SER (Fig. 13.3B). Imaging studies include a CT scan, which will demonstrate opacification of the involved sinuses (Figs 13.2A and 13.3A). An MRI should be done in the presence of suspected or impending intracranial or intraorbital involvement (Fig. 13.2C).

The treatment of chronic sphenoid sinusitis is endoscopic drainage of the sinus by widening the natural sphenoid ostium, which is often obstructed by inflamed, oedematous mucosa (Fig. 13.3C). In cases where there is concomitant involvement of PEC and the sphenoid sinus, a sphenoethmoidectomy may be necessary. For isolated sphenoid involvement a direct endonasal sphenoidotomy is the approach of choice (Fig. 13.3D).

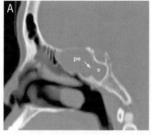 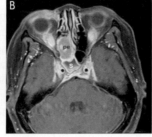 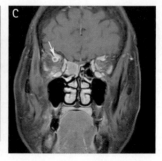

Figure 13.2   (A) Sagittal computed tomography (CT) scan of a 45-year-old woman presenting with right periorbital oedema. The scan shows complete opacification of the posterior ethmoid cells (pe) and the sphenoid sinus (s). The arrow is pointing to the anterior sphenoid wall. (B) T1-weighted axial magnetic resonance (MR) image of the patient in Figure 13.2A. The secretions within the posterior ethmoid cells show higher signals than the sphenoid sinus (s). (C) Contrast-enhanced T1-weighted coronal MR image of same patient. Note the thrombosed superior ophthalmic vein (arrow).

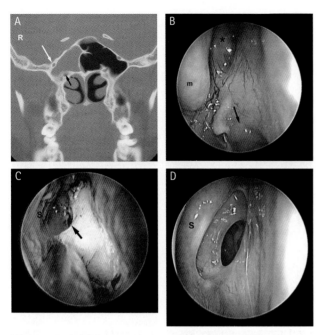

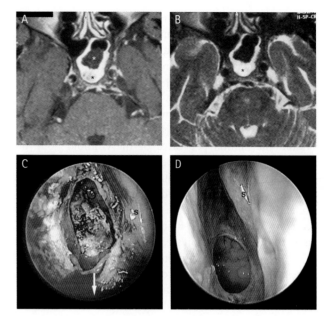

Figure 13.3 (A) Coronal computed tomography (CT) scan showing an opacified right sphenoid sinus in a patient who presented with right retro-orbital pain. The white arrow is pointing to the foramen transmitting the second branch of the trigeminal nerve (maxillary nerve) and the black arrow is pointing to the pterygoid canal carrying the vidian nerve. (B) Endoscopic view of the right sphenoethmoid recess in the same patient as in Figure 13.3A. Note the mucosal oedema overlying the sphenoid ostium (asterisk). Also seen is the right posterior choana (arrow). m, middle turbinate. (C) Intraoperative view of the right sphenoethmoidal recess in a patient undergoing endoscopic sphenoidotomy. The arrow is pointing to the sphenoid ostium. s, superior turbinate. (D) Endoscopic view of a right sphenoidotomy 4 weeks postoperatively. s, superior turbinate.

Figure 13.4 (A) T1-weighted axial magnetic resonance (MR) image with contrast showing hypodense opacity in the sphenoid sinus (white asterisk). Note the surrounding oedematous sphenoid mucosa (black asterisk). (B) T2-weighted axial MR image showing the lesion in the sphenoid sinus is almost signal void in contrast to the sphenoid mucosa (asterisk). (C) Intraoperative view of a fungal mass within the left sphenoid sinus (s, left superior turbinate; arrow is pointing to the posterior choana). Fungal culture yielded *Aspergillus*. (D) Endoscopic view of a left sphenoidotomy. Note the mucosal oedema within the sphenoid sinus has completely reversed to normal mucosal lining. s, superior turbinate.

Fungal disease

There are four different types of fungal sinus infection and each type can involve the sphenoid and/or posterior ethmoid sinuses.

NON-INVASIVE FUNGAL SINUSITIS

This is the accumulation of fungal elements and debris in a sinus cavity without mucosal invasion or significant inflammatory reaction (also termed mycetoma or 'fungal ball'). *Aspergillus* is the most common pathogen although other fungi can also infect the sinuses. The most common affected sinus is the maxillary sinus, although the sphenoid and ethmoids can also be involved. Symptoms from an isolated sphenoid fungal mass may be insidious or similar to chronic sphenoid bacterial sinusitis. The surgical treatment is endoscopic sphenoidotomy, which should be large enough to remove all the fungal debris (Fig. 13.4).

ALLERGIC FUNGAL SINUSITIS

Allergic fungal sinusitis is a non-invasive disorder, seen in immunocompetent individuals, that produces a severe inflammatory reaction. The criteria for diagnosis of this condition have undergone numerous revisions; however, most authors agree on the following: the presence in patients with chronic rhinosinusitis (confirmed by CT scan) of characteristic allergic mucin containing clusters of eosinophils and their by-products; and the presence of fungal organisms within that mucin detectable on staining or culture. In addition, most experts require the presence of type 1 (IgE-mediated) hypersensitivity to fungi, and nasal polyposis. *Aspergillus* species are believed to be the predominant cause of allergic fungal sinusitis. More recent series suggest that various dematiaceous (brown-pigmented) environmental moulds, including *Alternaria*, *Bipolaris*, *Cladosporium*, *Curvularia* and *Drechslera* species, can also be responsible. This condition occurs in young immunocompetent adults with chronic relapsing rhinosinusitis, unresponsive to antibiotics, antihistamines or corticosteroids. Although patients do not have underlying immunodeficiencies, 50–70 per cent are atopic. There is no male or female predominance.

Many patients with allergic fungal sinusitis have a history of chronic rhinosinusitis and have undergone multiple operations prior to diagnosis. Although there are no unique pathognomonic symptoms, patients often present with unilateral nasal polyposis and thick yellow–green nasal or sinus mucus. The nasal polyposis can be unilateral or bilateral and may form an expansive mass that causes bone necrosis of the thin walls of the sinuses. Should the lamina papyracea of the ethmoid bone be traversed it can cause proptosis. Polypoid material can also push the nasal septal into the contralateral airway. Severe mucosal oedema and mucopus may be evident on endoscopic examination (Fig. 13.5). The mucosal secretion contains bone-destructive enzymes that might cause the bone resorption seen in Figure 13.6. On CT scans (Fig. 13.6), there is often a characteristic serpiginous sinus opacification of more than one sinus, and also mucosal thickening and erosion of bone, but this does not represent tissue invasion. In addition, allergic fungal sinusitis may be suspected when a patient with nasal polyposis having no other known disease responds only to oral corticosteroids.

Other investigations include microscopic examination of the characteristic allergic mucin (either at the time of surgical debridement for chronic sinusitis or endoscopic examination for drainage) to determine the presence of eosinophils and fungal elements. Histological examination of sinus tissue is undertaken to rule out invasion. Radiographic studies help assess the extent of disease. Laboratory testing is also done for eosinophilia, total serum IgE, specific IgE against fungal antigens, and a positive skin prick test to fungal antigens. Fungal cultures are required to identify the responsible fungus.

The treatment of allergic fungal sinusitis includes surgical debridement to remove polyps and the allergic mucin-containing fungal debris, which has 'peanut butter' type of consistency (Fig. 13.5G) and is thought to be the cause of the immune reaction in the sinus mucosa. More than one surgical procedure may be required to accomplish this goal. Adjunctive medical management is also required because it is unlikely that all fungal elements can be removed and, in small studies, postoperative systemic corticosteroids resulted in reduced recurrence of disease. Many studies have noted a high recurrence rate.[6,7] Allergic aspergillosis has been likened to allergic bronchopulmonary aspergillosis, in other words it is a systemic reaction to an allergen in the respiratory tract.[8]

There is no published evidence that oral or topical antifungal treatment is of benefit in allergic fungal sinusitis although there are anecdotal reports of surgeons using preoperative itraconazole for 4 weeks. These reports claim that this can markedly reduce the extent of surgery that is required, and given along with a 6-week course of postoperative itraconazole, reduces the risk of recurrence. In addition oral corticosteroids reduce symptomatic recurrence but these are contraindicated in several conditions including diabetes, blood dyscrasias, immunodeficiency, glaucoma, osteoporosis and hepatitis.

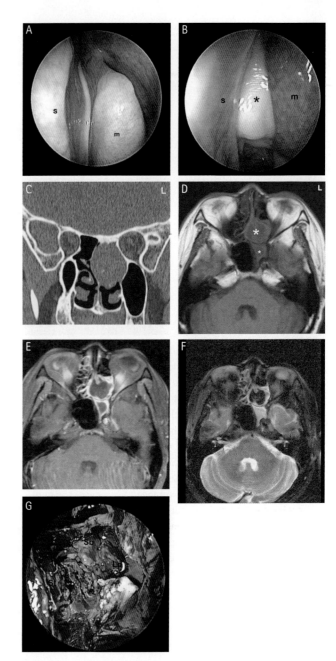

Figure 13.5 (A, B) Endoscopic examination of the left nasal cavity showing mucopus and gross (asterisk) oedema medial to the middle turbinate (m) in a patient with fungal infection of the posterior ethmoid cells. s, nasal septum. (C) Coronal computed tomography (CT) scan showing an expansile lesion in the posterior ethmoid cells (PEC). Note the speckled calcification within the lesion. (D) Non-contrast T1-weighted axial magnetic resonance (MR) image of the same patient showing a lesion with low signal from the PEC (large asterisk) and sphenoid sinus (small asterisk). (E) T1-weighted axial MR image with contrast showing mucosal enhancement surrounding the low signal mass. (F) T2-weighted axial MR image showing high signals from the sphenoid sinus as compared with the lesion in the PEC. (G) Intraoperative endoscopic view showing 'peanut butter like' thick fungal mucin in the PEC. Note the boundaries of the PEC: the lamina papyracea (Lp) laterally, skull base (Sb) superiorly and the superior turbinate (St) medially.

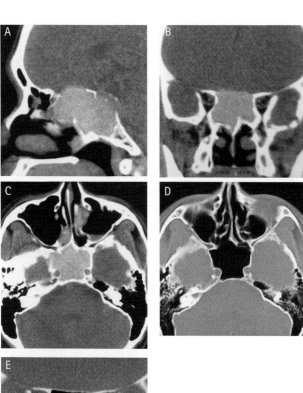

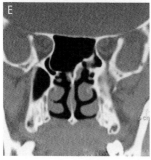

Figure 13.6 (A–C) Sagittal, coronal and axial computed tomography (CT) scans showing a lesion in the posterior ethmoid cells and sphenoid sinus eroding the skull base, sella turcica and the clivus. Intraoperatively this was seen to be thick fungal mucin. (D, E) Postoperative axial and coronal CT scans of the same patient 2 years postoperatively show complete resolution of the disease.

Topical steroids also help in reducing symptomatic recurrence. Monitoring total serum IgE and endoscopic examination have been proposed to aid early detection of recurrent disease.

CHRONIC INVASIVE FUNGAL SINUSITIS

Chronic invasive fungal sinusitis is a slowly progressive disease that is seen in both immunocompromised and immunocompetent individuals. Granulomatous invasive fungal sinusitis often presents with long-standing symptoms of nasal obstruction, unilateral facial discomfort and/ or enlarging mass, or with a silent proptosis.[9,10] Chronic invasive fungal sinusitis is caused by the species *Alternaria*, *Aspergillus*, *Bipolaris*, *Curvularia* and *Exserohilum*. Many of these organisms are ubiquitous in the environment,

being found in the air, in soil and on decomposing organic matter; others are plant pathogens.

The condition may begin as a paranasal sinus fungus ball and then become invasive, perhaps as a result of the immunosuppression associated with diabetes mellitus or corticosteroid treatment. If left untreated, the infection can spread to invade adjacent structures, including the orbit and brain. In patients with chronic invasive sinusitis, non-contrast CT scans will show a hyperdense mass within the involved sinus with associated erosion of the sinus walls. There is profuse fungal growth with localized tissue invasion, and non-caseating granulomas with giant cells. The granulomatous response is often intense enough to cause pressure necrosis of bone and can cause proptosis. Unless removed, the fungal mass can spread into the orbit and brain.

Chronic (invasive) fungal sinusitis requires long courses of itraconazole, unless the disease is of the acute fulminant type with blood vessel invasion, when intravenous amphotericin is indicated. Chronic invasive sinusitis is often advanced by the time of diagnosis, with posterior erosion out of the ethmoid sinus, or even cavernous venous thrombosis. It is important to distinguish a chronic expanding fungal disease comprising a mycetoma that can erode bone and expand into neighbouring areas from chronic invasive aspergillosis, which not only leads to bone loss on CT but, most importantly, penetration of soft tissues. Itraconazole has revolutionized the treatment of this condition and a 12-month course will often make surgery unnecessary and lead to a cure.[11] It is important to monitor liver function and morning cortisol before and after 1 month of treatment with itraconazole, and liver function monthly thereafter.

FULMINANT FUNGAL SINUSITIS

Acute fulminant (invasive) fungal sinusitis is a rapidly progressive disease that is most commonly seen in immunocompromised individuals or diabetic people with uncontrolled ketoacidosis. Immunocompetent individuals are seldom affected. The commonest causes of acute fulminant sinusitis are moulds of the order Mucorales, including the species *Rhizopus* and *Rhizomucor*. Other less frequent causes of fulminant sinusitis include *Aspergillus* species, particularly *A. flavus* and *A. fumigatus*.

The infection can spread from the nasal mucosa and sinus into the orbit and brain. The aetiological agents have a predilection for vascular invasion, causing thrombosis, infarction and ischaemic necrosis of tissues. Prolonged neutropenia and metabolic acidosis are well recognized as important risk factors for rhinocerebral mucormycosis and fulminant aspergillus sinusitis among patients with haematological malignancies, haematopoietic stem cell transplant recipients and individuals with diabetes mellitus. Other contributing factors include the use of corticosteroids and desferrioxamine and human immunodeficiency virus

(HIV) infection. In immunocompromised persons, acute invasive fungal sinusitis presents with fever, unilateral facial swelling, unilateral headache, nasal obstruction or pain, and a serosanguineous nasal discharge. Necrotic black lesions on the hard palate or nasal turbinate are a characteristic diagnostic sign. As the infection spreads into the orbit, periorbital or perinasal swelling occurs and progresses to disfiguring destruction of facial tissue. Ptosis, proptosis, ophthalmoplegia and loss of vision can occur.

The drug of choice in the immunocompromised or diabetic patient with acute invasive sinusitis is amphotericin B (at a dose of 1.0–1.5 mg/kg per day). If the disease fails to respond to the conventional formulation of amphotericin B, treatment should be changed to one of the lipid-based formulations of the drug at doses of 3–5 mg/kg or higher. This should be continued until the patient recovers, or for at least 2 weeks before reverting to conventional amphotericin B. Administration of lipid-based amphotericin B is also recommended for patients in whom the conventional formulation is contraindicated because of renal impairment and in those who develop side effects that would otherwise necessitate discontinuation of the drug.

Fungal sinusitis should be suspected when calcified foci are noted in an opaque sinus CT. This sign may be seen in 76 per cent of patients with aspergillosis of the paranasal sinuses.[12] These densities are attributed to calcium phosphate and calcium sulphate. In addition to calcium salts, there are considerably high levels of ferromagnetic elements such as iron, magnesium and manganese. These ferromagnetic elements are part of fungal metabolism and are thought to be responsible for the low signal intensities on MRI[13] (Figs 13.4 and 13.5E, F). Hence, a completely opaque sinus on CT may appear signal void on MRI, giving the impression of a normal air-filled sinus (Fig. 13.5F).

MUCOCOELE

A mucocoele is a closed sac lined by respiratory epithelium that forms a cavity lining in continuity. It most frequently involves the fronto-ethmoid region yet can also affect the sphenoid or posterior ethmoid sinuses. A mucocoele cavity has no drainage pathway so its secretions accumulate, raising the pressure, which gradually increases its size and it then exerts pressure on its surroundings. Expansion symptoms in the sphenoethmoid region can include discomfort, nasal obstruction, optic nerve compression and visual loss, third, fourth and sixth cranial nerve palsies, pituitary dysfunction and symptoms of increased intracranial pressure.[14] Endoscopic examination in a patient with sphenoid mucocoele may appear normal or may reveal expansion in the SER. Rarely, a nasal mass covered by smooth mucosa may be seen.

The diagnostic modalities of choice are CT and MRI; CT characteristics include expansion and bony resorption

of the involved sinus (Figs 13.7 and 13.8A), and MRI provides more information about the secretions contained within and the surrounding soft tissue involvement (Figs 13.8B and 13.9). The MRI findings vary depending on the protein content of the secretions within the mucocoele. Sinonasal secretions normally consist of 95 per cent water and 5 per cent solute. Virtually all the solids are macromolecular proteins. On MRI, sinonasal secretions usually show low signals on T1-weighted images and high signals on T2-weighted images. When a sinus is obstructed, water is reabsorbed with an increase in protein concentration. As the protein content rises from 5 per cent to about 25 per cent, both T1 and T2 relaxation times shorten resulting in high signals on T1-weighted images (Figs 13.8B and 13.9A) and relatively low signals on T2-weighted images (Fig. 13.9B). At 25–30 per cent protein content, there is cross-linking of protein molecules, giving rise to a solution of viscid consistency. With protein content between 35 per cent and 40 per cent, semisolid protein is formed, resulting in very low signals in T1 and T2-weighted images.

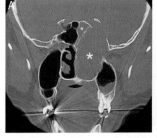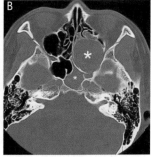

Figure 13.7   (A, B) Coronal and axial computed tomography (CT) scans showing a large mucocoele of the posterior ethmoid cells (large asterisk) causing decalcification of the surrounding bone. The opacification of the sphenoid sinus (small asterisk) is due to retained secretions as a result of obstruction of the sphenoid ostium.

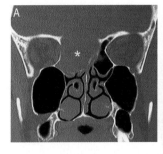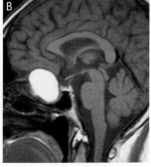

Figure 13.8   (A) Coronal computed tomography (CT) scan of a patient with a mucocoele of the right posterior ethmoid cells (asterisk). Note the skull base is almost completely eroded as a result of the expansile effect. (B) T1-weighted sagittal MR image of the patient in Figure 13.8A.

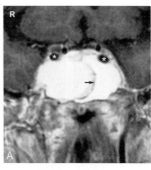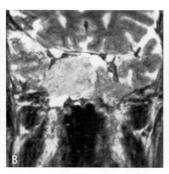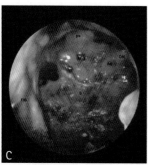

Figure 13.9   (A) T1-weighted magnetic resonance (MR) image in a patient who presented with sudden blindness of the right eye, showing a large mucocoele with bilateral sphenoid involvement. The arrow is pointing to the intersinus septum and the asterisks to the location of the cavernous carotid arteries. (B) T2-weighted MR image of the same patient as in Figure 13.9A. (C) Endoscopic view through the left nose showing a wide midline sphenoidotomy carried out in the patient in Figure 13.9A, B. Thick inspissated secretions were removed and the right optic nerve decompressed. The patient's vision recovered postoperatively. Structures that can be identified in the above figure are the posterior nasal septum (ns), planum sphenoidale (ps), sella turcica (s), the left optic nerve (on) and the left cavernous carotid artery (ca).

The management of mucocoeles is endoscopic wide marsupialization (Fig. 13.9C). The prognosis is excellent with low recurrence rates.

SPHENOETHMOIDAL RECESS POLYPS

Polyps in the SER are rare and arise from a variety of anatomical sites. Although most arise from the sphenoid sinus it is important to keep in mind adjacent sites as the possible origin of such polyps (Fig. 13.10). Often inflammatory in nature, these polyps may sometimes signify existing pathology within the sphenoid sinus.[15] We have reported a case of giant aneurysm arising from the petrous part of the internal carotid artery that presented as a polyp in the SER.[16]

TUMOURS AND TUMOUR-LIKE LESIONS

Primary benign lesions

Benign tumours or tumour-like lesions of the sphenoid sinus are uncommon. All forms of bone tumours such as osteomas and giant cell tumours are rarely encountered in the sphenoid sinus. In contrast, fibrous dysplasia is relatively more common. Fibrous dysplasia usually affects several bones of the cranium but is noted to affect the sphenoid sinus predominantly. The sphenoid sinus may be completely obliterated by fibro-osseous tissue (Fig. 13.11). Benign soft tissue tumours including adenomas and papillomas are also uncommon. These lesions show non-specific features and the diagnosis is based on endoscopic evaluation and confirmation after biopsy. Inverted papillomas are usually found arising from the lateral nasal wall but they may originate in the sphenoid sinus[17] (Fig. 13.12). The senior author has treated four patients with inverting papilloma arising within the sphenoid sinus. Infiltrative pituitary tumours arising within the sella, the sphenoid sinus, clival tumours or lesions from the petrous

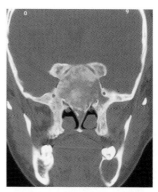

Figure 13.11   Coronal computed tomography (CT) scan of sphenoid sinus showing the classical 'ground glass' appearance in a patient with fibrous dysplasia.

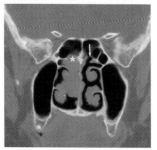

Figure 13.10   Coronal computed tomography (CT) scan of a patient with a right spheno-choanal polyp. The origin of the polyp as identified on the scan is from the mucosa of the right sphenoid ostium (asterisk). The arrow indicates the left sphenoid ostium.

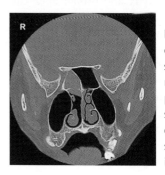

Figure 13.12   Coronal computed tomography (CT) scan of an 80-year-old man who presented with a polypoid lesion in the right sphenoethmoid recess. Biopsy of the lesion following the CT study showed this to be an inverting papilloma.

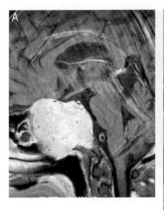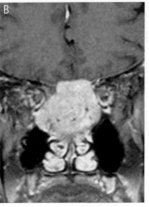

Figure 13.13 (A, B) Sagittal and coronal T1-weighted magnetic resonance (MR) image with contrast showing an enhancing mass occupying the entire sphenoid sinus. Biopsy of this mass proved this to be a non-secretory pituitary adenoma.

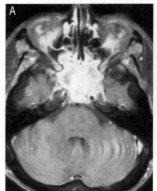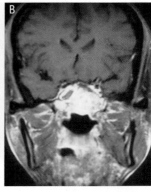

Figure 13.14 (A, B) Axial and coronal T1-weighted magnetic resonance (MR) image with contrast showing an enhancing mass within the sphenoid sinus in a young Chinese man. Biopsy showed this was an undifferentiated carcinoma consistent with nasopharyngeal carcinoma.

apex may present with a mass lesion within the sphenoid sinus (Fig. 13.13). In some cases, the tumour may prolapse through the sphenoid sinus ostium or erode the anterior sphenoid wall and present as a polypoid mass in the SER.

Primary malignant lesions

Primary tumours of the sphenoid sinus are rare. They are usually epithelial in origin such as squamous cell carcinoma arising in inverted papilloma, adenocarcinoma, squamous cell carcinoma or anaplastic carcinoma. Tumours in the sphenoid sinus are best assessed with MRI, as suprasellar extension or infiltration of the cavernous sinus can be readily and accurately mapped. Tumours of the salivary glands may also be found in the paranasal sinuses. These tumours include mucoepidermoid carcinoma and adenocystic carcinoma.

Extension of pathology to the sphenoid sinus

NASOPHARYNGEAL CARCINOMA

In contrast to primary tumours of the sphenoid sinus, secondary involvement of the sphenoid sinus by tumours of the surrounding region is relatively more common. Both benign and malignant tumours originating in the sella, skull base, the nasopharynx and orbital apex can extend into the sphenoid sinus. The most common tumour in the nasopharynx to involve the sphenoid sinus is nasopharyngeal carcinoma (NPC). The floor of the sphenoid sinus forms the roof of the nasopharynx and as such is commonly involved in NPC (Fig. 13.14). From the sphenoid sinus, the tumour may subsequently spread intracranially by direct suprasellar extension or by breaching the lateral sinus walls into the cavernous sinus. It is, therefore, not uncommon for these patients to have associated palsies of cranial nerves III, IV and VI.

CHORDOMA

Chordoma is a skull base tumour thought to arise from the remnants of the notochord. The notochord, which passes through the clivus, terminates just inferior to the sella turcica. More than a third of chordomas originate in the clivus. Imaging usually shows both bone destruction and an associated soft tissue mass in the skull base. On CT, the tumour shows bone destruction and a gross soft tissue mass. This tumour is associated with calcification and some of the hyperattenuation foci noted on CT may be related to bone remnants as a result of tumour invasion (Fig. 13.15).

On MRI scan the signal characteristics of clival chordomas are variable. The lesion is usually hypointense on T1-weighted images but may contain areas of high signals indicating haemorrhage or low signal areas suggesting cystic degeneration or calcification. The tumour also shows variable contrast enhancement (Fig. 13.15B). A variety of lesions in the orbital apex may also extend into

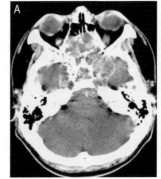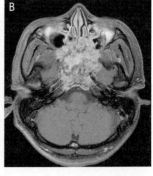

Figure 13.15 (A) Axial CT scan showing a soft tissue mass in the posterior ethmoid cells and sphenoid sinus with extensive surrounding bone destruction. (B) T1-weighted contrast enhanced axial magnetic resonance (MR) image of the patient in Figure 13.15A showing variable contrast enhancement. Biopsy of this lesion was consistent with clival chordoma.

the sphenoid sinus. These lesions include lymphomas, pseudotumours and haemangiomas. They usually have non-specific imaging findings. Imaging is crucial in the assessment of these lesions as biopsy confirmation can be obtained endoscopically.[18]

PITUITARY TUMOURS

Sellar lesions may erode the thin anterior sellar wall to invade the sphenoid sinus and present as a sphenoid lesion (Fig. 13.13). The most common pathology is a pituitary adenoma, but craniopharyngioma, pituitary malignancy and metastatic lesions to the sella may also involve the sphenoid sinus. Treatment of sellar lesions is primarily surgical with endoscopic resection becoming the standard of care in recent decades[19] (Fig. 13.16).

PLANUM SPHENOIDALE LESIONS

Meningioma, chordoma and aesthesioblastoma are the main pathologies located at this region. The tumour may encroach down on the sphenoid as well as the ethmoid sinuses or exert pressure upwards towards the parasellar structures causing symptoms similar to pituitary lesions.

CLIVUS REGION

Chordoma and metastatic disease are the most common pathologies in this area although other rare conditions such as lymphoma and osteomyelitis can also occur. The tumour can exert pressure either backwards on the brainstem or upwards on the sphenoid and sella.

TEMPORAL BONE APEX

Cholesterol granuloma as well as temporal bone osteomyelitis can expand medially to involve the sphenoid sinus. While treatment for cholesterol granuloma is endoscopic marsupialization, osteomyelitis is treated conservatively with long-term antibiotic therapy.

SURGICAL APPROACH TO THE POSTERIOR ETHMOIDS AND SPHENOID SINUS

Since the introduction of endoscopic sinus surgery in the mid-1980s, the endoscopic approach to the PEC and the sphenoid sinus has become increasingly popular. The illumination and magnification provided by the endoscopes remains unparalleled. The ability to visualize the sinuses with angled endoscopes enables a more complete intraoperative examination and extirpation of the disease. Whereas the advantages of endoscopic approach to the PEC and sphenoid sinus are clear, it is not without danger. Anatomical proximity of this region to the orbital apex, optic nerve and the carotid artery puts these structures at surgical risk. Inadequate understanding of the anatomy, improper instrumentation and overzealous

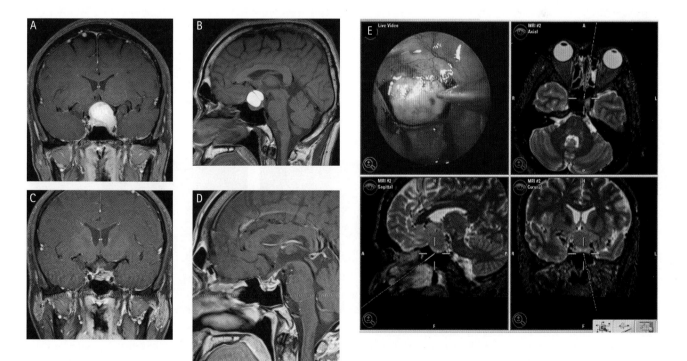

Figure 13.16   (A, B) T1-weighted contrast enhanced coronal and sagittal magnetic resonance (MR) images in a patient with bitemporal hemianopia showing a pituitary tumour. (C, D) Postoperative T1-weighted (with contrast) MR images showing the tumour has been completely removed. (E) Intraoperative images of the patient undergoing endoscopic removal of the pituitary tumour using image-guided navigation.

use of powered instrumentation in this region may lead to serious complications such as orbital haematoma, optic nerve injury and trauma to the cavernous sinus and the carotid artery.

General considerations

Preoperative imaging studies for sphenoethmoid pathology include CT and MRI. Computed tomography helps delineate the bony boundaries of the lesion and plan the surgical approach while MRI provides information regarding involvement of the optic nerve, orbital content and intracranial structures in the parasellar area. The latter is also indicated if there is bony erosion or intracranial extension of the pathology is suspected. Magnetic resonance angiography (MRA) and carotid artery angiography may be indicated in selected cases. If available the use of image-guided system (IGS) navigation is encouraged, for the surgeon not to operate by but to confirm their position.

It is important to understand and map out the relationship of the posterior ethmoid with the sphenoid sinus; in particular, the presence or absence of a sphenoethmoid cell should be clearly documented and considered in planning the endoscopic approach. Depending on whether the pathology is isolated (either in the posterior ethmoid or the sphenoid sinus) or involves both sinuses, the appropriate endoscopic approach is selected.

Endoscopic approach to the posterior ethmoid complex

Exposure of the posterior ethmoid complex is a direct extension of an anterior ethmoidectomy. Following the resection of the uncinate process and bulla ethmoidalis,

the lamina papyracea and basal lamella of the middle turbinate are identified.

The basal lamella is perforated to enter the posterior ethmoid cells. The exact location where the basal lamella is perforated is critical, not only to avoid skull base injury but also to retain the posterior third of the middle turbinate to ensure its postoperative stability. An imaginary line is drawn from the roof of the maxillary sinus to the middle turbinate. The basal lamella is perforated at the point where this line meets the middle turbinate (Fig. 13.17A).

The opening in the basal lamella is enlarged inferiorly to identify the free anterior margin of the superior turbinate, which forms the medial boundary of the posterior ethmoid cells (Fig. 13.17B). The inferior and lateral aspect of the basal lamella is removed to the extent necessary to expose and delineate the inferior aspect of the superior turbinate and its insertion onto the lateral nasal wall. The sphenoid ostium is located medial to the superior turbinate in the SER. The PEC are lateral to the superior turbinate (Fig. 13.17C).

All ethmoid cells posterior to the basal lamella are systematically removed while identifying the lamina laterally, the middle turbinate and the superior turbinate medially, and the skull base superiorly. The posterior third of the middle turbinate is retained in order to preserve middle turbinate stability.

The transition from the posterior ethmoid cells into the sphenoid sinus requires a clear understanding. It is extremely important for the surgeon to remember that the sphenoid sinus is located inferior and medial to the most posterior cell of the PEC and does not lie directly posterior to it. As mentioned earlier in this chapter, this relationship is particularly important when a sphenoethmoid cell is present. In the presence of a large sphenoethmoid cell, the optic nerve and the cavernous carotid artery may be in direct relationship with the PEC. Bleeding, mucosal oedema,

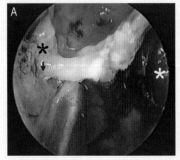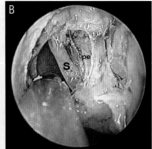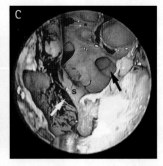

Figure 13.17   (A) Endoscopic view of the basal lamella. The ethmoid bulla has been removed and a wide middle meatal antrostomy created (white asterisk). The black asterisk shows the location where the basal lamella will be perforated and the arrow shows the direction in which the opening will be widened to identify the superior turbinate. (B) The opening in the basal lamella has been widened inferiorly and medially to identify the superior turbinate (s). The posterior ethmoid cells (pe) are lateral to the superior turbinate and the sphenoethmoid recess medial to it. (C) The inferior third of the superior turbinate (s) has been partially removed to expose the sphenoid ostium (white arrow). The posterior ethmoid cells have been opened and the optic nerve (black arrow) and the posterior ethmoid neurovascular bundle (asterisk) identified.

polyps and other sinus pathology can obscure the surgical field leading to difficulty in intraoperative identification of these structures and making them susceptible to surgical trauma. It is therefore, extremely important to identify the sphenoethmoid cell on preoperative CT study and plan the entry into the sphenoid sinus.

Endoscopic approach to sphenoid sinus

The sphenoid sinus may be approached in many ways. The selection of the most appropriate approach depends on the location and extent of the pathology and the presence or absence of a sphenoethmoid cell with or without pathology.

TRANSETHMOID APPROACH

This is the approach of choice when pathology involves both the posterior ethmoids and the sphenoid. In this approach the anterior wall of the sphenoid sinus is perforated to gain entry into the sphenoid sinus. To ensure a safe entry to the sinus, it is important to determine the orientation of the anterior sphenoid sinus wall, which varies depending on the presence or absence of a sphenoethmoid cell. Following a posterior ethmoidectomy, as described above, the following four structures are identified:

- the lamina papyracea laterally
- skull base superiorly
- superior turbinate medially
- horizontal portion of the middle turbinate inferiorly.

These structures form a 'rectangular box'-like relationship and orientation to each other. The anterior wall of the sphenoid sinus is at the back of this box. It is important to remember that the plane and orientation of the anterior sphenoid wall vary, depending on the presence or absence of a sphenoethmoid cell. When a sphenoethmoid cell is present, the anterior sphenoid wall is displaced from a more coronal to an oblique orientation. In fact, in an extensive sphenoethmoid cell formation the anterior sphenoid wall may be oriented in an almost horizontal plane. In such a configuration, it is best to identify the sphenoid ostium in the SER and extend the sphenoid ostium to create a sphenoidotomy.

In the absence of a sphenoethmoid cell, the 'rectangular box' may provide a guide to a transethmoid sphenoidotomy. A line connecting the superior medial corner and the inferior lateral corner divides the box into superolateral and inferomedial triangles. Perforation of the anterior sphenoid wall, in the inferomedial triangle, provides safe entry into the sphenoid sinus. The superolateral triangle contains the optic nerve and the carotid artery, and overzealous instrumentation in this area should be avoided (Fig. 13.18).

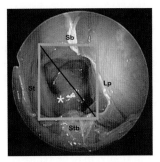

Figure 13.18   Endoscopic view of the posterior ethmoid boundaries (in a cadaver dissection) showing the 'box-like configuration'. The four sides of the box are the lamina papyracea (Lp) laterally, the skull base (Sb) superiorly, the superior turbinate (St) medially and the lamella of the middle turbinate inferiorly. The box is divided into a superolateral triangle and an inferomedial triangle by a line (black line) drawn from the superomedial angle of the box to the inferolateral angle. To make a transethmoid entry into the sphenoid sinus it is safer to enter it by creating an opening in the inferomedial triangle (asterisk). The superolateral triangle is closely related to the skull base and the optic nerve.

DIRECT ENDONASAL APPROACH

The sphenoid sinus can be directly approached through its natural ostium if the disease process involves the sphenoid exclusively. The sphenoid ostium is identified in the SER and widened (sphenoidotomy) to address the pathology within. The maxillary and ethmoid sinuses are not addressed and dissection is carried out medial to the middle turbinate. Depending on the extent of the pathology, the sphenoidotomy may be unilateral or bilateral.

Unilateral sphenoidotomy

Retracting the posterior inferior part of the middle turbinate laterally, the superior turbinate is identified. The natural sphenoid ostium is located behind its inferior third, in the SER, about 15 mm superior to the superior arch of the posterior choana. In the presence of sphenoid pathology, the sphenoid ostium may be obscured by mucosal oedema and may not be readily identified. In such a situation, probing the SER gently with a seeker or a 7-size suction may assist in its identification. In the presence of extensive mucosal oedema, the use of a microdebrider to remove the oedematous mucosa may help in the localization of the sphenoid ostium. Once identified, the opening is then enlarged (sphenoidotomy) and the sphenoid sinus entered.

The size of the sphenoidotomy will be determined by the type and extent of the pathology (Fig. 13.3B–D). Resection of the superior turbinate is not necessary in most cases. However, if required, the inferior third of the superior turbinate may be removed with nasal scissors or through-cutting forceps. This allows for extension of the sphenoidotomy laterally. In extending the sphenoidotomy inferiorly, it must be remembered that the posterior division of the sphenopalatine artery runs across the medial wall of the sphenoid sinus, from a lateral to medial direction. The direct endonasal approach is ideal for isolated sphenoid pathology such as chronic sinusitis, mucocoeles or fungal disease (Figs 13.4C, D and 13.9C).

Bilateral sphenoidotomy

In the presence of bilateral sphenoid pathology, bilateral sphenoidotomy, as described above, is indicated. The intersinus septum, if any, may be removed to convert the sphenoid sinus into a single cavity. No attempt should be made to remove the accessory septations as these may insert onto the optic nerve or the carotid artery.

The above described approaches will suffice in most cases of sphenoid pathology. In endoscopic transsphenoidal approach to the sella and the surrounding region, a wider access to the sphenoid sinus is necessary for adequate instrumentation allowing the 'four handed' technique.

Midline wide sphenoidotomy

The bilateral sphenoidotomies are connected in the midline by removing about 1 cm of the posterior nasal septum to create an opening that extends superiorly to the roof of the sphenoid, inferiorly to the floor of the sphenoid sinus and laterally to the superior turbinate on either side. This wide sphenoidotomy permits a panoramic view of the sphenoid sinus and is often used for access to the sella turcica, clivus and the petrous apex (Fig. 13.19). Removal of the posterior nasal septum facilitates the introduction of instruments from both nostrils and enables two surgeons to work together using both hands. This allows introduction of up to four separate instruments, two through each nostril. For a wider access, necessary in some patients with

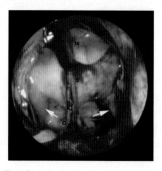

Figure 13.19 This figure shows the endoscopic approach to the sella turcica for pituitary surgery. The anterior wall of the sphenoid sinus has been removed on both sides. The superior turbinates on either sides form the lateral boundaries of the sphenoid opening, which extends superiorly to the planum sphenoidale and inferiorly to the floor of the sphenoid. About 1 cm of the posterior nasal septum is removed to enable unimpeded instrumentation from both sides. The wide opening provides excellent access to the sella (s), tuberculum sella (ts) and clivus (c) and allows two surgeons to work together to perform surgery beyond the sphenoid sinus. The approach is totally endoscopic and is referred to as the 'bimanual endoscopic technique'.

large tumours requiring an extended approach, the entire posterior bony nasal septum may be removed to facilitate instrumentation.

Sphenoid marsupialisation

In this procedure the floor of the sphenoid sinus, which is a common wall with the roof of the nasopharynx, is endoscopically removed and a flap of nasopharyngeal wall mucosa is placed within the sinus. This eliminates the sinus floor, partially obliterates the sinus cavity, diminishes the sinus size and opens it completely allowing it to drain freely into the nasopharynx.[20]

TRANSPTERYGOID APPROACH

A lateral recess of the sphenoid sinus (LSR) is often seen in an extensively pneumatized sphenoid sinus. The LSR, lateral to the vidian and maxillary division of the trigeminal nerves and posterosuperior to the pterygoid process, is sometimes the site of pathology such as cerebrospinal fluid (CSF) leaks and tumours. Access to this aerated pouch through the sphenoid sinus is difficult and merits a more aggressive transpterygoid approach, which involves exposure of the pterygopalatine fossa (PPF) and lateral displacement of the PPF contents. Removal of the medial pterygoid plate, which forms the posterior wall of the PPF, enables better exposure of the LSR. A complete ethmoidectomy is performed followed by a sphenoidotomy. The middle meatal antrostomy is widened posteriorly as far as the posterior wall of the maxillary sinus. The sphenopalatine foramen (SPF) is next identified at the point of entry into the nasal cavity. The sphenopalatine artery is identified and clipped. The anterior lip of the SPF is removed with a 1 mm Kerrison punch and extended laterally to remove the posterior wall of the maxillary sinus to expose the periosteum of the PPF. The contents of the PPF are retracted laterally, exposing the posterior wall of the PPF, which is formed by the medial pterygoid plate. The medial pterygoid plate is removed while preserving the vidian and trigeminal nerves until the entire lateral recess can be visualized using a 0° endoscope and instrument manipulation inside the recess is enabled. Particular care is taken in the region of the lateral sphenoid wall, since the carotid artery and the cavernous sinus are right next to it.

This approach is ideal for encephalocoeles located very laterally in the LSR (Fig. 13.20). Of the eight cases of encephalocoeles in the LSR successfully repaired by the senior author, four had failed a subfrontal approach to repair the encephalocoele and the skull base defect.[21]

TRANSSEPTAL APPROACH

The transseptal approach to the sphenoid sinus was traditionally used to approach the sella in the microscopic era. It provides a safe midline approach to the sphenoid

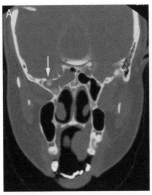
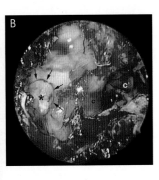

Figure 13.20   (A) Computed tomography (CT) cisternogram showing a defect in the right lateral recess of the sphenoid sinus in a patient with a cerebrospinal fluid leak following a road traffic accident. The patient had undergone two unsuccessful repairs of the defect, which included a craniotomy and an endoscopic approach. (B) Intraoperative endoscopic view of the transpterygoid approach to the right lateral recess of the sphenoid sinus showing the encephalocoele (asterisk) and the skull base defect (arrows). Other structures identified are the right cavernous carotid artery (black c), sella (s) and the clivus (white C). A three-layer repair of the defect led to a successful outcome.

sinus. The technique involves a hemitransfixion incision, elevation of a mucoperichondrial flap on the side of the incision, identification of the bony cartilaginous junction, dislocation of cartilage from the bony nasal septum and elevation of mucoperiosteal flaps on both sides of the bony nasal septum as far back as the sphenoid keel to identify the sphenoid ostia on both sides. The bony posterior nasal septum is removed exposing the sphenoid keel in the midline. The anterior wall of the sphenoid sinus is removed by widening the sphenoid ostia inferior and medially and superiorly and medially. The approach provides excellent access to the sphenoid sinus in the midline and has been used not only to deal with sphenoid pathology but also for access to the sella turcica.[22]

When used for pituitary surgery, the transseptal approach has the disadvantage that two surgeons are trying to work through a narrow tunnel created by the mucoperiosteal flaps. The wide sphenoidotomy approach, described above, is preferred for pituitary surgery.

COMPLICATIONS

Complications of endoscopic surgery of the posterior ethmoid cells and sphenoid surgery include CSF leak, bleeding and orbital injury. The sinus anatomy, adjacent structures, disease entity and the specific approach used determine the potential complications. Preoperative evaluation of imaging studies with special attention to anatomical variants may assist in anticipating and avoiding complications.

Bleeding associated with sphenoid surgery is usually due to mucosal trauma or injury to the posterior septal branch of the sphenopalatine artery, which may occur if the sphenoidotomy is extended inferiorly. Carotid artery injury is potentially fatal but fortunately rare. Management of carotid artery injury is outside the scope of this chapter but it is advised that all surgeons performing sphenoid surgery should have a plan in place should this complication occur. Ophthalmic complications can result from injury to the optic nerve, globe or extraocular muscles leading to blindness, ophthalmoplegia and diplopia (Fig. 13.21).

A CSF leak during transethmoid sphenoid surgery may result from injury to the skull base. If recognized intraoperatively, repair must be accomplished at primary surgery. Undiagnosed CSF leaks may lead to meningitis and intracranial abscess (Fig. 13.22).

Septal perforation may occur particularly with the transseptal approach. Numbness of the upper lip, teeth and cheeks may result from injury to the second branch of the trigeminal nerve particularly during transpterygoid access to the LSR.

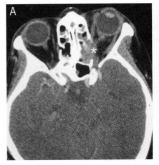
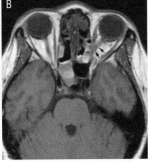

Figure 13.21   (A) Axial computed tomography (CT) scan of a patient who woke up blind in the right eye following endoscopic sinus surgery. The scan shows a breach of the posterior part of the lamina papyracea (asterisk) and the orbital apex.
(B) T1-weighted (with contrast) axial magnetic resonance (MR) image showing complete truncation of the optic nerve (arrows) of the patient in Figure 13.21A.

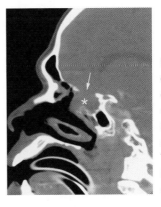

Figure 13.22   Sagittal computed tomography (CT) scan of a patient who underwent endoscopic sinus surgery 8 years prior to his current admission for meningitis. The scan shows a large skull base defect (arrow) with an encephalocoele (asterisk).

REFERENCES

1. Sethi DS, Stanley RE. Endoscopic anatomy of the sphenoid sinus and sella turcica. *J Laryngol Otol* 1995; **109**: 951–5.

2. Jho HD, Ha HG. Endoscopic endonasal skull base surgery. Part 1 – The midline anterior fossa skull base. *Minim Invasive Neurosurg* 2004; **47**: 1–8.

3. Renn WH, Rhoton AL Jr. Microsurgical anatomy of the sellar region. *J Neurosurg* 1975; **43**: 288–98.

4. Fujii K, Chambers SM, Rhoton AL Jr. Neurovascular relationship of the sphenoid sinus – A microsurgical study. *J Neurosurg* 1979; **50**: 31–9.

5. Sethi DS. Isolated sphenoid lesions: diagnosis and management. *Otolaryngol Head Neck Surg* 1999; **120**: 730–6.

6. Kupferberg SB, Bent JP, Kuhn FA. The prognosis of allergic fungal sinusitis. *Otolaryngol Head Neck Surg* 1997; **117**: 35–41.

7. Kuhn FA, Javer AR. Allergic fungal sinusitis: a four year follow-up. *Am J Rhinol* 2000; **14**: 149–56.

8. Schubert MS. Allergic fungal sinusitis. *Otolaryngol Clin North Am* 2004; **37**: 301–26.

9. de Carpentier JP, Ramamurthy L, Denning DW *et al.* An algorithmic approach to aspergillus sinusitis. *J Laryngol Otol* 1994; **108**: 314–18.

10. Clancy CJ, Nguyen MH. Invasive sinus aspergillosis in apparently immunocompetent hosts. *J Infect* 1998; **37**: 229–40.

11. Browning AC, Sim KT, Timms JM *et al.* Successful treatment of invasive cavernous sinus aspergillosis with oral itraconazole monotherapy. *J Neurophthalmol* 2006; **26**: 103–6.

12. Zinreich SJ, Kennedy DW, Malat J *et al.* Fungal sinusitis: Diagnosis with CT and MR imaging. *Radiology* 1988; **169**: 439–44.

13. Som PM, Dillon WP, Curtin HD *et al.* Hypointense paranasal sinus foci: Differential diagnosis with MR imaging and relation to CT findings. *Radiology* 1990; **176**: 777–81.

14. Sethi DS, Lau DPC, Chan C. Sphenoid sinus mucocele presenting with isolated oculomotor nerve palsy. *J Laryngol Otol* 1997; **111**: 471–3.

15. Sethi DS, Lau DPC, Lincoln WJ *et al.* Isolated sphenoethmoid recess polyps. *J Laryngol Otol* 1998; **112**: 660–3.

16. Singh H, Thomas J, Hoe WLE *et al.* Giant petrous carotid aneurysm: persistent epistaxis despite internal carotid artery ligation. *J Laryngol Otol* 2008; e18. Epub 13 June 2008.

17. Peters BW, O'Reilly RC, Wilcox TO *et al.* Inverted papilloma isolated to the sphenoid sinus. *Otolaryngol Head Neck Surg* 1995; **113**: 771–8.

18. Sethi DS, Lau DPC. Endoscopic management of orbital apex lesions. *Am J Rhinol* 1997; **11**: 449–55.

19. Sethi DS, Leong JL. Endoscopic pituitary surgery. *Otolaryngol Clin North Am* 2006; **39**: 563–83.

20. Donald P. Radical sphenoidectomy with nasopharyngeal flap. *Oper Tech Otolaryngol Head Neck Surg* 2003; **14**: 195–8.

21. Forer B, Sethi DS. Endoscopic repair of CSF leaks in the lateral sphenoid sinus recess. *J Neurosurg* (in press).

22. Sethi DS, Pillay PK. Endoscopic surgery for pituitary tumors. *Oper Tech Otolaryngol Head Neck Surg* 1996; **7**: 264–8.

14

Management of recalcitrant sinusitis, including allergic fungal sinusitis and Samter's triad

MARC A TEWFIK, ERIK K WEITZEL, PETER-JOHN WORMALD

INTRODUCTION

The management of polypoid chronic rhinosinusitis (CRS) can be extremely challenging, even for the experienced rhinologist. This is particularly true for severe recalcitrant CRS, which has not responded to an initial functional endoscopic sinus surgery (FESS). With possible contributions from factors such as allergy, ciliary dysmotility and microbial agents, the underlying pathogenesis may be quite distinct from patient to patient. Other variables include differences in patterns of tissue trauma and repair – in instances when endoscopic sinus surgery is attempted – and the situation becomes further complicated. However, what has become clearer in the recent literature is that patients with severe disease appear to be symptomatically better for longer periods following more aggressive surgery. The present chapter seeks to review the management of these challenging patients, with an emphasis on surgical techniques, by discussing the evidence and rationale for performing more extensive surgery.

EVIDENCE FOR PERFORMING MORE EXTENSIVE SINUS SURGERY

The principle that extensive sinus surgery is best for patients with severe mucosal disease is illustrated in patients with eosinophilic mucus CRS, where simply creating a wide antrostomy is not sufficient to treat severe maxillary sinus disease. Leaving polyps and eosinophilic mucus within the sinus contributes to a rapid recurrence of disease.[1] This may be due to ongoing exposure to fungus within the mucus,

or toxic substances such as major basic protein released by the eosinophils. Polyps and thick tenacious mucus in the sinuses therefore require thorough and complete removal. The senior author was able to show, in a study of patients with severely diseased maxillary sinuses, that those who underwent canine fossa trephination and clearance of the sinuses had significantly improved long-term outcomes with regard to disease recurrence and symptom scores as compared with patients who underwent maxillary clearance by transmaxillary ostial methods alone.[1]

Other well-conducted studies build a strong argument suggesting that more extensive FESS leads to significantly better outcomes in terms of ethmoidectomy as well as frontal sinus surgeries. Jankowski et al. carefully documented and evaluated the efficacy of two surgical techniques for similar disease states of severe nasal polyposis.[2] One technique involved a more targeted functional approach to performing ethmoidectomy, and the other a more radical 'nasalization' or complete FESS, with removal of all bony lamellae and mucosa within the labyrinth. Significantly better outcomes were noted with the more radical FESS in terms of recurrence rate, need for revision surgery, endoscopic examination, radiological outcomes, and functional benefit (specifically in nasal obstruction, anterior and posterior rhinorrhoea, although olfaction showed no difference).[2]

Several studies have shown a clear benefit from dissection of the frontal recess in polypoid CRS patients. Hosemann et al. retrospectively evaluated their outcomes of complete FESS with frontal recess clearance in 110 patients with CRS.[3] Overall 70 per cent of patients reported a significant improvement in their symptoms. By carefully analysing their failures, they found that the frontal ostium stenosis rate was affected by the extent of ostial enlargement and the severity of the underlying disease. Frontal ostia enlarged to a minimum dimension of 5 mm or greater became obstructed in 16 per cent of cases, compared with obstruction in 30 per cent of cases where the ostium was less than 5 mm. Following this trend, the authors found that with a minimum dimension of 2 mm, 50 per cent of frontal ostia went on to complete stenosis. They additionally found that patients with Samter's triad and pronounced polyposis showed a trend towards a higher rate of ostial stenosis. These authors concluded that a greater postoperative frontal ostium size leads to better long-term outcomes.

A retrospective study by Weber *et al.* further supports the notion that a larger frontal sinus ostium provides a better outcome.[4] This group analysed 1286 patients undergoing frontal sinus surgery, including Draf I, II and III procedures. They found that there was progressive improvement in the rate of subjective and objective outcomes as the surgeries become more extensive. The best results were seen with Draf III operations (equivalent to the modified endoscopic Lothrop [MEL] procedure or frontal drill-out) irrespective of poor prognostic status.[4]

A retrospective review of our practice aimed to evaluate the outcomes of different frontal surgical approaches for polypoid CRS patients (unpublished data). Our surgical algorithm involves a staged and progressive approach moving initially from a frontal recess clearance to the MEL procedure in recalcitrant cases. We found two major factors that identified patients who were likely to require revision surgery: the presence of fungus in the sinuses and aspirin (acetyl-salicylic acid [ASA]) sensitivity. Patients with fungal disease include those with allergic fungal sinusitis (AFRS) and non-allergic fungal sinusitis.[5] In our series, fungus was nearly four times more prevalent in patients requiring revision surgery than in those who did not require revision surgery. In addition, ASA sensitivity was over five times more common in patients with recurrent disease than in favourable responders to primary FESS. Patients who underwent the MEL procedure had a lower rate of recurrent polyposis requiring surgery, as well as a significantly longer symptom-free period than those who underwent revision FESS. When Samter's triad patients were analysed, the mean postoperative Lund–Kennedy endoscopy scores at 6 months in aspirin-sensitive patients were nearly twice those of patients not sensitive to aspirin. This study complements previous findings that the presence of eosinophilic mucus, a marker of severe inflammation, is associated with extensive sinus disease and a more recalcitrant clinical course compared with patients who do not have eosinophilic mucus in their sinuses.[5,6] The revision rate for the MEL procedure over a 5-year period has been 12 per cent and all of these cases have responded to revision MEL.

The success of the MEL procedure is most likely due to two main factors; the maintenance of physiological mucociliary clearance and the large size of the frontal sinus neo-ostium. Mucociliary clearance is largely unaffected following a MEL procedure because the lateral and posterior portions of the frontal ostium where the normal pattern of mucociliary clearance occurs remain intact.[4,7] Hence, following a MEL procedure, mucosal secretions formed in the frontal sinuses move from the superior aspect of the frontal sinus laterally and then pass through the neo-ostium onto the ostiomeatal complex and common drainage pathway (Fig. 14.1).

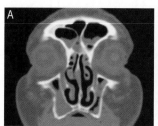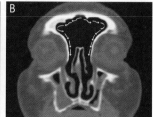

Figure 14.1   (A) Unoperated frontal sinus demonstrating mucosal disease. (B) After frontal drill-out, the direction of mucociliary flow (arrows) remains similar to the normal preoperative condition.

The maximum diameter of the neo-ostium may be the most important factor in the success of the MEL procedure, even in the group with a poor surgical prognosis. Following a frontal recess clearance, recurrent disease is first seen in the region of the frontal sinus ostium. Despite full clearance, the region of the frontal recess is still relatively narrow and predisposes to early obstruction. This is manifested initially by oedema followed by mucosal cobblestoning and culminating in polyp formation. Although the exact pathogenesis is not understood, it is conceivable that the obstruction may be associated with colonization with bacteria and fungi and biofilm formation. A biofilm is a multicellular community of bacteria that are embedded in a self-produced exo-polysaccharide matrix and irreversibly attached to a surface. These factors may lead to an exacerbation of the mucosal inflammation by several methods that may involve secondary infection and immunological mechanisms including innate and superantigen-driven responses. The intense inflammatory response may recruit more lymphocytes and eosinophils, resulting in further epithelial injury and ineffective wound healing and remodelling.

The existence of biofilms on the sinus mucosa of patients with CRS is well described, and there is increasing evidence that biofilms affect the postoperative evolution of these patients. In a retrospective analysis by our department of 40 sinus surgical patients, bacterial biofilms were detected in 50 per cent of these.[8] This subset of patients had significantly worse preoperative radiological scores, postoperative symptoms and outcome measures. The only other factor that was statistically related to an unfavourable outcome was the presence of fungus at the time of surgery. This provides further evidence that biofilms may play an active role in perpetuating inflammation in CRS patients, and may explain the recurrent and resistant nature of this disease.

The beneficial effect of a large neo-ostium with a MEL procedure may be twofold. First, the large neo-ostium minimizes the obstruction to mucociliary drainage of the sinus caused by fluctuations in mucosal thickness. Second, the large neo-ostium allows for effective postoperative debridement and irrigation with saline and topical medications. Together, these measures may be the key to help control the inflammation and be responsible for the reduced recurrence rates seen in polyp patients following a MEL procedure.

PREOPERATIVE WORK-UP OF RECALCITRANT RHINOSINUSITIS

The preoperative assessment is discussed in detail in Chapter 5. Briefly, the work-up seeks to identify mucosal, systemic and environmental factors responsible for poor outcome. Findings specific to the maxillary sinus include the presence of accessory ostium and mucus recirculation, as identified on endoscopy, or a Haller (infraorbital) cell causing ostiomeatal obstruction. Once the decision to operate has been made, the preoperative imaging must be scrutinized carefully in order to detect high-risk situations. In patients selected to undergo revision maxillary sinus surgery, it is critically important to determine the integrity of the lamina papyracea. Recognition of this situation is of utmost importance, as the use of the microdebrider to clear disease overlying the dehiscence could result in orbital penetration with disastrous consequences. In this instance, polyps should be carefully cleared using cold steel instruments, such as through-biting Blakesley forceps.

The preoperative assessment of the frontal sinus includes:

- extent of frontal sinus and recess involvement
- size of the natural frontal ostium
- presence of osteitis and neo-osteogenesis
- anatomy of the frontal recess and cells obstructing the course of the drainage pathway
- coexisting pathology, including frontal osteoma.

MEDICAL MANAGEMENT

An adequate trial of maximal medical therapy should be given preoperatively and documented in the clinical record. This is discussed in detail in Chapter 3.

Systemic steroids may be beneficial in the preoperative period to reduce the size and vascularity of polyps in patients with significant nasal polyposis. A preliminary study found that 30 mg of prednisone administered daily for 5 days preoperatively resulted in a significantly improved surgical field grading score during endoscopic sinus surgery.[9] Empirical treatment regimens range from 30 mg to 50 mg of prednisone daily for between 5 and 7 days preoperatively. However, further studies are necessary to clarify the optimal dose of steroids, length of treatment and groups of patients who would benefit from this treatment.

SURGICAL MANAGEMENT

Goals in revision sinus surgery

The causes of recalcitrant rhinosinusitis requiring revision surgery can broadly be divided into technical factors associated with previous surgery, and recurrent sinus disease.

The technical factors associated with previous surgery are:

- retained uncinate process or persistent ethmoid cells on computed tomography (CT)
- unrepaired septal deviation or persistent Haller cell impairing maxillary sinus drainage
- missed ostium sequence with recirculation of mucus
- synechia formation causing obstruction of nasal passage or sinus outflow
- lateralization of the middle turbinate with or without adhesions between the middle turbinate and lateral nasal wall
- significantly denuded bone, with subsequent osteitis and bony hypertrophy impairing sinus outflow
- suspected mucocoele formation.

Recurrent sinus disease includes:

- recurrent nasal polyps refractory to maximal medical management
- persistent isolated sinusitis that is symptomatic
- recurrent AFRS
- concurrent nasal polyposis and an intolerance or contraindication to oral cortisone.

The surgical algorithm begins with a thorough endoscopic clearance of polyps and mucus from all affected sinuses. This includes complete dissection of all bony septations blocking the frontal recess, frontal ostium and frontal sinus, thorough clearance of the maxillary and ethmoid sinuses and creating a large sphenoidotomy. The aims of surgery are to remove polyps and mucus from the diseased sinuses, preserve mucosa and to provide an anatomically patent and functional sinus ostia and drainage pathways.

In patients who have complete opacification of the maxillary sinuses, canine fossa trephinations may also be required. This procedure has been shown to have almost no significant long-term morbidity, superior access to the anterior half of the maxillary sinus, and potential for complete debridement without mucosal stripping.[1,6,10] Preservation of the mucosal lining is critical for rapid regeneration of a functional epithelial lining and minimizing the formation of synechiae.

In patients with frontal sinus involvement, special attention is given to meticulous clearance of the frontal recess by removal of any obstructing polyps, mucus and remaining cells so that the frontal ostium and frontal sinus is visualized adequately. Polypoid CRS patients who have recurrent frontal sinus disease (Fig. 14.2) despite having a full frontal recess clearance and maximum medical treatment are offered a MEL procedure. There is little to be gained from further conservative surgery as it can be assumed that the pathological process causing ongoing nasal polyp formation is not capable of being managed with the size of the natural ostium achieved with frontal recess clearance.

Several anatomical considerations also play a role in the decision to perform a MEL procedure, which may be contemplated early in the treatment algorithm of selected patients. Patients who have extensive disease with a naturally very narrow frontal ostium will often do poorly with 'standard FESS'. When the ostium is less than 3×3 mm, obstruction occurs easily in the postoperative period[3] (Fig. 14.3). In addition, the MEL procedure may be the best option to adequately manage patients with complex frontal recess cell configurations that narrow the natural frontal ostium including an intersinus septal cell

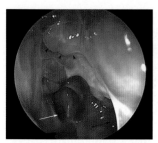

Figure 14.2   Oedema and polyp formation in the area of the frontal recess (arrowheads) after a standard functional endoscopic sinus surgery (FESS). The maxillary (black arrow) and sphenoid (white arrow) ostia are also demonstrated.

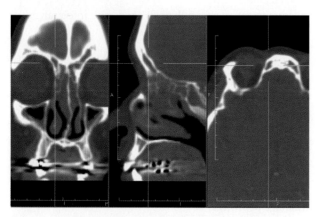

Figure 14.3   Three-dimensional computed tomography (CT) reconstruction demonstrating a very narrow frontal recess drainage pathway in a patient with small frontal sinuses; patients with such anatomical configurations tend to fair poorly after frontal recess clearance alone.

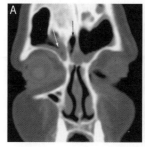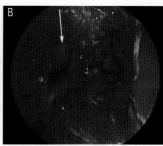

Figure 14.4   (A) Coronal computed tomography (CT) scan showing a large intersinus septal cell (black arrow) narrowing and pushing the frontal ostium laterally (white arrow). (B) Intraoperative view showing how this cell (black arrow) obstructs and narrows the right frontal ostium (white arrow).

or type 3 and type 4 frontoethmoidal cells (see Chapter 12). An example of an intersinus septal cell with a firm cell roof that could not be fractured is presented in Figure 14.4A. This will often push the ostium laterally and markedly narrow it (Fig. 14.4B). Furthermore, patients with polypoid CRS who have neo-osteogenesis in the region of the frontal ostium do very poorly and are best managed by a MEL procedure.

Revision maxillary sinus surgery including canine fossa trephination

MIDDLE MEATAL ANTROSTOMY

An antrostomy diameter of approximately 10×10 mm, created by the anterior and inferior dissection of the maxillary ostium, is usually sufficient to accurately examine the sinus with an angled scope, and to remove all the diseased material. In cases of accessory or iatrogenic sinus ostia located in the area of the posterior fontanelle (Fig. 14.5), or if the ostium has been missed in previous surgery,

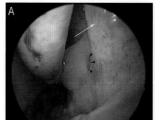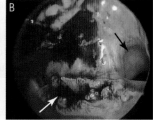

Figure 14.5   (A) Intraoperative view of an accessory ostium (arrowheads) in the posterior fontanelle of the left maxillary sinus, demonstrating mucus recirculation; note that the natural maxillary ostium is obscured by the uncinate process (white arrow). (B) Following partial uncinectomy in the same patient, view of the left natural maxillary ostium anteriorly (black arrow), as well as an accessory ostium in the posterior fontanelle (arrowheads), and cut edge of the uncinate process (white arrow), using a 30° endoscope. These ostia were subsequently joined surgically (not shown).

it is necessary to surgically join the posterior ostium to the natural maxillary sinus ostium in order to prevent the recirculation of mucus. This can be done by inserting a backbiter into the accessory ostium and dissecting forwards to the natural ostium; any excessive tissue edges can be carefully microdebrided thereafter. Enlargement of the maxillary sinus ostium into the posterior fontanelle is reserved for patients with severe disease, including extensive polyp formation within the maxillary sinus, or large amounts of thick and viscid secretion, such as fungal mucus. In such situations a wide meatal antrostomy allows copious sinus irrigation and the delivery of topical therapy.

Following an uncinectomy, it is useful to grade the extent of disease affecting the maxillary sinus at the time of surgery. This will aid in the intraoperative decision-making process. A 70° endoscope is used to visualize the maxillary sinus contents through the natural ostium, and the level of disease is graded according to Table 14.1. Grade 1 (Fig. 14.6A) and grade 2 (Fig. 14.6B) are reversible with adequate clearance of mucus and aeration of the maxillary sinus, but grade 3 disease is irreversible (Fig. 14.6C). Therefore, the polyps, and especially the thick eosinophilic mucus, should be cleared so that re-epithelialization and re-ciliation will occur.

Extensive maxillary sinus disease can be a difficult problem to tackle endoscopically, especially in the anterior and inferior regions of the antrum. In patients with extensive polyposis and/or eosinophilic mucin, mucopyocoeles and foreign material, it is essential to remove as much of the disease burden as possible to improve the resolution of symptoms. Access by way of the natural ostium of the maxillary sinus will only allow the posterior lateral wall, the posterior region of the roof, and the posterior wall of the maxillary sinus to be cleared of pus, fungal debris and polyps.

CANINE FOSSA TREPHINATION

Canine fossa trephination is now our procedure of choice for anterior approaches to the maxillary sinus. Using this

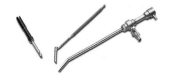

Figure 14.7   The canine fossa trephination kit (Medtronic ENT) consisting of: an endoscope sheath (right) with a protruding blade, which allows retraction of soft tissues during dissection on the anterior face of the maxilla; a re-usable drill guide (centre); and 5 mm re-usable drill bit (left) that fits the microdebrider handpiece.

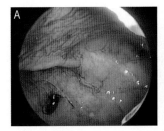 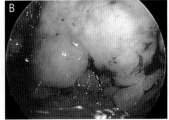 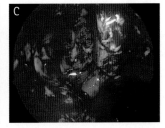

Figure 14.6   The following pictures of the right maxillary sinus were taken after a maxillary antrostomy has been performed and illustrate the grades of disease. (A) Grade 1: normal or slightly oedematous mucosa. (B) Grade 2: oedematous mucosa with small polyps, which are reversible with medical treatment, provided there is no significant eosinophilic mucus. (C) Grade 3: extensive polyps and tenacious mucus completely filling the maxillary sinus, requiring canine fossa trephination.

Table 14.1   Endoscopic grading of the diseased maxillary sinus with associated computed tomography (CT) findings and suggested management

Grade	Endoscopic findings	CT findings	Suggested surgery
1	Normal or slightly oedematous mucosa	Minimal mucosal thickening and ostiomeatal complex obstruction	Uncinectomy alone with visualization of the natural ostium
2	Oedematous mucosa with small polyps, without significant eosinophilic mucus	Moderate mucosal oedema and/or opacification (uniform consistency, air bubbles or fluid levels)	Enlargement of the maxillary ostium to ~1 × 1 cm, with suction clearance of the sinus
3	Extensive polyps and tenacious mucus	Double densities and complete maxillary opacification*	Canine fossa trephination with complete clearance of polyps and mucus, and creation of a large antrostomy

*Not all completely opacified maxillary sinuses will need trephination if the contents of the sinus are easily removed with suction.

technique, a 5 mm hole is accurately drilled through the anterior maxillary face under direct visualization. In order to accomplish this, the canine fossa trephination kit (Fig. 14.7) contains an endoscope sheath with a protruding blade, which allows retraction of soft tissues during dissection on the anterior face of the maxilla. In addition, the kit contains a re-usable drill guide and 5 mm re-usable drill bit that fits the microdebrider handpiece.

A brief description of the surgical technique is as follows. The endoscope sheath is placed on a 0° scope, the lip is held up and the gingivobuccal sulcus infiltrated with lidocaine and adrenaline (epinephrine). A 6 mm vertical incision is made, and a suction Freer elevator is used to elevate the soft tissues off the anterior face of the maxilla in a subperiosteal plane. The extension on the endoscope sheath is used to hold away soft tissues, and the dissection is continued to expose the area located at the intersection of the mid-pupillary line and a horizontal line running along the lower border of the nasal alae (Fig. 14.8). If a branch of the anterior superior alveolar nerve is seen, the dissection is carried a little further to avoid injury to the nerve.

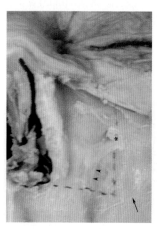

Figure 14.8   The landmarks for canine fossa trephination, as demonstrated in a cadaver specimen, at the intersection between a vertical line through the pupil and a horizontal line through the floor of the nose; note that the infraorbital nerve (asterisk) is seen emerging from its foramen, and the anterior superior alveolar nerve (arrowheads) and middle superior alveolar nerve (black arrow) are also seen.

The canine fossa drill bit (Medtronic ENT) is attached to the microdebrider handpiece and irrigation is attached. The canine fossa drill guide (Medtronic ENT) is placed perpendicular to the anterior face of the maxilla, at the junction of the two lines described above. Image guidance can be used as an adjunct to verify correct entry location. A 5 mm diameter hole is drilled through the bone (Fig. 14.9), and a Frazier suction is used to remove any bone dust from the hole and surrounding soft tissues. The 4 mm microdebrider blade is then placed through the trephine into the maxillary sinus in the closed position, and a 70° endoscope is passed transnasally to the maxillary antrostomy in order to confirm the position of the blade (Fig. 14.10).

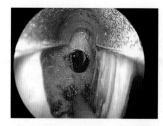

Figure 14.9   A 5 mm hole is drilled into the anterior face of the maxilla, as viewed through a 0° endoscope with the protruding blade of the endoscope sheath used to retract the premaxillary soft tissues.

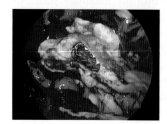

Figure 14.10   Endoscopic view through a left maxillary antrostomy using a 70° endoscope, illustrating the microdebrider blade having been passed though the canine fossa trephination in the anterior maxilla and embedded in thick mucus prior to activation.

The first step is to enlarge the maxillary antrostomy as this improves visualization into the sinus with the 70° scope. The surgeon can then remove polyps and thick mucus from the sinus under direct vision. Angled suction devices are used for the lateral and retrolacrimal recesses and anterior face of the maxillary sinus. The endoscope can also be placed through the trephine into the sinus to inspect and ensure the complete removal of disease material. It is important to note that only polypoid tissue and mucus are removed, and denudation of bone is avoided to ensure rapid re-epithelialization and re-ciliation in the postoperative period.

Revision frontal sinus surgery including the modified endoscopic Lothrop procedure

FRONTAL RECESS CLEARANCE

The primary approach to the frontal sinus is discussed in detail in Chapter 12. The frontal recess clearance begins by creating an axillary flap. The anterior wall of the agger nasi cell is removed with a Hajek–Koeffler punch flush with the frontal process of the maxilla. The remaining frontal recess dissection includes complete removal of all cells that encroach on the frontal ostium, thereby maximizing the natural ostium of the frontal sinus without drilling the frontal beak (Fig. 14.11).

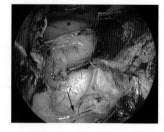

Figure 14.11   Right frontal ostium after clearance of all obstructing cells and polyps with visualization of the frontal sinus (asterisk); note the anterior ethmoid artery (arrow) on the skull base.

If the frontal drainage pathway is not visualized easily at this point, then frontal sinus mini-trephination is also performed. This is often the case with severe mucosal disease, complex frontal recess anatomy, or where the operative field is very bloody. At the end of the frontal recess dissection, the surgeon should be able to clearly visualize the skull base, including the anterior ethmoid artery, the frontal ostium and the roof of the frontal sinus (see Fig. 14.11). There should be no residual cell structures on the lamina papyracea or on the medial aspect of the frontal beak.

MODIFIED ENDOSCOPIC LOTHROP PROCEDURE

The effectiveness of the MEL procedure relies on the creation of the widest possible diameter of the frontal neo-ostium. Preoperatively, the maximum diameter can be determined on an axial scan at the level of the olfactory bulb. In most patients we are able to achieve a diameter of 22 × 18 mm. The surgical steps have been fully described elsewhere[11,12] and in Chapter 12. In brief, the procedure begins with a septal window that removes the high anterior septal cartilage and bone. Using the fluorescein-stained saline flushed via mini-trephines as a guide, the frontal process of the maxilla is drilled using a 3.2 mm cutting bur. The lateral limit of the dissection is determined by exposing small areas of the undersurface of skin. Once the frontal sinus is entered bilaterally, the frontal beak is removed until the anterior wall of the frontal sinus runs smoothly into the nasal cavity without any ridge (Fig. 14.12).

The maximum posterior limit is achieved by identifying the first olfactory neurone that forms the anterior boundary of the olfactory fossa (Fig. 14.13A). Second, drilling with the aid of image guidance allows for the gradual removal of bone under the olfactory bulb, thereby clearly defining the 'T' shaped anterior projection of the cribriform plate (Fig. 14.13B). Failure to achieve the maximum dimension of the frontal sinus ostium is generally due to inadequate reduction of the bone over the olfactory bulb and is predictable when a 'banana' shape is evident instead of a more desirable oval shape. Studies in our department have shown that the average neo-frontal ostium stenoses over the course of 1 year by about 33 per cent after which it is

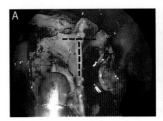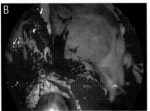

Figure 14.13   (A) The frontal 'T' (dashed lines) is exposed and the olfactory mucosa reflected posteriorly to expose the first olfactory neurone (arrow). (B) View after removal of bone overlying the olfactory bulb, down to the level of the first olfactory neurone (arrow).

generally stable.[13] If a crescent-shaped ostium is created rather than an oval opening, the anteroposterior diameter is small and a narrowing of 25 per cent is sufficient to cause obstruction and disrupt the mucociliary clearance.

POSTOPERATIVE CARE

Patients who have undergone either canine fossa trephination or frontal sinus mini-trephinations usually do not require suturing of the incisions. Patients who have undergone canine fossa trephination are advised to rinse their mouths with saline after meals during the first few postoperative days, until the incisions have sealed. The frontal sinus cannulae are left in place for 5 days postoperatively. Frontal sinus saline douches are begun within 2 hours of completion of surgery in order to wash out any blood clots from the frontal ostium. Immediately prior to removal of the cannulae, 5 mL of steroid and antibiotic cream (not ointment) are injected into each frontal sinus. Nasal saline irrigation is begun on the day after surgery, and all patients receive broad-spectrum antibiotics for 5–10 days. The first postoperative visit and debridement is performed at 2 weeks.

CONTROVERSIES

Enlargement of the maxillary ostium

It is currently unclear whether creating a wide meatal antrostomy is detrimental to the long-term health of the maxillary sinus. Some authors would argue that there are two approaches to dealing with the maxillary ostium: leave it alone or maximize it entirely. The reason for this stance is the belief that a 1 × 1 cm ostium is apt to stenose and create a worse problem for the patient than the one they started with. For this reason, it is suggested that the antrostomy should be opened into the posterior fontanelle whenever there is disease present within the sinus. Cho and Hwang[14] have reported success using the endoscopic maxillary mega-antrostomy (EMMA) without the feared

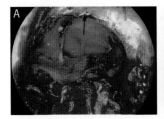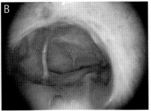

Figure 14.12   (A) The anterior walls of the frontal sinus move smoothly into the nasal cavity without a ridge as the beak has been completely removed (arrow), thereby maximizing the size of the neo-frontal ostium. (B) Postoperative view after 2 years.

complication of 'empty nose syndrome' in patients with severe recalcitrant maxillary sinus disease. With this technique, the antrostomy is extended through the posterior half of the inferior turbinate down to the floor of the nose. Furthermore, Videler et al.[15] have advocated the use of the Denker procedure, namely removing the lateral nasal wall, including the inferior and middle turbinates, in patients with recurrent problems after ESS.

Other reasons for not enlarging the maxillary antrostomy include significantly decreasing the nitric oxide concentration in the maxillary sinus and nasal cavities.[16] Nitric oxide is known to stimulate ciliary motility, and is believed to play an important role in the innate immune defences of the nasal mucosa to bacteria, viruses and fungi.[17] However, it is not known whether a lower concentration of nitric oxide in the nasal cavity and sinuses actually predisposes to recurrent infections and this still needs to be studied. Another consequence of removal of the posterior fontanelle during enlargement of the middle meatal antrostomy may be the drainage of secretions from the frontal and anterior ethmoid sinuses into the maxillary sinus. For these reasons, it is our view that enlargement of the maxillary sinus ostium into the posterior fontanelle should be reserved for patients with more severe disease.

Indications for primary modified endoscopic Lothrop procedure

At present there are no clear guidelines as to which patients would benefit from primary frontal drill-out, without first attempting a routine FESS with frontal recess clearance. As we have suggested in this chapter, certain patient factors are predictive of surgical failure; these include the presence of eosinophilic or fungal mucus and a high preoperative Lund–MacKay score. In addition, anatomical factors such as a narrow frontal sinus ostium lead to a greater likelihood of complete postoperative ostial stenosis.

Should certain patients therefore be offered a primary modified endoscopic Lothrop procedure? It can be argued that patients with a combination of narrow anatomy and severe disease should be offered the more radical surgery from the start. However, there are no good prospective randomized studies in the current literature to answer this question. Most authors would argue that there is a benefit to staging frontal sinus surgery, with an initial frontal recess clearance, since this provides two chances to completely clear out the ethmoid cells and reduce the disease burden medically in between surgeries. This has also been our philosophy in the overwhelming majority of patients. The only exceptions to this rule at present are those patients with unusual frontal sinus anatomy, including certain type 4 frontoethmoidal cells, and erosive sinus pathology involving either the posterior table, extreme lateral, or supraorbital regions of the frontal sinus that are not accessible through a complete frontal ostium dissection.

CONCLUSION AND SUMMARY

Even if initial surgical management is optimal, there are several potential reasons for disease persisting within the sinus that will require further surgical intervention. The goal of the clinical evaluation and diagnostic imaging studies is to determine the underlying factors that contribute to sinus disease and that will help define who will best respond to which surgical procedure.

Revision maxillary sinus surgery seeks to improve the means by which medical management will work by reducing disease load and improving the maxillary sinus drainage pathway in part by providing access for topical medication. This is done by removing recurrent nasal polyps or hypertrophic sinonasal mucosa from the maxillary sinus and ensuring an adequate maxillary antrostomy. The canine fossa trephination technique is a highly effective way to reduce disease load in the severely diseased maxillary sinus, whether in revision surgery or in the primary setting. Recent modifications to this technique have been successful in reducing the rate of associated complications.

Effective surgical management of the frontal sinus in polypoid CRS depends on the complete removal of nasal polyps and achieving a widely patent drainage pathway. In most situations this goal is accomplished with complete clearance of the frontal recess. The MEL procedure is particularly beneficial in cases of recurrent polypoid disease and pathologically narrowed anatomical configurations of the frontal outflow tract. Furthermore, recognition of the high-risk subgroups of polypoid CRS patients enables appropriate risk stratification for recurrence and the need for subsequent surgery. Patients with eosinophilic mucus CRS, Samter's triad, and those with high Lund–MacKay scores would be more likely to benefit from the MEL procedure and thus, deserve early consideration for it when their disease recurs following clearance of the frontal recess.

KEY MESSAGES

- When assessing the patient with symptoms suggestive of persistent or recurrent sinus disease it is important to identify mucosal and systemic factors that can contribute to a poor outcome.
- Eosinophilic mucus and high Lund–MacKay scores are risk factors that predispose patients to requiring further surgery.
- More aggressive (extensive) FESS leads to better clinical outcomes with polypoid CRS.
- The goal of surgery is to provide well-ventilated, epithelialized and disease-free sinuses that are more easily accessible to topical medical therapy.
- The canine fossa trephination technique is a highly effective way to reduce disease load in the severely diseased maxillary sinus, whether in revision surgery or in the primary setting.

- Successful surgical management of the frontal sinus is the most challenging aspect of FESS; the MEL procedure (also known as Draf III or frontal drill-out) is an excellent option for symptomatic patients with surgically recalcitrant polypoid CRS.
- The MEL procedure has a considerably lower rate of recurrent polyposis than frontal recess surgery alone.
- Continued medical management is required after surgery, and protocols should be in place to manage bacterial or fungal colonization.

REFERENCES

1. Sathananthar S, Nagaonkar S, Paleri V *et al.* Canine fossa puncture and clearance of the maxillary sinus for the severely diseased maxillary sinus. *Laryngoscope* 2005; **115**: 1026–9.
2. Jankowski R, Pigret D, Decroocq F *et al.* Comparison of radical (nasalisation) and functional ethmoidectomy in patients with severe sinonasal polyposis. A retrospective study. *Rev Laryngol Otol Rhinol (Bord)* 2006; **127**: 131–40.
3. Hosemann W, Kuhnel T, Held P *et al.* Endonasal frontal sinusotomy in surgical management of chronic sinusitis: a critical evaluation. *Am J Rhinol* 1997; **11**: 1–9.
4. Weber R, Draf W, Kratzsch B *et al.* Modern concepts of frontal sinus surgery. *Laryngoscope* 2001; **111**: 9.
5. Pant H, Kette FE, Smith WB *et al.* Eosinophilic mucus chronic rhinosinusitis: clinical subgroups or a homogeneous pathogenic entity? *Laryngoscope* 2006; **116**: 1241–7.
6. Robinson SR, Baird R, Le T *et al.* The incidence of complications after canine fossa puncture performed during endoscopic sinus surgery. *Am J Rhinol* 2005; **19**: 203–6.
7. Rajapaksa SP, Ananda A, Cain T *et al.* The effect of the modified endoscopic Lothrop procedure on the mucociliary clearance of the frontal sinus in an animal model. *Am J Rhinol* 2004; **18**: 183–7.
8. Psaltis AJ, Weitzel EK, Ha KR *et al.* The effect of bacterial biofilms on post-sinus surgical outcomes. *Am J Rhinol* 2008; **22**: 1–6.
9. Sieskiewicz A, Olszewska E, Rogowski M *et al.* Preoperative corticosteroid oral therapy and intraoperative bleeding during functional endoscopic sinus surgery in patients with severe nasal polyposis: a preliminary investigation. *Ann Otol Rhinol Laryngol* 2006; **115**: 490–4.
10. Singhal D, Douglas R, Robinson S *et al.* The incidence of complications using new landmarks and a modified technique of canine fossa puncture. *Am J Rhinol* 2007; **21**: 316–19.
11. Wormald PJ. *Endoscopic sinus surgery*, 2nd edn. New York: Thieme, 2007.
12. Wormald PJ. Salvage frontal sinus surgery: the endoscopic modified Lothrop procedure. *Laryngoscope* 2003; **113**: 276–83.
13. Tran KN, Beule AG, Singal D *et al.* Frontal ostium restenosis after the endoscopic modified Lothrop procedure. *Laryngoscope* 2007; **117**: 1457–62.
14. Cho DY, Hwang PH. Results of endoscopic maxillary mega-antrostomy in recalcitrant maxillary sinusitis. *Am J Rhinol* 2008; **22**: 658–62.
15. Videler WJ, Wreesmann VB, van der Meulen FW *et al.* Repetitive endoscopic sinus surgery failure: a role for radical surgery? *Otolaryngol Head Neck Surg* 2006; **134**: 586–91.
16. Kirihene RK, Rees G, Wormald PJ. The influence of the size of the maxillary sinus ostium on the nasal and sinus nitric oxide levels. *Am J Rhinol* 2002; **16**: 261–4.
17. Schlosser RJ, Spotnitz WD, Peters EJ *et al.* Elevated nitric oxide metabolite levels in chronic sinusitis. *Otolaryngol Head Neck Surg* 2000; **123**: 357–62.

15

What is new in managing the maxillary sinus?

SCOTT M GRAHAM

INTRODUCTION

Contemporary surgery of the maxillary sinus focuses almost exclusively on manipulations of the natural ostium for the treatment of medically resistant disease. Options for the surgeon include a complete or partial uncinectomy, simple exposure of the natural ostium and a variety of degrees of surgical manipulations of the ostium. Some surgeons even make decisions about the fate of the middle turbinate based on its capacity for lateralization and ostial occlusion. Septal surgery or reduction of a concha bullosa may aid surgical exposure of the maxillary sinus ostium. More recent options of balloon ostioplasty, approached either transnasally or via the canine fossa, stretch, tear or dilate the ostium and may fracture or displace the uncinate. Older interventions such as antral puncture, inferior meatal window and the Caldwell–Luc operation are used only for the most select of indications.

Different techniques

In deciding which operation is best suited to a particular patient it would seem reasonable to look to the published literature for guidance. While the literature is replete with descriptions of techniques of ostioplasty and even includes information about patency rates there is little describing the indication for a particular procedure and even less comparing one technique with another. Instead of relying on surgical evidence we are left relying on what has mostly seemed to work before. At the time of the widespread introduction of endoscopic sinus surgery in the late 1980s, maxillary ostioplasty was a relatively standard technique. An uncinectomy was performed by the surgeon's preferred technique and the natural ostium was enlarged, often significantly so.[1] It seemed that this procedure was performed almost as a matter of routine – if you, as a patient, were getting a 'FESS', then you were getting a substantial increase in the size of your maxillary sinus ostium. For the most part there was not a nuanced approach to maxillary sinus surgery, it was almost as if 'one size fitted all'. This sort of approach produced good patency rates of the neo-ostium and was perhaps technically easier than endoscopic surgery on the other paranasal sinuses. There were also those churlish enough to suggest that part of its popularity, in the USA, at least, related to the fact that it was a separately reimbursable event.

The minimalist strategy

Critics of maxillary ostioplasty argued that the convoluted sequestered anatomy of the maxillary sinus ostium, tucked away from the main airflow in the nose, serves a useful purpose and that routine enlargement of the maxillary sinus ostium might actually adversely change the sinus's bacterial flora and make it more susceptible to infection. Out of the perceived shortcomings of 'conventional' maxillary sinus ostioplasty have arisen a variety of more minimalist interventions complete with acronyms such as MIST. Catalano[2] describes surgery on the 'pre-chambers' or 'transition spaces' of the sinuses, with identification but not enlargement of the maxillary sinus ostia. He reported good results for this procedure for mostly limited disease in 85 patients followed for an average of nearly 2 years.

Critics of these more minimalist interventions, which would seem best suited to minimal disease, have argued that a more determined attempt at maximal medical treatment might successfully treat minimal disease and obviate the need for minimal access surgery. Proponents of the importance of bone involvement in chronic sinusitis[3] complain that such minimalist procedures leave potentially involved bone untreated. Taken as a whole these controversies are, of course, not close to resolution. What is perhaps clear is simply the obvious: that not every patient needs the same operation and that an effort should be made to tailor the surgical intervention to the needs of the patient. Additional complexity is added to the decision-making process by the relative weight given to preoperative imaging and intraoperative findings. For example would you perform an antrostomy on a patient with substantial disease on a preoperative computed tomography (CT) scan but with very little to find at the time of surgery? These discrepancies are less likely to occur if you do not rely on a single CT for operative planning. Furthermore, surgery should only be considered, again obviously, after extensive medical treatment has failed.

Does size matter?

For certain indications a large antrostomy would seem helpful. With extensive nasal polyps a large antrostomy permits removal of polyps from the maxillary sinus and also permits access of medication to the sinus postoperatively. Antro-choanal polyps have often accomplished a significant 'auto-antrostomy', although not always through the natural ostium (Fig. 15.1). A large antrostomy in this situation allows endoscopic access to the base of polyp and its point of attachment in many situations. Biopsy of infratemporal fossa or pterygopalatine fossa masses via the posterior wall of the maxillary sinus or manipulation of masses in this area such as angiofibromas is most conveniently achieved via a large antrostomy. Likewise endoscopic orbital decompression is best performed via a large antrostomy, either to allow surgical manipulations of the floor via the antrostomy in selected patients or to reduce the potential for postoperative nasal obstruction from fat prolapse after medial wall decompression.

Perhaps the commonest indication for maxillary antrostomy is to improve ventilation of the sinus in the hope of re-establishing more normal mucociliary clearance. Brumund et al.[4] reported the influence of ostial size on maxillary sinus ventilation in the xenon sheep model. An uncinectomy, small antrostomy and large antrostomy were performed endoscopically in the sheep maxillary sinus and verified by CT scan. Xenon

perfusion studies showed no benefit from uncinectomy alone. A small and large antrostomy provided a significant increase in ventilation over baseline, with no incremental further improvement provided by a large antrostomy over a smaller one.

SPECIAL SITUATIONS

Diffuse polyposis

Despite performing a large antrostomy and using a curved microdebrider blade it may not be possible to remove all of the polypoid material from the maxillary sinus. Anteromedial disease in particular can be difficult to reach and polyps and fungal debris in this location can be overlooked. Sathanathar et al.[5] have championed the utility of introducing the microdebrider through a canine fossa puncture to enhance the thoroughness of surgery. The position of the microdebrider tip can be viewed through the middle meatal antrostomy. They reported 'significantly better symptom control' in 25 patients undergoing this technique compared with 12 patients who had undergone more routine treatment. The potential for injury to branches of the anterior superior alveolar nerve as it ramifies over the anterior wall of the maxilla needs to be considered in any evaluation of this technique. Robinson et al.[6] in a cadaver study suggested that the risk of nerve injury could be minimized if the canine fossa antrostomy was performed at the intersection of imaginary lines drawn from the mid-pupil and the floor of the pyriform aperture. However, in a separate publication, Robinson et al.[7] reported on 21 patients who had undergone this technique. The authors found complications including cheek swelling, facial pain, cheek pain, dental numbness and facial tingling. Most complications rapidly resolved although a few patients had persisting complaints.

In a well-performed, prospective randomized study from South Korea, Lee et al.[8] reported no benefit from a canine fossa procedure over the more conventional use of middle meatal antroscopy. Equally importantly, the authors found a 54 per cent incidence of canine fossa puncture complications, all of which resolved at 3 months. Many of the advantages of the canine fossa puncture can be obtained with few of its disadvantages by placing the microdebrider into the maxillary sinus through the inferior meatus. Although this does not provide as direct access, significant further dissection can be performed (D S Sethi, personal communication, 2007). This is the technique I have found most helpful.

Orbital decompression

Surgery of the maxillary sinus for orbital decompression is most often performed for thyroid eye disease. Most recent attention has focused on endoscopic decompression

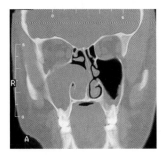

Figure 15.1   Coronal computed tomography (CT) scan showing a right antro-choanal polyp with an auto-antrostomy.

of the medial wall with a so called 'mega-antrostomy'. Transantral orbital decompression, however, remains a time-honoured technique still used in some centres.[9]

'Mega'-antrostomies are performed by enlarging the maxillary sinus ostium at the expense of each of its dimensions except for anteriorly.[10] Superiorly the ostium is enlarged to the orbital floor, inferiorly the ostium is enlarged down to the inferior turbinate and posteriorly the ostium is enlarged back to the posterior wall of the maxillary sinus. The anterior aspect of the antrostomy is left undisturbed, obviating the potential for nasolacrimal injury and reducing the potential for circumferential stenosis. This provides surgical access to the orbital floor medial to the infraorbital nerve. With the creation of the antrostomy, prolapsing fat is unlikely to result in postoperative maxillary sinus obstruction (Fig. 15.2). However, increasingly a 'balanced' decompression of the orbit is being performed. The medial and lateral walls of the orbit are decompressed and no surgery is performed on the floor. In balanced orbital decompression no antrostomy is performed.[11]

Silent sinus syndrome

Patients with the 'silent sinus syndrome' usually present to their ophthalmologist with apparent proptosis. In reality the affected eye is enophthalmic due to orbital floor erosion (Fig. 15.3A). Imaging reveals a unilateral opacified hypoplastic maxillary sinus with erosion of the floor of the orbit. Maxillary antrostomy in this situation is doubly difficult. The uncinate is retracted and collapsed against the lamina and many a well-intentioned uncinectomy in this situation has turned into an orbitotomy. It is likely that retrograde dissection of the uncinate with a back-biting instrument is the safest way to perform the uncinectomy in this situation. The lack of height differential between the top of the inferior turbinate and the eroded enophthalmic orbital floor may also enhance the difficulty of the surgery.

An antrostomy alone is usually performed at the first procedure. This usually produces subsequent resolution of the enophthalmos without the need for orbital floor grafting and augmentation[12] (Fig. 15.3B).

ANTRAL LAVAGE

Antral lavage was one of the mainstays of maxillary sinus treatment in the pre-endoscopic era. Today it is used much less frequently but still has occasional utility in isolated maxillary sinus disease. This provides the 'gold standard' for microbiological analysis. It may also have some utility, perhaps as an initial procedure in conjunction with adenoidectomy, in the paediatric population. Antral lavage can be accomplished via the canine fossa or inferior meatus. In postoperative patients, endoscopically directed aspirates of sterile saline installed via the middle meatus provide useful information in refractory maxillary sinus disease.

TOPICAL ANTIBIOTICS FOR REFRACTORY MAXILLARY SINUSITIS

In refractory maxillary sinusitis direct topical antral instillation of culture-directed antibiotics can be considered. Most experience has been gathered using topical aminoglycosides in patients with cystic fibrosis.[13] The application of the aminoglycoside solution is most easily performed in patients with prior antrostomies. In patients without previous antral surgery an indwelling catheter such as a Jazbi tube can be used. In one study, magnetic resonance imaging was used to analyse the maxillary sinuses of adult cystic fibrosis patients admitted to hospital for the treatment of exacerbations of their pulmonary disease. With the other side serving as a control, one maxillary sinus was cannulated and lavaged daily, initially with saline, followed by tobramycin in a dose of 40 mg twice a day for 10 days. This produced a significant lasting improvement in maxillary sinus aeration over the control side (Fig. 15.4A, B).

BALLOON OSTIAL DILATION

Dilation of the maxillary sinus ostium by inflatable balloons has certainly been one of the major 'novel' approaches

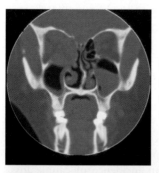

Figure 15.2   Coronal computed tomography (CT) scan after combined orbital decompression for thyroid eye disease. (Reproduced with permission from *Clin Otolaryngol*.[10])

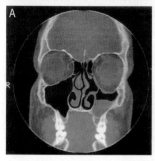
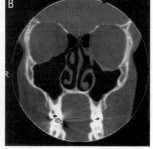

Figure 15.3   (A) Coronal computed tomography (CT) showing left silent sinus syndrome variant. (Reproduced with permission from *Am J Rhinol*[12].) (B) Coronal CT showing left silent sinus syndrome variant after maxillary sinus antrostomy. (Reproduced with permission from *Am J Rhinol*[12].)

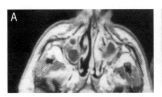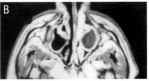

Figure 15.4 (A) Axial magnetic resonance (MR) image of maxillary sinus disease in a patient with cystic fibrosis. (Reproduced with permission from *J Laryngol Otol*[13].) (B) Axial MR image of the maxillary sinus after antral instillation of tobramycin, showing a clear right maxillary sinus. (Reproduced with permission from *J Laryngol Otol*[13].)

to the maxillary sinus in recent years. As the balloon inflates it dilates or tears the maxillary sinus ostium and fractures or displaces the uncinate process. Throughout the sinuses balloon transnasal ostial dilation has been generally associated with favourable reported results and a good safety profile. Initial studies relied on fluoroscopic confirmation of balloon position. More recently light catheter technology has been utilized. Increasingly the use of balloon dilation in the maxillary sinus ostium is sometimes more technically challenging than in the frontal or sphenoid sinus. Its use in the maxillary sinus is also the most conceptually challenging of its anatomical applications. Many patients undergo so called 'hybrid' procedures where the ethmoid – not addressed by balloon technology – is separately dissected. Most surgeons would find uncinate retention an impediment to smooth ethmoidectomy. In a recent publication of 2-year follow-up results from a multicentre study it is interesting to note that of the seven sinuses requiring revision, five were maxillary sinuses.[14]

Even more recently, transantral endoscopically guided balloon dilation of ostiomeatal complex has been reported.[15] In approximately 70 per cent of subjects this was performed under local anaesthesia with sedation. The authors note that a particular advantage of this technique is that 'intranasal obstacles' are avoided as the instrumentation is introduced via the canine fossa. In this initial publication of 30 patients from three centres, improvement in the Sinu-Nasal Outcome Test (SNOT)-20 scores were reported at 1 week, 3 months and 6 months. To be included in this study, patients must have failed 'robust, albeit non-uniform medical management'. Further reading of the study reveals that 47 per cent of the participants received antibiotics for 1–3 weeks prior to the procedure. The number of patients who had undergone the procedure after a single week of antibiotics was not specified.

MORE RADICAL SURGERY

Although the focus in much of the English-speaking world has been on repeat middle meatal surgery for recalcitrant

disease, certain centres in Europe have championed a role for more radical surgery in cases of repeated endoscopic failure. French authors have suggested 'nasalization' of the sinuses in these circumstances and groups from the Netherlands[16,17] have described their experience with their version of the Denker procedure. The nose and sinuses, except for the frontal sinus, are converted into a single cavity.

The goals of more radical surgery are clearly different from endoscopic functional procedures. There is no reasonable prospect of the return of mucociliary clearance and so the aims of surgery become ventilation, a reduction in secretory surface area, the removal of potentially osteitic bone and ready access for endoscopic cleaning. The middle and inferior turbinates are removed. No cases of the so-called 'empty nose syndrome' have been described after this substantial resection. The prospect of creating 'empty nose syndrome' may be of some medicolegal concern in the USA.

Wreesmann *et al.*[16] reported surgery of this magnitude in 82 patients over a 10-year period. This was 'last resort' surgery for patients who often had adverse prognostic variables such as Samter's triad and cystic fibrosis. Generally good results were reported. Videlar *et al.*[17] prospectively studied 24 patients, 3 per cent of their surgical practice, who underwent Denker's procedure. Most of the patients had polyps and had had a median of six surgeries prior to having Denker's procedure. The authors concluded that radical surgery was a 'viable option' for patients in this difficult-to-treat group.

CONCLUSION

For a long time the maxillary sinus has been comparatively ignored in contemporary rhinological literature. Its treatment has been almost regarded as 'standard' and perhaps not worthy of more detailed examination. Recent advances are changing this situation and contemporary maxillary sinus surgery embodies the obvious but important goal of tailoring the operative approach to the individual patient's disease.

REFERENCES

1. Stammberger H, Posawitz W. Functional endoscopic sinus surgery: concept, indications, and results of the Messerklinger Technique. *Eur Arch Otorhinolaryngol* 1990; **247**: 63–76.

2. Catalano P, Roffman E. Outcome in patients with chronic sinusitis after the minimally invasive technique. *Am J Rhinol* 2003; **17**; 17–22.

3. Khalid AR, Hunt J, Perloff JR *et al.* The role of bone in chronic rhinosinusitis. *Laryngoscope* 2002; **112**: 1951–7.

4. Brumund KT, Graham SM, Beck KC *et al.* The effect of maxillary sinus antrostomy size on xenon ventilation in

the sheep model. *Otolaryngol Head Neck Surg* 2004; **131**: 528–33.

5. Sathanathar S, Naggonkar S, Paleri V *et al.* Canine fossa puncture and clearance of the maxillary sinus for the severely diseased maxillary sinus. *Laryngoscope* 2005; **115**: 1026–9.

6. Robinson S, Wormald PJ. Patterns of innervation of the anterior maxilla: a cadaver study with relevance to canine fossa puncture of the maxillary sinus. *Laryngoscope* 2005; **115**: 1785–8.

7. Robinson SR, Baird R, Le T *et al.* The incidence of complications after canine fossa puncture performed during endoscopic sinus surgery. *Am J Rhinol* 2005; **19**: 2, 203–6.

8. Lee Y, Lee SH, Hong HS *et al.* Is the canine fossa puncture approach really necessary for the severely diseased maxillary sinus during endoscopic sinus surgery? *Laryngoscope* 2008; **118**: 1083–7.

9. Seiff SR, Tovilla JL, Carter SR. Modified orbital decompression for dysthyroid orbitopathy. *Ophthalm Plast Reconstr Surg* 2000; **16**: 62–8.

10. Graham S, Carter KD. Combined-approach orbital decompression for thyroid-related orbitopathy. *Clin Otolaryngol Allied Sci* 1999; **24**: 109–13.

11. Graham SM, Brown CL, Carter KD *et al.* Medial and lateral orbital wall surgery for balanced decompression in thyroid eye disease. *Laryngoscope* 2003; **113**: 1206–9.

12. Thomas RD, Graham SM, Carter KD *et al.* Management of the orbital floor in silent sinus syndrome. *Am J Rhinol* 2003; **17**: 97–100.

13. Graham SM, Launspach JL, Welsh MJ *et al.* Sequential magnetic resonance imaging analysis of the maxillary sinuses: implications for a model of gene therapy in cystic fibrosis. *J Laryngol Otol* 1999; **113**: 329–35.

14. Weiss RL, Church CA, Kuhn FA *et al.* Long term outcome analysis of balloon catheter sinusotomy: Two year follow-up. *Otolaryngol Head Neck Surg* 2008; **139**: 538–46.

15. Stankiewicz J, Tami T, Truitt T *et al.* Transantral, endoscopically guided balloon dilatation of the ostiomeatal complex for chronic rhinosinusitis under local anesthesia. *Am J Rhinol Allergy* 2009; **23**: 321–7.

16. Wreesman VB, Fokkens WJ, Knegt PP. Refractory chronic sinusitis: evaluation of symptoms improvement after Denker's procedure. *Otolaryngol Head Neck Surg* 2001; **125**: 495–500.

17. Videlar WJM, Wreesman VB, Van der Muelen FW *et al.* Repetitive endoscopic sinus surgery failure. A role for radical surgery? *Otolaryngol Head Neck Surg* 2006; **134**: 586–91.

16

Paediatric issues in sinus surgery

NICHOLAS JONES

NASAL SYMPTOMS

Rhinorrhoea, snoring, mouth breathing, nasal obstruction and hyponasal speech are very common symptoms in childhood. Children with these symptoms should not be labelled as having either having 'rhinitis' or 'sinusitis' but rhinosinusitis, as the nasal mucosa is a continuous lining which runs between the nasal passages and the paranasal sinuses in continuity, and one is rarely affected without the other. This is illustrated by Gwaltney's findings that 95 per cent of subjects with a history of a recent viral upper respiratory tract infection, with no preceding problems, had changes in their sinuses on computed tomography (CT)[1] (Fig. 16.1). One fundamental problem is the lack of

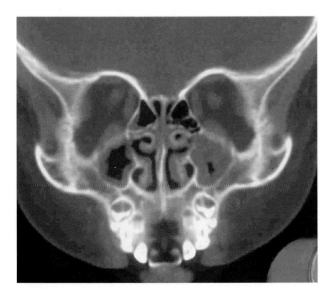

Figure 16.1   A coronal computed tomography (CT) scan of a child with incidental mucosal changes.

agreement about the definition of 'sinusitis' in children, as it is neither a clinical or a pathological distinct entity, and it is likely that factors which cause prolonged nasal secretion and/or mucosal hypertrophy are very pertinent to their management. Wald said in 1995, 'The primacy of infection as the pathophysiologic explanation for continued inflammation of the paranasal sinuses is quite unlikely', and that remains the case today.[2]

The main recognized factors that influence the pattern of paediatric symptoms are the frequency of upper respiratory tract infections, the relatively immaturity of the immune system in children, the prevalence of allergic rhinitis and adenoidal hypertrophy. Infection on its own is not an adequate explanation for the protracted inflammation that some children have in their paranasal sinuses.

It is worth explaining to parents that 2–5-year-old children average eight upper respiratory tract infections a year.[3] In a Dutch study,[4] parents of 228 per 1000 children reported that their child had had a cold or flu during the single 3-week study period. Awareness of these figures alone will often do much to reassure parents.

In an acute viral rhinitis there is often fever, malaise and possibly cough with a serous nasal discharge at first, which then becomes mucopurulent before settling spontaneously in approximately 10 days. However, up to 13 per cent of children aged 1–3 years will have symptoms for more than 15 days[5] (Fig. 16.2). Children under the age of 3.5 years rarely blow their nose and stagnant secretions collect in the nasal airway, only for those in the nasal vestibule to become colonized with nasal commensals that discolour them. If they are sucked out (not to be recommended as this will alarm the child with a loud sucking noise!), the middle meatus and sinuses examined and the secretions cultured, the majority of children will be found to have no evidence of infection in their sinuses.

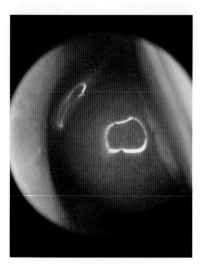

Figure 16.2 Mucosal changes in a 5-year-old child 2 weeks after an upper respiratory tract infection. No evidence of allergy or active infection was found and the symptoms resolved spontaneously.

Most acute bacterial sinus infections have been shown to be due to *Streptococcus pneumoniae*, *Haemophilus influenzae* and *Moraxella catarrhalis,* and amoxicillin is the first choice drug unless the child has been treated within the previous month, the area has a high prevalence of β-lactamase-resistant *H. influenzae* or if there are any associated complications of sinusitis. Culturing purulent secretions is unlikely to contribute to management. A French bacteriological study of purulent secretions obtained under endoscopic control from the sinus ostia or cavity in 394 patients with chronic rhinosinusitis and 139 controls showed no difference in the positive culture rate between these two groups.[6] The majority of bacterial infections resolve spontaneously.

The prevalence of allergic rhinitis in children is approximately 20 per cent. While most parents recognize hay fever or seasonal allergic rhinitis, few are aware that many children who have allergic rhinitis have symptoms all the year round because they are allergic to perennial allergens such as house dust mite or pet allergens (Fig. 16.3). Adenoidal hypertrophy is common with a tendency to spontaneous involution by 8–10 years (Fig. 16.4).

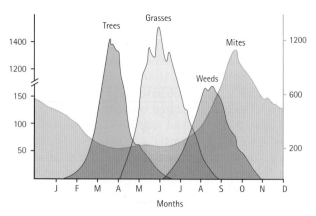

Figure 16.3 Monthly prevalence of some seasonal and perennial allergens.

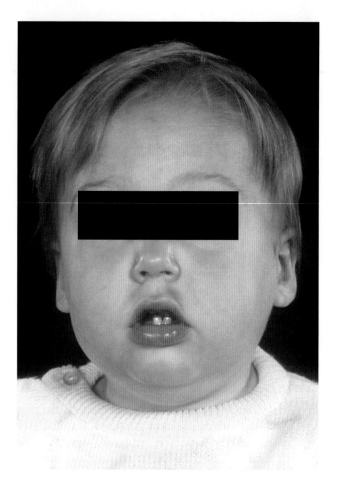

Figure 16.4 A child might be labelled as having adenoid hypertrophy when their nasal obstruction is due to a perennial allergic rhinitis.

The symptoms and signs that parents mention include snuffles in a baby, snoring, mouth breathing, feeding problems, bad breath, cough and hyponasal speech. It is often striking how concerned parents are while the child often appears unconcerned about their symptoms. Facial pain and headache are rare symptoms in children with rhinosinusitis.

How persistent have symptoms to be before they become noteworthy? One useful question is: 'Does the child have any periods when their nose is clear, or do they have persistent symptoms week after week?'. If there are periods when the nose is clear it is more likely that the child fits into the category of having multiple upper respiratory tract infections (Fig. 16.5). If their nose is never clear then it is worth asking about symptoms which indicate that perennial allergic rhinitis may be part of the problem. Ask if they have asthma, sneeze a lot, have itchy eyes or is there a family history of seasonal asthma or rhinitis, as these features are associated with allergic rhinitis (Fig. 16.6). Another common factor contributing to persisting symptoms is adenoidal hypertrophy, but it is difficult to differentiate this from perennial allergic rhinitis

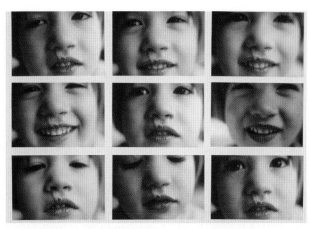

Figure 16.5   These photographs taken on separate occasions make the point that a child who has periods when their nose is clear is probably having intermittent upper respiratory tract infections.

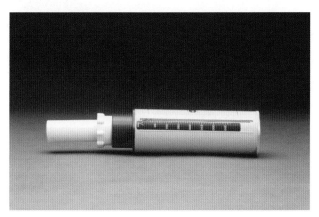

Figure 16.6   Over 80 per cent of children with asthma have allergic rhinitis.

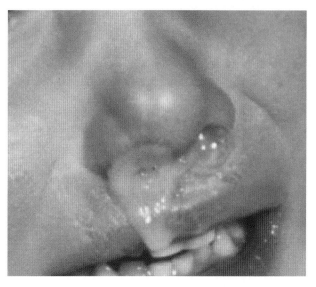

Figure 16.7   A foreign body should be excluded in any child with a persistent unilateral purulent nasal discharge.

CLINICAL SIGNS

The signs that are associated with the broad label of rhinosinusitis (and many of the other aforementioned conditions) include a blocked and running nose in a child who mouth breathes. The colour of the nasal discharge is clear in the early stages of a viral rhinosinusitis and soon becomes yellow, which does not necessarily imply a current infection as it is often stained by white cells in the recovery phase (non-infective) of a viral or bacterial infection or by eosinophils in an allergic rhinitis. Purulent rhinitis alone is not equivalent to sinusitis.[7] It is said that very pale or boggy bluish turbinate mucosa is indicative of an allergic rhinitis but this is an unreliable sign and does not allow differentiation between the allergic, infective or postinfective state.

Nasal polyps in children are uncommon. The term 'nasal polyp' is not a diagnosis but a sign of inflammation of the lining of the nose that can be due to a range of important diseases. Unilateral polyps are often due to an antrochoanal polyp (Fig. 16.8) but other pathology

on the basis of symptoms alone. A child who mouth breathes is often labelled as having adenoidal hypertrophy but a child with turbinate hypertrophy due to allergic rhinitis can look the same (Fig. 16.4). If snoring is a major problem it is worth asking if the child regularly stops breathing for more than 10 seconds, even when they do not have an active respiratory tract infection, as this raises the possibility that they may have sleep apnoea, which will need further investigation. For some unknown reason parents often omit to mention apnoeic episodes but there is obvious recognition and relief when these symptoms are described to parents whose children have them.

With a unilateral nasal discharge a foreign body should be excluded. There is often some excoriation around the nostril (Fig. 16.7). Gastro-oesophageal reflux has been implicated as a possible contributing factor in rhinosinusitis, but this has yet to be proven as both conditions are common and their coexistence may be coincidental. Nasal symptoms do not cause eating problems that would directly reduce a child's intake, although a loss of sense of smell reduces their ability to taste.

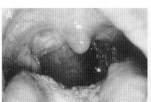
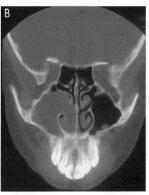

Figure 16.8   (A) An antrochoanal polyp visible in the posterior oropharynx. (B) Computed tomography (CT) scan of a right antrochoanal polyp.

such as an encephalocoele (Fig. 16.9), inverted papilloma, haemangioma, angiofibroma (Fig. 16.10), nasal glioma (Fig. 16.11) and malignancy must be excluded (Fig. 16.12). Bilateral polyps are usually associated with cystic fibrosis (Fig. 16.13) but primary ciliary dyskinesia, immunodeficiency or chronic infection may be responsible. A sizable minority are idiopathic. It is important to exclude any systemic underlying cause so this can be addressed.

Antrochoanal polyps result from mucosal retention cysts in the maxillary sinus that have prolapsed either through the infundibulum or accessory ostia (see Fig. 16.8A). The best way of reducing the chance of recurrence is to remove the mucosa around their base so that scar tissue forms. The management of paediatric polyposis is often disappointing because apart from those with an antrochoanal polyp they have a high rate of recurrence.

Mucosal hypertrophy can cause mouth breathing and snoring whether it is due to allergic, infective or postinfective rhinosinusitis, but so can adenoid and tonsillar hypertrophy. As long as there is no remarkable sleep apnoea, these symptoms cause no harm and usually settle by 8–10 years of age. Adenoid hypertrophy usually

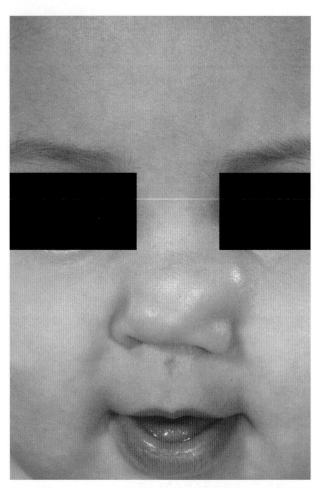

Figure 16.11   A left-sided glioma of the lateral nasal wall.

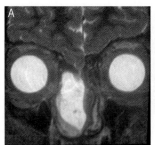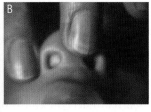

Figure 16.9   (A) A magnetic resonance image of a right encephalocoele in a 3-year-old child. (B) A right nasal 'polyp' in a neonate that was an encephalocoele.

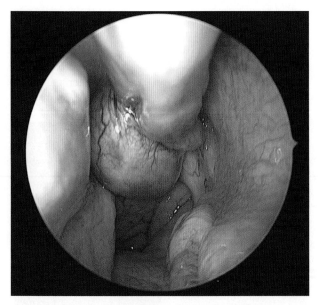

Figure 16.10   Endoscopic view of a left angiofibroma.

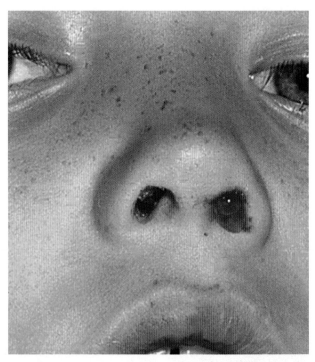

Figure 16.12   Bloody mucoid discharge from a left-sided rhabdomyosarcoma of the paranasal sinuses.

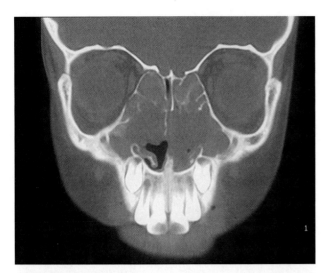

Figure 16.13   Characteristic coronal computed tomography (CT) changes in a child with cystic fibrosis. Note the absence of bony landmarks with opacification of all the sinuses.

resolves spontaneously around 7–9 years (Fig. 16.14). The adenoid can be examined using an angled mirror but a strong gag reflex or a frightened child may prevent this from being done. It often helps to tell a child that you want to look at their teeth as they understand this and will open their mouths. A lateral soft tissue plain radiograph is the most reliable method of assessing adenoid size but in any event this is unlikely to influence the management in most children. Signs such as 'dark rings around the eyes' and pallor are weak and not indicative of any worrying disease.

INVESTIGATIONS

If allergy is suspected, skin tests can be carried out in children after about the age of 5 years. The skin prick test involves the most minimal discomfort, as only the epidermis should be breached and it should be so superficial that there is no bleeding. This test has very good specificity and moderately good sensitivity. It not only helps the clinician but illustrates to the parents and the older child the allergens that are responsible. It illustrates that surgery will not cure this aspect of the problem. The main perennial allergens are from the house dust mite and pet proteins. If the prospect of a skin test is unacceptable and allergy is suspected then a trial of a safe topical nasal steroid taken daily for 6 weeks can make the diagnosis more likely if the symptoms return when the spray stops. An alternative is to test for specific IgE, especially in children who are taking antihistamines or those who have eczema or dermatographism.

Nasal endoscopy has little to offer in a child under approximately 8 years as visibility is often restricted and it can upset the child. Plain sinus radiographs have no place in the routine management of rhinosinusitis, as a 'thickened mucosa' is a non-specific finding and may occur in asymptomatic patients. So are plain sinus radiographs obsolete? They do have a role in the management of acute maxillary and frontal sinusitis which is unresponsive to medical treatment prior to drainage. They may also help where a radio-opaque foreign body is sought.

Computed tomography may provide better images but it has its problems: the dose of radiation, the need for sedation, but, most important of all, the limited significance of CT image findings. In addition, CT is not much better at diagnosing rhinosinusitis than plain sinus radiographs. This point is demonstrated by the prevalence of mucosal changes found incidentally in asymptomatic control groups (see Fig. 16.1, p. 139). In asymptomatic children there is a high prevalence rate of mucosal thickening or opacification on CT of approximately 50 per cent.

Anatomical variations appear to play little if any role in the prevalence of paediatric sinusitis and this was shown by Willner et al.,[8] who found that anatomical 'abnormalities' appear to be a range of normal variations that did not correlate with disease. Culture swabs of the nasal airway are frequently contaminated by commensals from the nasal vestibule. Obtaining an antral specimen for culture requires general anaesthesia and an antral wash-out, which in itself has not been shown to be of therapeutic benefit at 3 months.

TREATMENT

In children who do not respond to conservative management or who repeatedly fail to improve, even

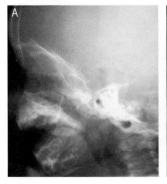
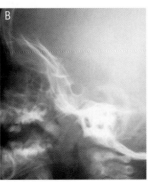
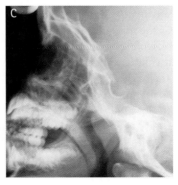

Figure 16.14   (A–C) These lateral soft tissue radiographs of the same patient were found incidentally and they demonstrate the natural involution of the adenoid that occurs around 7–9 years of age.

temporarily, with medical management, it is worth considering whether there is an immunological defect. The majority of children with an immunodeficiency who have severe sinusitis have inadequate humoral defences rather than cell-mediated problems. As many immunodeficiency diseases are hereditary it is worth asking about first-degree relatives, or whether the patient has also had recurrent pneumonias, cellulitis, candidiasis, chronic diarrhoea or failure to thrive.

Reduced immunoglobulins to pneumococcal, *Haemophilus* or tetanus antigens are markers of reduced immunity.[9] Vaccination can be given and then the antibody titres retested after 1 month to see if they are in the normal range. If not, referral to an immunologist is indicated. The commonest immunodeficiency due to a lack of antibodies is common variable immunodeficiency (CVID), in which there is a reduction in IgG subclasses although the number of B lymphocytes is usually normal. In X-linked agammaglobulinaemia, disorders of IgG subclass deficiency and CVID, treatment with immunoglobulins may be effective whereas antibiotics on their own are not. Prolonged courses of antibiotics with anaerobic cover are needed. Measurements of CD4 lymphocytes and neutrophil function tests occasionally uncover other abnormalities that may present with recurrent unresponsive sinusitis.

If a child has persistent lower as well as upper respiratory tract problems it is worth testing their peak flow in case they have asthma. If they develop bronchiectasis, persistent purulent sinusitis and middle ear effusions (persistent discharge through a grommet) or aural discharge through a perforation, primary ciliary dyskinesia should be considered. Stagnant mucus may be seen in the nose in the absence of an enlarged adenoid or unilateral choanal atresia (Fig. 16.15). The most simple and practical test of ciliary function is the saccharine clearance test, which is done by placing a quarter of a saccharine tablet under the anterior end of the inferior turbinate. However, this is crude in comparison with a brushing or biopsy looking at ciliary movement or the electron microscopic appearance. Any biopsy should be taken from an area of healthy looking mucosa, otherwise a false abnormal biopsy will be obtained. An alternative if the nasal mucosa cannot be rendered healthy, even for a short period to enable it to have a biopsy when it is not infected, is to do a tracheal biopsy.

One of the main reasons for a baby or child having a runny nose is that ciliary function is impaired for up to a few weeks after a viral upper respiratory tract infection. The best way to clear the nose of mucus under these circumstances is nose blowing or saline sprays or douching. Unfortunately most children under the age of 3.5 years are poor at blowing their nose. Saline sprays are effective at cleaning the nose and may improve mucociliary clearance. The saline mechanically removes mucus and helps patient comfort. Saline sprays may also help reduce the tenaciousness of secretions, and they can be repeated as frequently as needed to clear the nose without causing any harm.

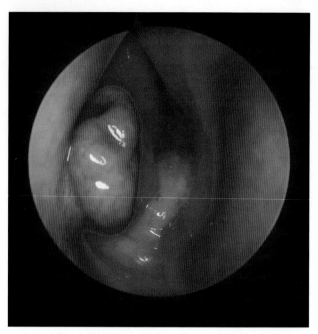

Figure 16.15 Stagnant mucus in the floor of the nose that raises the question whether the child has an enlarged adenoid, unilateral choanal atresia or primary ciliary dyskinesia.

Studies of the natural history of persistent rhinorrhoea unresponsive to treatment have produced the useful information that by the age of 7 over 95 per cent had resolved without any further action.[10] One of the most disputed questions is whether antibiotics make any difference. Several studies have found no difference between those treated with antibiotics and a control group when the subjects are followed up for more than 12 weeks.

In children with perennial allergic rhinitis with a single allergy to house dust mite, rigorous allergen avoidance may provide some help although the evidence base for this is not strong. Alteration in diet does not usually help, although occasionally parents report that avoiding milk products has reduced nasal discharge. For symptoms of nasal obstruction due to allergy, regular age-appropriate topical nasal steroids work best. Antihistamines help the symptoms of sneezing and itching and clear the rhinorrhoea. The second and third generations of H1 receptor antagonists are preferable because they cause far less sedation than previous antihistamines and they can be taken as required.

COMPLICATIONS OF INFECTIVE RHINOSINUSITIS

The complications of infective sinusitis occur rarely and their incidence is unpredictable. They include periorbital cellulitis, a periorbital or frontal subperiosteal abscess and intracranial infections. Any periorbital swelling warrants admission, parenteral antibiotics, detailed assessment and monitoring of vision, and CT scanning if there is a suspicion of involvement of the post-septal compartment or if the patient fails to respond within 24–36 hours. Contemporary guidelines for the management of orbital cellulitis advise against the use of CT in the first instance if there is no chemosis, proptosis, painful or decreased extraocular movements, an afferent pupillary defect or visual impairment. If any of these features are present, or if they develop, or there is no clinical response to the appropriate antibiotic after 48 hours, CT is warranted.[11] If there is a post-septal collection of pus, it needs to be drained as compression in this area due to a subperiosteal abscess can cause blindness.

Intracranial infection secondary to infective sinusitis is rare and sporadic. The unusual intracranial complications of sinusitis occur most frequently just before, or in, the early teens and usually present with an altered mental state, headache, fever, seizures, vomiting, unilateral weakness/hemiparesis or a cranial nerve sign.[12] These justify an urgent MRI or CT scan. The importance of imaging before a lumbar puncture cannot be overemphasized as otherwise the brainstem can be compressed if there is raised intracranial pressure from an abscess and a lumbar puncture is done. Of particular note is the finding that almost 50 per cent of patients in a consecutive series who presented with intracranial sepsis secondary to bacterial sinusitis had periorbital cellulitis or a frontal swelling.[13] Therefore it is important to recognize that because a collection of pus presents anteriorly it precludes any intracranial involvement. Intracranial infections secondary to rhinosinusitis occur sporadically and although it appears that this cannot be prevented,[13] early recognition and treatment is essential to reduce any subsequent morbidity or mortality. *Streptococcus milleri* and *Staphylococcus aureus* are the most common organisms cultured.

ENDOSCOPIC SINUS SURGERY

Endoscopic techniques can reduce surgical morbidity and achieve better symptomatic control than conventional surgery in cystic fibrosis, allergic fungal sinusitis, antrochoanal polyp, mucocoeles and repair of cerebrospinal fluid (CSF) leaks, intracranial complications (Fig. 16.16), mucocoeles or mucopyocoeles, a periorbital abscess (Fig. 16.17), traumatic injury to the optic canal, fibrous dysplasia causing optic nerve decompression (Fig. 16.18), dacryocystitis, choanal atresia (Fig. 16.19), unilateral fungal sinusitis, some meningoencephalocoeles and some neoplasms.

Few studies of endoscopic sinus surgery in children treated for rhinosinusitis report more than an 80 per cent improvement in symptoms and when these results are compared with the reported improvement that occurs without any treatment,[14,15] surgery does not compare favourably.

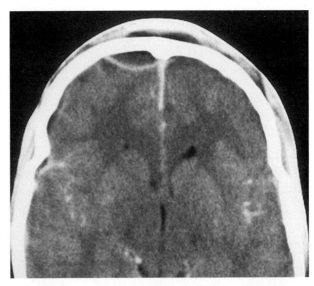

Figure 16.16   A subgaleal and extradural abscess secondary to sinusitis.

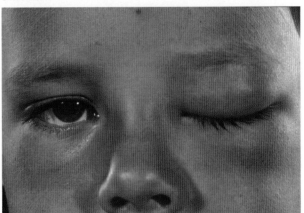

Figure 16.17   A left periorbital abscess.

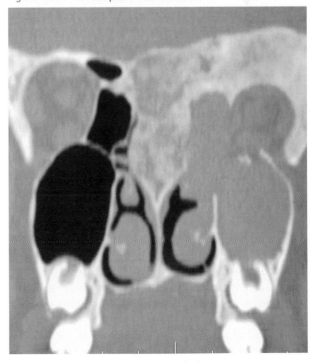

Figure 16.18   Left-sided fibrous dysplasia.

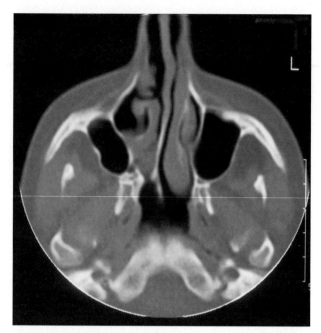

Figure 16.19 An axial computed tomography (CT) scan showing right choanal atresia.

ANTROCHOANAL POLYP

An antrochoanal polyp is composed of a cystic part that fills the maxillary sinus and a solid part that has prolapsed into the nasal airway. The interstitium is oedematous but the eosinophilia that is seen in most other inflammatory polyps is absent. Many appear to originate from a mucus retention cyst that expands until it prolapses through the maxillary ostium or an accessory ostium to extend into the nasopharynx. Evidence of atopy, or a predisposition to type I hypersensitivity (skin prick test positive or a raised IgE) is not more prevalent in patients with unilateral polyps and does not seem to play a role in the pathogenesis of most paediatric patients with unilateral nasal polyps.[16] Only two bilateral cases have been reported in the literature.[17] A large, single nasal polyp can be seen which may be visible at the back of the oropharynx. Computed tomography shows a uniform hypoattenuating mass, occasionally with some remaining air in the roof of the sinus.

Simple avulsion is associated with a high rate of recurrence. The best way to minimize the likelihood of recurrence is to remove the whole base of an antrochoanal polyp. Historically, avulsion or a Caldwell–Luc approach was used to remove an antrochoanal polyp but the frequency of postoperative facial pain has made this unpopular. With the use of the endoscope it is possible not only to open the maxillary sinus but to visualize the base of the polyp using a 45°, 70° or 120° endoscope.[18] A range of curved instruments, including the Heuwieser antrum grasping forceps, allow the whole base of the polyp to be removed, thus reducing the chance of recurrence. If the polyp is based on the anterior wall a large maxillary sinusotomy, a range of curved grasping forceps and perseverance are

required. It is important to avoid damaging the roots of growing teeth in children. Sometimes an antrochoanal polyp is so large that the bulk of it has to be delivered transorally.

SUMMARY

The symptoms associated with rhinosinusitis are usually self-limiting and become progressively less common in older children. There is no evidence that the majority of children who have persistent symptoms attributed to rhinosinusitis develop into adults with chronic sinus disease (the exceptions are those with cystic fibrosis, ciliary dyskinesia and immune deficiencies). Therefore, any treatment that is recommended while the child's immune resistance is maturing or an enlarged adenoid is shrinking should have few side effects or be associated with few complications. This would hold true even if funds available for medical and surgical treatments were unlimited.

First-line treatment should involve harmless measures such as teaching nose blowing, saline sprays, short courses of topical decongestants and probably most of all, an explanation to the parents. Allergen avoidance in children with coexisting allergic mucosal disease will help, as will regular topical nasal steroids for symptoms of obstruction and non-sedative antihistamines for itchy eyes, sneezing and rhinorrhoea. Children with an allergic nasal airway have an increased chance of having asthma and vice versa. If antibiotics are given for persistent purulent rhinorrhoea or postnasal drip they should be given with the expectation that reinfection is likely to occur within the next few weeks. The place of radiology in the management of children with rhinosinusitis is very limited and is confined to the few who develop the complications of sinusitis or in whom a tumour or atypical infection is suspected.

The adage of '*primum non nocere*' or 'do no harm' should underlie the management of paediatric sinusitis.

REFERENCES

1. Gwaltney JM, Phillis CD, Miller RD *et al.* Computed tomographic study of the common cold. *N Engl J Med* 1994; **330**: 25–30.
2. Wald ER. Chronic sinusitis in children. *J Pediatr* 1995; **127**: 339–47.
3. Wald ER. Sinusitis in children. *N Engl J Med* 1992; **326**: 319–23.
4. Bruijnzzeels MA, Foets M, Van Der Wouden JC *et al.* Everyday symptoms in childhood: occurrence and general practitioner consultation rates. *Br J Gen Pract* 1998; **48**: 880–4.
5. Wald ER, Guerra N, Byers C. Upper respiratory tract infections in young children: duration of and frequency of complications. *Pediatrics* 1991; **87**: 129–33.

6. Klossek JM, Dubreuil L, Richet H *et al.* Bacteriology of chronic purulent secretions in chronic rhinosinusitis. *J Laryngol Otol* 1998; **112**: 1162–6.

7. Newton DA. Sinusitis in children and adolescents. *Prim Care* 1996; **23**: 701–17.

8. Willner A, Choi SS, Vezina LG *et al.* Intranasal anatomic variations in pediatric sinusitis. *Am J Rhinol* 1997; **11**: 355–60.

9. Cooney T, Jones NS. Investigation for immunodeficiency in patients with recurrent infections. *Clin Otolaryngol* 2001; **26**: 184–8.

10. Otten FWA, van Aarem A, Groote JJ. Long-term follow-up of chronic maxillary sinusitis in children. *Int J Pediatr Otorhinolaryngol* 1991; **22**: 81–4.

11. Howe L, Jones NS. Guidelines for the management of periorbital cellulitis/abscess. *Clin Otolaryngol* 2004; **29**: 725–8.

12. Giannoni C, Sulek M, Friedman EM. Intracranial complications of sinusitis: a pediatric series. *Am J Rhinol* 1998; **12**: 173–8.

13. Jones NS, Walker J, Punt J *et al.* Intracranial complications of sinusitis: can they be prevented? *Laryngoscope* 2002; **112**: 59–63.

14. Otten FWA, van Aarem A, Grote JJ. Long-term follow-up of chronic therapy resistant purulent rhinosinusitis. *Clin Otolaryngol* 1992; **17**: 32–3.

15. Otten FWA, Grote JJ. Treatment of chronic maxillary sinusitis in children. *Int J Pediatr Otorhinolaryngol* 1988; **15**: 269–78.

16. Schramm VL, Effron MZ. Nasal polyps in children. *Laryngoscope* 1980; **90**: 1488–95.

17. Basu SK, Bandyopadhay SN, Bora H. Bilateral antrochoanal polyps. *J Laryngol Otol* 2001; **115**: 561–2.

18. Sato K, Nakashima T. Endoscopic sinus surgery for chronic sinusitis and antrochoanal polyp. *Laryngoscope* 2000; **110**: 1581–3.

Sinus surgery and olfaction in chronic rhinosinusitis

DANIEL B SIMMEN

INTRODUCTION

Chronic rhinosinusitis, especially with nasal polyposis, is the most common cause for olfactory impairment among patients presenting to an ENT specialist.[1] Olfactory disorders are often not taken seriously because they are viewed as affecting the 'lower senses' – those involved with the emotional life – instead of the 'higher senses' that serve the intellect.[2] 'Sense of smell? …. I never gave it a thought' – one does not normally give it a thought but when it is lost, it is like being struck blind or deaf.

In the clinical setting too, surgeons unfortunately often underestimate the extent of the importance of sense of smell for their patients. In fact, it is a sense that often escapes the notice of both surgeons and patients. The reason may be that the loss of this sense often creeps up on the patient slowly or because the patient does not recognize that this loss is responsible for their reduced enjoyment of food. However, the rewards for patients in preserving or restoring their sense of smell are enormous, the value of this sense often only being appreciated after it is lost. The sense of smell also impacts on our interaction with the environment and therefore its loss can have a direct influence on human behaviour and lead to an appreciable decrease in the quality of life.[3,4] In modern rhinology many symptoms can be managed by medical treatment alone but an impaired or lost sense of smell is not always easy to restore. Thus improving this symptom is one of the main goals of the modern management of chronic rhinosinusitis (CRS). In the postoperative period deterioration in this symptom is the first sign of any increase in inflammatory oedema of the nasal mucosa as this has an immediate impact on the sense of smell.

Rhinosinusitis with nasal polyposis has the potential to impair olfaction in several ways (Fig. 17.1). Inflammation of the nasal mucosa leads to constriction of the airways (ortho- and retronasal airflow) and therefore reduced access of the odorant flow to the neuroepithelium (conduction). The composition of the mucous layers is altered and this can affect both access and binding of olfactory molecules to the receptor sites. Proteins secreted by diseased mucosa may alter or damage the function of the neuroepithelium in a direct way. Ongoing inflammation may lead to histological changes that prevent the regeneration of

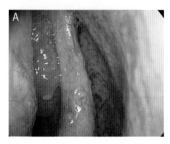 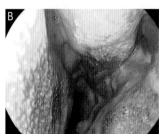 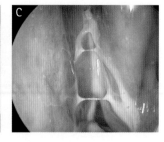

Figure 17.1 (A) Nasal polyps, (B) polypoid mucosa and marked oedema and (C) purulent mucus in the left olfactory cleft reducing the airflow to the olfactory cleft (conduction).

neuroepitheleum.[1,5] Therefore, any medical and surgical treatment strategy for a rhinitis-induced olfactory disorder should focus on these issues.

IMPAIRED OLFACTION – AN IMPORTANT PRIMARY SYMPTOM IN CHRONIC RHINOSINUSITIS

A patient with nasal disease may have any of a large array of symptoms. However there are four main symptoms that are always worth asking about:

- nasal obstruction
- sense of smell
- secretions
- pain or pressure.

It is important to rank these symptoms in the order of priority for the patient. This not only helps to make a diagnosis, but it focuses the surgeon's mind on how best to meet the patient's needs and chief complaint. We need to make sure that patients understand that it is usually not possible to fully rid them of their polyps or eradicate all their symptoms. We explain to our patients that their symptoms are like a person trying to get from the ground floor of a skyscraper to the top floor to get a good view. On the ground floor the patient feels 'blocked' with a poor sense of smell. Medical treatment can get them up a few flights of stairs, and oral steroids may get them near the top in a lift, but the lift often comes down again. Surgery together with medical treatment will help them to get a better sense of smell for a longer period, but it will not necessarily get them to the top floor (Fig. 17.2).

Many patients complain of having a poor sense of taste, being unaware that the problem is a reduced sense of smell, which needs to be clarified. The sense of taste can only discern salty, sweet, bitter, or sour. In order to taste or smell anything else, you require a functioning olfactory epithelium. Ask the patient whether their loss of the sense of smell is total or partial. If it is total, you should enquire whether it occurred immediately after a head injury, following an influenza-like illness, or slowly in conjunction with other nasal symptoms, such as in CRS. A history of head injury must raise suspicion that the olfactory nerves were severed as they pass through the cribriform plate. If it followed an influenza-like illness and is absolute, then it is likely that it is secondary to a neuropathic influenza viral infection.

Many patients say that their loss of sense of smell is absolute, but on closer questioning they will mention that they recently did notice a smell of burning toast or some perfume or taste some food using descriptive terms other than salt, sweet, bitter or sour. This indicates that there is some functioning olfactory mucosa. In these patients, it is likely that they have some mucosal disease, and it is possible that their sense of smell can be improved by reversing this. A minority of patients have a distorted sense

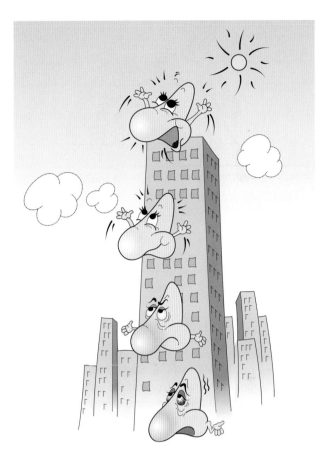

Figure 17.2   Skyscraper analogy illustrating the effect of rhinosinusitis on quality of life.

of smell and it is worth referring to a specialist text for more information on this topic.[6–8]

CLINICAL OLFACTORY TESTING – A PRIMARY GOAL IN MODERN RHINOLOGY

Chronic rhinosinusitis can impair orthonasal as well as retronasal olfactory acuity (Fig. 17.3). A major proportion of patients have normal retronasal olfactory perception but a markedly impaired orthonasal perception.[9] In evaluating a patient who may have a possible olfactory disorder, clinicians have several tools at their disposal. The patient's history, physical exam and olfactory testing as well as taste testing are all necessary to obtain the information that is relevant to diagnosing the aetiology of their possible hyposmia. Diagnostic radiology has a contributory role in the diagnosis of smell disorders with computed tomography (CT) showing the presence of an anterior skull base fracture in some patients with anosmia following head trauma or rarely an anterior skull base meningioma. Magnetic resonance imaging (MRI) can show an absent or hypoplastic olfactory bulb, for example in Kallmann's syndrome (hypogonadotrophic hypogonadism and olfactory dysplasia), invasion by an anterior skull base tumour, post-traumatic encephalomalacia or cortical changes associated with dementia.

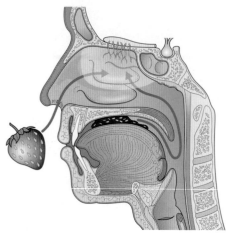

Figure 17.3   Orthonasal olfactory sensation is often altered in chronic rhinosinusitis whereas the retronasal detection is often only minimally altered.

Since the sense of olfaction can differentiate between thousands of different odorants, it is impossible to assess the whole sensory system with a few simple tests. Depending on the information needed, specific tests can be used to measure certain facets of the olfactory system. In rhinology, quantitative assessment of smell is important because hyposmia or anosmia due to conductive olfactory loss is a frequent symptom in rhinological diseases such as severe allergic rhinitis or CRS.[6–8] These tests are usually detection threshold tests that involve measurement of the lowest concentration of a stimulus (odour) that can be discerned, thus combining the quantitative and qualitative aspects of olfaction.

Qualitative disorders, the so-called dysosmias (for example cacosmia or parosmia), are much more difficult to measure. Nevertheless, specific tests for the assessment of qualitative disorders have also been developed. Qualitative tests can discriminate between two test stimuli to see whether they are the same or different or, alternatively, they can involve multidimensional scaling, in which pairs of smells are rated. Often eight vials containing four odorants are used. Qualitative tests can also serve as identification tests, and in these response alternatives are often needed as many people have a problem naming even familiar odours.

Olfactory tests do remind the surgeon to counsel the patient about hyposmia as a potential complication of nasal surgery[10] and to mention that the patient should *not expect* their smell to return.

PREOPERATIVE SCREENING OF THE PATIENT – WHAT THE SURGEON SHOULD KNOW

Subjective screening tests for the sense of smell

Subjective tests are frequently used to assess olfaction because they can be done quickly and easily in a compliant patient. Several simple chemosensory tests can be done in the physician's office. In a specialized ENT set-up today, a validated screening test and a documented result are desirable. In the past decade, few validated screening tests for olfaction have been developed worldwide and they can be used by the physician or self-administered by the patient. The tests can be grouped into three categories:

- screening tests of olfaction
- qualitative olfaction tests
- quantitative olfaction tests.

SCREENING TESTS OF OLFACTION

These are designed to detect whether a patient has an impaired sense of smell or not (identification test). These tests should be quick to administer, reliable and cheap. A common known example is the use of bottles containing a certain odorant, such as coffee, chocolate or perfume, to simply have an overview of the problem. Each nostril should be tested separately to ascertain whether the problem is unilateral or bilateral – 'lateralization screening'. In recent years, more sophisticated tests have been developed that are both reliable and convenient to use. The University of Pennsylvania Smell Identification Test (UPSIT) or the Smell Identification Test (Sensonics) is a well-known example that is frequently used in the USA; it is a scratch and sniff test with microencapsulated odorants.[11] Other examples are the 12-item Brief Smell Identification Test (Sensonics),[12] Japanese Odor Stick Identification Test (OSIT),[13] Scandinavian Odor Identification Test (SOIT),[14] and Smell Diskettes for the screening of olfaction (Novimed; Fig. 17.4). The last test presents eight odorants in reusable diskettes to the patient and also includes pictorial representations that use a forced multiple choice procedure for the patient to perform.[15] Another example is the Sniffin' Sticks test, which uses a pen-like device for odour identification[16] and finally there is a brief three-item smell identification test,[17] which is highly sensitive in identifying olfactory loss in patients with chemosensory complaints.

All the listed test batteries have been validated (some with a cultural bias), documented in the literature, and are used as a first-line investigation in olfactory disorders. Any of these tests can, and ideally should, be used to document olfactory function before any form of nasal surgery. However, a supra-threshold screening test can only reliably distinguish between normal and absent smell function as quantifying the response is very subjective. For further evaluation of smell dysfunction, a quantitative investigation should be carried out.

Nasal airflow patterns and olfaction – impact on the surgical technique

The airflow pattern defines the pathway into the olfactory region where the molecules diffuse through the aqueous

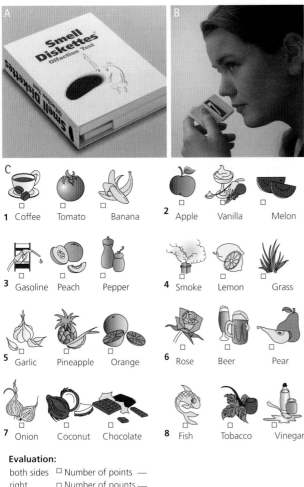

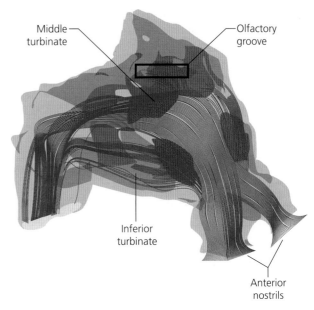

Figure 17.5 Airflow in the healthy nose model. In computational fluid dynamics (CFD) and the study of the human healthy nose model, the main inspiratory air streamlines are found to occur in the middle of the airway, between the inferior and middle turbinates and the septum. There is only a small airflow breath through the dorsal region (including olfactory groove) with a low velocity (0.34 m/s) and wall shear stress (0.04 Pa). (Courtesy of Professor De-Yun Wand, National University of Singapore.)

Figure 17.4 (A) Smell Diskettes for screening olfaction. (B) One of the eight odorants that are presented to the patient in reusable diskettes. (C) Pictorial representation in a forced multiple choice fashion.

mucus layer to stimulate the olfactory sensory neurones. The signal is then transported from the olfactory sensory neurones to the olfactory bulb and from there to the central nervous system. Every surgeon should understand the physiology of nasal airflow and the profound impact that surgery can have on it. Recent studies that have compared CT scans and MR images of nasal anatomy with measurements of olfaction in individual subjects have found a correlation between specific anatomical areas and olfactory performance (Fig. 17.5). Anatomical changes in the olfactory region and the nasal valve area will strongly affect airflow patterns and odorant transport through the olfactory region and affect olfactory function.[18]

The olfactory region of the nose is ventilated towards the end of inspiration, when air speed declines significantly, causing turbulence in the olfactory cleft between the middle turbinate and septum. During expiration the distribution of flow is much more even and the olfactory region is aerated early on and throughout the breathing cycle. The olfactory mucosa is therefore not directly exposed to the high velocity airstream during inspiration but rather to a much weaker 'secondary flow', prolonging the contact time of olfactory active particles with the olfactory sensory neurones.[19] Modern technology using a nasal CT scan from an individual patient and converting it into a three-dimensional nasal model can then be used to predict airflow and odorant transport, and this could possibly become an important guide for the treatment of CRS with nasal polyposis to optimize airflow and improve olfactory function (Fig. 17.6).[18]

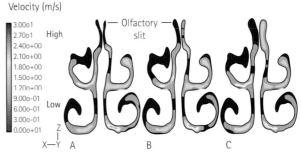

Figure 17.6 Contour plot of velocity magnitude: (A) narrowed olfactory slit, (B) original airflow model and (C) widened olfactory slit. (Courtesy of Professor De-Yun Wand, National University of Singapore.)

A further consideration is that olfactory sensory neurones do not work well if the mucosa around them is dry. This is thought to be because the olfactory molecules have to dissolve or diffuse through the mucus. This has implications in sinus surgery as nasalization, or the aggressive removal of turbinate tissue, may not only result in the removal of olfactory mucosa but can lead to the mucosa drying out with subsequent loss of the sense of smell.

Location of the olfactory epithelium

We still do not know the exact distribution of the functioning olfactory epithelium, so the surgeon should preserve potential olfactory mucosa at all cost (Fig. 17.7). The distribution of olfactory mucosa and functional neuroepithelium has been recently investigated by Leopold *et al.* with an electro-olfactogram and anatomically located biopsies. They concluded that the distribution of the olfactory mucosa is much more anterior to the lateral nasal wall and septum than was previously assumed.[20] The most likely location of functional olfactory epithelium is the dorsoposterior region of the nasal septum and the superior turbinate but, surprisingly, also more ventrally and anteriorly on both septum and turbinates.[21]

Volatile chemicals can be inhaled into the nasal cavity orthonasally through the nostrils or can enter retronasally via the mouth during swallowing.[9,22]

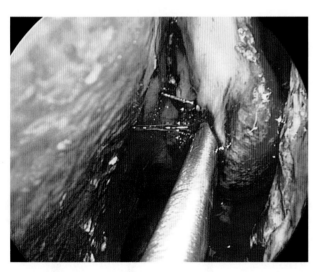

Figure 17.7   Intraoperative endoscopic view into the olfactory cleft in a patient with chronic rhinosinusitis and nasal polyps.

MEDICAL MANAGEMENT OF DISORDERED SMELL IN CHRONIC RHINOSINUSITIS

Hyposmia and anosmia are common symptoms in patients with CRS and polyposis. The more extensive the disease, the more likely the patient's sense of smell will be reduced. Before embarking on surgery, a trial of medical treatment

should take place. Even a proportion of patients with nasal polyps that fill the nasal vestibule can be successfully managed with medical treatment alone. In any event, it is useful to try to obtain an estimate of the 'olfactory reserve' that the patient has, so that they can be given an estimate as to how much, if any, their sense of smell might improve with surgery – followed by maintenance medical treatment (Fig. 17.8). This is particularly relevant if the patient does not achieve any sense of smell after maximum medical treatment as this may be a warning that they have no functioning olfactory mucosa.

Historically, medical treatment has often been started with local measures and then escalated. However, in a patient with hyposmia and nasal polyposis it is often helpful to give maximum medical treatment with oral steroids initially to minimize any nasal symptoms and then try to maintain this situation with topical treatment. Systemic steroids should be avoided in those with a history of risk factors, such as gastric ulceration, poorly controlled hypertension, diabetes, osteoporosis and psychosis. Patients should be warned of side effects, the most common being a change in mood, possibly with a disrupted sleep pattern, and stomach discomfort. Short courses are best to minimize any effect on the hypothalamic–pituitary–adrenal axis, and steroids are best taken in the morning when normal cortisol levels are highest. For patients with hyposmia or anosmia related to nasal polyps, oral steroids usually have an appreciable and gratifying result.

It needs to be stated that the term 'nasal polyps' is not a diagnosis but a sign of diseased mucosa whose pathology can vary. The aetiology of CRS with or without nasal polyps is contentious[4] and does not usually appear to be the result of an unresolved acute sinusitis, so much so that the preface to a text on the subject started by saying 'One of the most intriguing aspects of CRS is the growing appreciation that for most patients this is not an infectious disease'.[23] The treatment of idiopathic nasal polyposis is largely empirical. Treatment is centred on systemic and topical steroids, with 12 studies showing significant benefit compared with three that showed none.[4] Systemic steroids work well and although there have been no placebo-

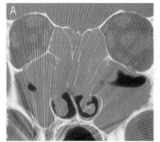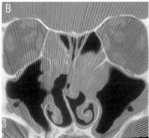

Figure 17.8   Computed tomography (CT) scan (A) before and (B) after medical management to estimate the olfactory reserve in a patient with chronic rhinosinusitis and nasal polyps.

controlled studies, other studies have shown a relationship between dose and response. No studies have quantified the benefit of medical treatment on olfaction in nasal polyps. In one study, patients were treated with systemic steroids and topical steroids and were then randomized to functional endoscopic sinus surgery (FESS) done on one side with the other remaining untouched. They were then given topical nasal steroids for another 12 months.[24] Their sense of smell was tested on each side separately. Surgery did not produce any added improvement although it helped nasal patency more, and a quarter required surgery on the unoperated side.[24]

In a randomized study of patients with CRS and polyps who remained symptomatic after 6 weeks of intensive medical treatment and then went on to receive either surgery or medical treatment, both groups had an improvement in their symptoms at 6 and 12 months with the only difference being that the surgical group had a larger nasal volume.[25] In another randomized study patients were either given oral steroids or endoscopic sinus surgery and both groups were given follow-up topical nasal steroids. At 6 and 12 months the Medical Outcome Survey Short Form 36 (SF-36) scores improved in both groups but the surgical group did better for nasal obstruction, sense of smell and polyp size at 6 months but only for polyp size at 12 months.[26] The European Position Paper on Rhinosinusitis and Nasal Polyps (EP3OS) concluded that 'In the majority of patients, appropriate medical treatment is as effective as surgical treatment. Sinus surgery should be reserved for patients who do not respond satisfactorily to medical treatment.'[4]

SINUS SURGERY AND OLFACTION IN CHRONIC RHINOSINUSITIS

A patient whose sense of smell returns after oral steroids, only to rapidly deteriorate thereafter in spite of maintenance treatment with topical nasal steroids, is the patient whose sense of smell may benefit from surgery. A patient with anosmia who has had previous surgery is unlikely to regain any sense of smell if systemic steroids have not helped as this indicates that there is unlikely to be a useful reserve of functioning olfactory mucosa. However, a patient with anosmia who has not had surgery previously and did not respond to oral steroids may still regain their sense of smell after a frontoethmoidectomy and gently lateralizing the middle turbinate. It is vital that the middle and superior turbinate are treated with meticulous care in these patients when the olfactory cleft is opened surgically (Fig. 17.9). We advise against suturing the middle turbinate to the septum as this closes the olfactory cleft. Lateralizing the middle turbinate after a frontoethmoidectomy may restrict direct endoscopic examination of the frontal recess after surgery but it rarely causes stenosis if the mucosa in this area is preserved.

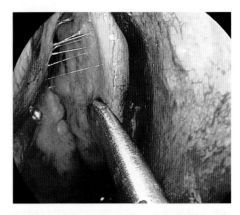

Figure 17.9   Lateralizing the middle turbinate after a fronto-sphenoethmoidectomy to expose the olfactory cleft to the airstream.

TAILORING THE SURGERY TO THE EXTENT OF THE PROBLEM

There is a price to be paid for the extensive removal of tissue. That price may be the loss of olfactory mucosa, frontonasal stenosis, altered sensation, dryness and an increased risk of violating the boundaries of the paranasal sinuses. Surgery is primarily aimed at improving ventilation of the sinuses and restoring paranasal mucociliary clearance. The removal of tissue alone does not cure mucosal disease. After a trial of maximum medical treatment including systemic and topical steroids it is possible to assess the 'olfactory reserve'. This will indicate the olfactory potential as long as the olfactory mucosa is preserved and the olfactory cleft opened.

Overzealous trimming of mucosa and turbinates results in an unphysiological distribution of airflow and much less airflow passing into the olfactory cleft. Endoscopic sinus surgery can affect the nasal airflow pattern because of the 'arched' main stream of airflow that passes the middle meatus with small eddy currents around the olfactory cleft. After surgery to the middle meatus, marked improvement in the nasal airway can potentially be achieved, especially in a narrow or congested nose. Furthermore, the gentle lateralization of the middle turbinate after sinus surgery helps to open up the olfactory cleft and allows much better air–mucosa contact in this area, which may help olfaction (Fig. 17.10).[1,5,18,19]

A COMMENT ON THE MANAGEMENT OF THE MIDDLE AND SUPERIOR TURBINATES

One of the main differences between this text and others is our concern for the sense of smell and our respect for turbinate and therefore olfactory tissue. Some authors have advocated resection of the middle turbinate to help access and with the aim of reducing the incidence of adhesions. We do not do this as we try to preserve all the olfactory

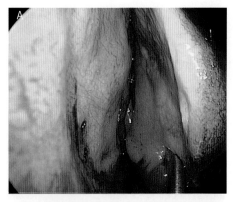

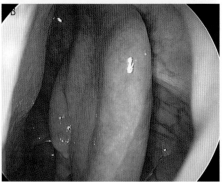

Figure 17.10 (A) Intraoperative view of lateralization of the middle turbinate to expose the olfactory cleft. (B) Postoperative view 1 year after the operation, with ongoing medical treatment with topical steroids.

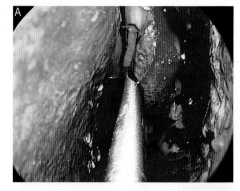

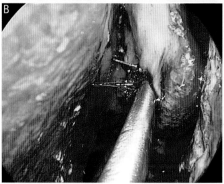

Figure 17.11 Intraoperative endoscopic view of (A) lateralization of the middle turbinate to check the patency of the maxillary sinusotomy (B) below the level of the middle turbinate.

mucosa on the medial surface of the ethmoturbinates and the septum.

The patient who has had anosmia or severe hyposmia may not 'miss' their sense of smell after surgery as it was poor in the first place. This has led surgeons to become complacent about the sense of smell, particularly in those with late-onset asthma and polyps medial to the middle turbinate, where the results of surgery have been mixed (70 per cent with hyposmia improve but this rarely lasts for longer than 6 months even in the presence of continued medical treatment). However, if a patient's sense of smell is restored their quality of life is much improved and they are extremely grateful. By preserving 'all' the mucosa in the olfactory area on the septum and the turbinates, as well as opening the olfactory cleft, this can be done.

The middle and superior turbinates should gently be lateralized after a complete sphenoethmoidectomy to open up the olfactory cleft. Atraumatic lateralization of the turbinates is only possible after making space for them. This reduces the mucosa/mucosa contact in this area and it allows better access for topical nasal steroids (Fig. 17.10). Although it is difficult to resist the temptation to remove or debulk polyps medial to the middle turbinate, it is best to preserve this mucosa. A course of preoperative steroids will help reduce the size of the polyps. Only remove polyps that come from the posterior ethmoid under the superior

turbinate and *not the polyps that originate from the septum or the middle turbinate.*

If a surgeon displaces the middle turbinate in this way they must also carry out a middle meatal antrostomy at a level below the inferior edge of the middle turbinate. In this way if the middle turbinate lateralizes the maxillary ostia can still drain and the maxillary sinusotomy and the frontal recess as well as the ethmoids can still be visualized with a 45° endoscope (Fig. 17.11). The middle turbinate should remain relatively stable as long as it is only gently lateralized and the base or inferior horizontal component of the ground lamella is preserved. Even when it is very mobile we would prefer to lateralize rather than for it to adhere to the septum and run the risk of making olfaction worse.

When the olfactory cleft is opened even large polyps medial to the middle turbinate resolve, so surgeons should not worry about leaving them behind. As stated above no polyps should be removed from the middle turbinate to preserve the olfactory mucosa. It is easy to remove them, but it is not easy to put back the olfactory epithelium that is removed with them.

IMPACT OF ENDOSCOPIC SINUS SURGERY ON OLFACTORY FUNCTION IN CHRONIC RHINOSINUSITIS

There is a strong suggestion in the literature that the degree of olfactory loss is correlated with disease severity.

Severe loss is usually associated with the presence of nasal polyposis.[27] In addition, patients with marked eosinophilia and aspirin intolerance experience a greater loss of their olfactory function.[28] Although many patients with Samter's triad often receive nasal surgery, in part to improve the sense of smell, relatively little research has been done to investigate the postoperative outcome. Our clinical impression is that these patients' sense of smell is difficult to preserve for any length of time in spite of maximum surgery and medical treatment. We need a better understanding of the disease to make more progress.[4]

Over many years little objective sensory testing has been done to investigate both the impact of CRS with nasal polyposis on olfactory function, and also the outcome of endoscopic sinus surgery.[3] Recent studies have included a quantitative assessment of smell.[28] The best improvements were obtained in patients with marked polyposis, eosinophilia and aspirin intolerance even though these patients started from a lower baseline. Neither age or presence of allergy or asthma, nor the number of previous surgical interventions had a significant impact on the outcome of surgery in terms of olfactory function. Overall in CRS with and without nasal polyps, only 1 out of 5 patients experienced a measurable improvement of olfactory function. These results were obtained 6–12 months after surgery. Currently information about the long-term results is lacking, as is information about the impact of medical treatment in maintaining olfaction. Clearly this is an area where there is a need and some potential for some improvement. This chapter has outlined our strategy to help patients preserve or regain their sense of smell and we are in the process of collecting long-term data to corroborate these ideas.

KEY MESSAGES

- Olfactory dysfunction is most commonly caused by CRS with nasal polyposis.
- Smell is a sense that is all too often forgotten and may escape the notice of both surgeons and patients.
- Optimizing the medical treatment of mucosal disease is important in providing symptomatic relief either on its own or in conjunction with surgery.
- Routine preoperative smell testing is advisable in assessing patients prior to surgery.
- Olfactory function correlates with disease severity.
- Far less or no surgery is needed if medical treatment has been successful.
- In severe olfactory loss in CRS with nasal polyposis, on average, the objective measures of olfaction improve significantly after endoscopic sinus surgery – particularly if the olfactory cleft is widened.
- Patients with polyposis and eosinophilia experience the greatest improvement in olfactory scores, perhaps because they start from a lower baseline.

- Impairment of smell might be the first sign of recurrence of nasal disease and helps to motivate the patient to comply with long-term medical treatment.

REFERENCES

1. Dalton P. Olfaction and anosmia in rhinosinusitis. *Curr Allergy Asthma Rep* 2004; **4**: 230–6.
2. Van Toller S. Assessing the impact of anosmia: review of a questionnaire's finding. *Chem Senses* 1999; **24**: 705–12.
3. Doty R, Mishra A. Olfaction and its alteration by nasal obstruction, rhinitis and rhinosinusitis. *Laryngoscope* 2001; **111**: 409–23.
4. Fokkens WJ, Lund VJ, Mullol J *et al*. European position paper on rhinosinusitis and nasal polyposis. *Rhinology* 2007; **20** Suppl: 1–88.
5. Kern CR. Chronic sinusitis and anosmia. Pathologic changes in the olfactory mucosa. *Laryngoscope* 2000; **110**: 1071–7.
6. Jones NS, Rog D. Olfaction: a review. *J Laryngol Otol* 1998; **11**: 11–24.
7. Estrem SA, Renner G. Disorders of smell and taste. *Otolaryngol Clin North Am* 1987; **20**: 133–47.
8. Seiden AM, Duncan J. The diagnosis of a conductive olfactory loss. *Laryngoscope* 2001; **111**: 9–14.
9. Landis BN, Frasnelli J, Reden J *et al*. Differences between orthonasal and retronasal olfactory functions in patients with loss of the sense of smell. *Arch Otolaryngol Head Neck Surg* 2005; **131**: 977–81.
10. Briner HR, Simmen D, Jones N. Impaired sense of smell in patients with nasal surgery. *Clin Otolaryngol* 2003; **28**: 417–19.
11. Doty RL, Shaman P, Kimmelman CP *et al*. University of Pennsylvania smell identification test: A rapid quantitative olfactory function test for the clinic. *Laryngoscope* 1984; **94**:176–8.
12. Doty RL, Marcus A, Lee WW. Development of the 12-item cross-cultural smell identification test (CC-SIT). *Laryngoscope* 1996; **106**: 353–6.
13. Hashimoto Y, Fukazawa K, Fujii M *et al*. Usefulness of the odour stick identification test for Japanese patients with olfactory dysfunction. *Chem Senses* 2004; **29**: 565–71.
14. Nordin S, Nyroos M. Applicability of the Scandinavian odour identification test: a Finnish-Swedish comparison. *Acta Otolaryngol* 2002; **122**: 294–7.
15. Briner HR, Simmen D. Smell diskettes as screening test of olfaction. *Rhinology* 1999; **37**: 145–8.
16. Kobal G, Hummel T, Sekinger B *et al*. 'Sniffin' Sticks': screening of olfactory performance. *Rhinology* 1996; **34**: 222–6.
17. Jackman A, Doty R. Utility of a three-item smell identification test in detecting olfactory dysfunction. *Laryngoscope* 2005; **115**: 2209–12.
18. Lee HP, Poh HJ, Chong FH *et al*. Changes of airflow pattern in inferior turbinate hypertrophy – a computational fluid dynamics model. *Am J Rhinol Allergy* 2009; **23**: 153–8.

19. Simmen DB, Scherrer JL, Moe K *et al.* A dynamic direct visualization model for the study of nasal airflow. *Arch Otolaryngol Head Neck Surg* 1999; **125**: 1015–21.

20. Leopold DA, Hummel T, Schwob JE *et al.* Anterior distribution of human olfactory epithelium. *Laryngoscope* 2000; **110**: 417–21.

21. Feron F, Perry C, Mc Grath JJ *et al.* New techniques for biopsy and culture of human olfactory epithelial neurons. *Arch Otolaryngol Head Neck Surg* 1998; **124**: 861–6.

22. Shepert GM. The human sense of smell: are we better than we think. *Biology* 2004; **2**: 572–5.

23. Ferguson BJ, Seiden AM. Chronic rhinosinusitis. *Otolaryngol Clin North Am* 2005; **36**: 1–1393.

24. Blomqvist EH, Lundbald L, Anggard A *et al.* A randomized controlled study evaluating medical treatment versus surgical treatment in addition to medical treatment of nasal polyposis. *J Allergy Clin Immunol* 2001; **107**: 224–8.

25. Ragab SM, Lund VJ, Scadding G. Evaluation of the medical and surgical treatment of chronic rhinosinusitis: a prospective, randomised, controlled trial. *Laryngoscope* 2004; **114**: 923–30.

26. Alobid I, Benitez P, Bernal-Sprekelsen M *et al.* Nasal polyposis and its impact on quality of life: Comparison between the effects of medical and surgical treatments. *Allergy* 2005; **60**: 452–8.

27. Apter AJ, Mott AE, Frank ME *et al.* Allergic rhinitis and olfactory loss. *Ann Allergy Asthma Immunol* 1995; **75**: 311–16.

28. Pade J, Hummel T. Olfactory function following nasal surgery. *Laryngoscope* 2008; **118**: 1260–4.

18

Postoperative management

VIJAY R RAMAKRISHNAN, JAMES N PALMER

GOALS

The postoperative management of patients may be of equal importance to patient outcome as the surgery itself. Attention to detail in postoperative management will optimize the results of the surgery, but it requires attention, time and skill. With such attention, the most common postoperative complications (bleeding, crusting, infection, synechiae, ostial stenosis and middle turbinate lateralization) may be minimized.

The postoperative management of the patient begins preoperatively and then continues in the operating room, and until the patient's symptoms have stabilized and the endoscopic examination becomes normal. The time period for this varies from patient to patient, but often lasts up to 2 years.

PERIOPERATIVE SETTING

Planning for the postoperative result begins with the preoperative environment. Medical treatment aimed at decreasing inflammation will reduce perioperative bleeding and reduce the likelihood of surgical complications as well as improve postoperative success. In the setting of active infection, culture-directed antibiotics should be used preoperatively or at the time of surgery to decrease inflammation. The use of antibiotics is not indicated for the unattainable goal of sinus sterilization, where the presence of polyps or stagnant inspissated mucopus makes this unlikely. Systemic steroids are administered preoperatively in patients with polyps with the goal of decreasing inflammation. A typical preoperative regimen for a patient with polyps would consist of 40 mg of prednisone in a man of average build, 30 mg in a woman, given orally for 5 days leading up to the surgery.

The medical management of patients with diabetes or hypertension has to be monitored, and other interactions and contraindications taken into consideration. Medication and herbal supplements known to cause coagulopathy or platelet dysfunction are stopped beforehand, e.g. aspirin, clopidogrel, gingko biloba extract. Abstinence from tobacco use is ideal. Tobacco has been shown to have deleterious effects on epithelial cell turnover and ciliary function, two crucial components of recovery after sinus surgery (Fig. 18.1). Multiple studies have demonstrated poorer surgical outcomes, higher rates of revision and decreased endoscopic improvement in patients who smoke.[1-3] Normal sinonasal epithelium has a cell turnover and

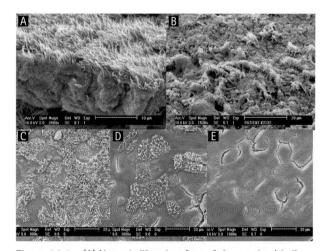

Figure 18.1 (A) Normal ciliated surface of sinonasal epithelium with 1 per cent regeneration. (B) After surgery, 20 per cent regeneration rate is normal. (C) Normal development of cilia in air–liquid interface cultures at 1 week. (D, E) Sparse to no development of cilia when it attempts regeneration in the presence of tobacco smoke extract.

new cilia formation rate of 1 per cent. Immediately after surgery or severe infection, that turnover rate increases to 20 per cent. Unfortunately, tobacco smoke exposure impairs ciliary function. Therefore, smoke exposure in the postoperative period is far more damaging to the sinonasal epithelium than in the non-operated patient, and may help explain the extremely poor outcomes seen from sinus surgery when it is carried out in tobacco smokers.

At the onset of surgery, intravenous dexamethasone is administered for its antiemetic and potential anti-inflammatory effects, and it may alleviate fatigue encountered in the postoperative period. Prophylactic antibiotics are not routinely used, as sterilization of the paranasal sinuses is not achievable. It should be noted that use of preoperative intravenous antibiotics may interfere with the result of any culture taken during endoscopic surgery. In the setting of orbital or intracranial penetration, intravenous antibiotics are administered due to the introduction of bacteria into otherwise sterile environments. Ampicillin with a β-lactamase inhibitor is preferred for orbital prophylaxis, and a third-generation cephalosporin such as ceftriaxone for intracranial prophylaxis, given its excellent cerebrospinal fluid penetration. Cultures are obtained wherever possible, and antibiotics are then prescribed on the basis of culture and bacterial sensitivity.

IMMEDIATE POSTOPERATIVE SETTING

On completion of the surgical dissection, consideration must be given to haemostasis, the management of the turbinates and the need for spacers or stents. For mucosal oozing, consider the use of topical oxymetazoline, adrenaline (epinephrine), thrombin or microfibrillar collagen, a fine form of oxidized cellulose (Surgicel Fibrillar). Several haemostatic formulations are in development, but previous formulations have created scarring and inflammation. Nasal packing or spacers may be used for haemostasis and can also serve to maintain the position of the middle turbinate and simplify postoperative debridement. Studies have documented patient discomfort with the use of nasal packs.[4] However, nasal packs with a *smooth* surface, and their removal, rate quite low on visual analogue scales of patient discomfort.[5]

We routinely use middle meatal spacers and thin Silastic frontal sinus stents. The middle meatal spacers are fashioned from Merocel sponges placed in a non-latex glove finger, and sutured in place through the anterior septum to prevent risk of dislodgement or aspiration. The glove finger is used to help reduce patient discomfort during removal. The gloved sponges serve a haemostatic function, prevent accumulation of blood, mucus, and fibrinous debris in the surgical cavity, and retain a wide middle meatus for ease of postoperative care and examination[6] (Fig. 18.2).

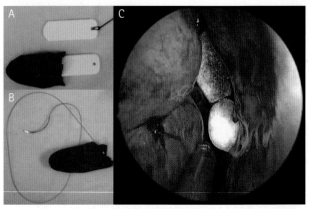

Figure 18.2   A middle meatal spacer keeps the middle turbinate medialized and decreases blood and debris accumulation in the middle meatus. (A) Merocel sponge placed inside non-latex finger cot to prevent ingrowth of mucosa into the cells of the sponge. (B) Finger cot closed over sponge with suture, needle used to tether spacer to the septum. (C) Spacer in place, inflated with saline and sewn to the septum. Average removal time is 1 week.

In the past, the use of frontal sinus stents has been routinely condemned by several surgeons for being responsible for poor postoperative results, particularly when the stents produced pressure on bone or mucosa, as they were thought to damage mucosa and enhance fibrosis. Such stents were often cylindrical, applied pressure to the surrounding tissue and were often left in place for 6 weeks to 6 months. We believe that there are two reasons for this strategy to fail. First, because of the pressure they can apply, and second, that bacterial biofilms can form on frontal recess stents in as short a time as 4 weeks (Fig. 18.3). Our current plan after frontal recess dissection is to fashion a stent or dressing in a 2 × 4 cm 'liberty bell' configuration from a thin Silastic sheet (0.5 mm). Side-to-side 90° giraffe forceps are used to gently place the stent in the frontal recess and unfurl the edges in the frontal sinus (Fig. 18.4). The frontal sinus stent is placed to limit the amount of fibrinous exudates that can provide a matrix for fibrous tissue to form in the frontal recess, and after the stent has been removed it makes debridement of this area substantially simpler to do in the office. It applies minimum pressure to the surrounding mucosa.

Prior to extubation, an orogastric tube is passed and the gastro-oesophageal contents are suctioned. Deep extubation is preferred to minimize straining and coughing. A smooth wake-up is favourable to minimize the bleeding caused by an increase in venous pressure particularly when mucosal inflammation is severe, and it is necessary for extended approaches that involve cerebrospinal fluid (CSF) leaks, intracranial or intraorbital dissection. The use of total intravenous anaesthesia (TIVA) and the administration of intravenous dexamethasone prior to surgery can help reduce coughing, nausea and vomiting postoperatively. In addition, the use of a laryngeal mask airway (LMA) eliminates tracheal irritation and coughing,

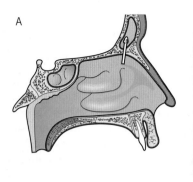
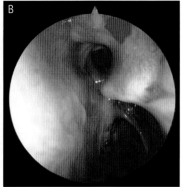
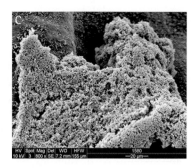

Figure 18.3   Previous (and often problematic) use of frontal sinus stents. (A) Schematic of stent placement through frontal recess into frontal sinus. (B) Cylinder-shaped collar of scar formation at the 6-week removal point. (C) Scanning electron microscopy image of bacterial biofilm formation on stent after only 4 weeks of placement.

and it is preferred over an endotracheal tube in the appropriate patient. A good working relationship with the anaesthesiologist is extremely helpful.

In the recovery room, the head of the bed is elevated to at least 30°, a moustache-type gauze dressing is placed beneath the nose if mild bleeding occurs, and an ice pack may be placed across the face or neck for comfort. Humidified oxygen is delivered via face tent as needed. Visual and mental status examinations are performed if indicated.

ROUTINE POSTOPERATIVE INSTRUCTION

On discharge, patients are instructed to restrict some of their activities. They are advised to abstain from heavy lifting and strenuous activity, and avoid aggressive nose blowing. A regular diet is resumed at the patient's discretion. Patients are instructed to perform gentle nasal saline irrigation twice a day beginning on postoperative day 1, and to use nasal saline sprays liberally. Patients are provided with a narcotic analgesic and are instructed to use stool softeners as needed to prevent constipation associated with the narcotic medication. Pain medication may quickly be tapered to paracetamol as needed. Salicylates and non-steroidal anti-inflammatory analgesics

are avoided for approximately 2 weeks. Patients are instructed to check their temperature and notify the office if it is greater than 37.5 °C (101.5 °F). Risk of toxic shock syndrome is low, but should be considered in the case of postoperative fever and rash.

MANAGEMENT OF POSTOPERATIVE EPISTAXIS

A small amount of bleeding may occur in the days after surgery, even if packing or spacers are used. In the normotensive patient without coagulopathy, topical oxymetazoline spray may be sufficient. If topical oxymetazoline is unable to control the bleeding an endoscopic examination is done. If the site of bleeding can be localized, focal unipolar or bipolar cautery is preferred over any broad topical therapy. If a single site cannot be localized, consider topical haemostatic materials, such as collagen, gelatin, hyaluronic acid, or cellulose-based formulations. One must be aware that certain agents, such as FloSeal, may increase the risk of short-term granulation and subsequent formation of adhesions.[7,8] Of the existing haemostatic formulations, we prefer a slurry of microfibrillar collagen which may be introduced via a 14-gauge or 16-gauge angiocatheter. Very rarely, arterial ligation or angiography with embolization is necessary.

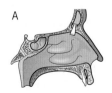
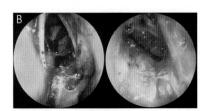
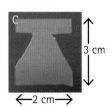
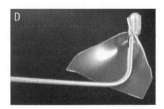

Figure 18.4   Alternative frontal sinus stent/dressing. (A) Schematic of placement of stent/dressing. (B) Dressing *in situ* covering most of cut edges of mucosa in the frontal recess (left panel) and immediately on removal (right panel). (C) The dressing is made from cut 0.5 mm Silastic sheet and (D) placed with giraffe forceps.

MEDICAL THERAPY

Medical therapy plays the key role in the acute and long-term management of the postoperative sinus patient. Postoperative medical therapy is slightly different for three surgical categories: chronic sinusitis, chronic sinusitis with nasal polyps or significant inflammation, and skull base or orbital surgery. However, the mainstay for all three is medical therapy that includes saline irrigation, topical and systemic corticosteroids, and culture-directed antibiotics.

After sinus surgery, mucociliary function is inhibited to some degree for at least 6–12 weeks.[9] Gentle saline irrigation is instituted twice daily beginning on day 1 to aid the clearance of secretions during this time period, and reduce crusting and oedema. Solutions may be mixed by the patient or purchased in prepared formulations. We prefer large volumes of isotonic saline, with a minimum of 500 mL irrigated twice daily. Patients are encouraged to use an irrigation apparatus that may be cleaned regularly. Depending on the patient's disease, topical antibiotics, antifungals, steroids, mucolytics or surfactants may be added to the solution. The importance of not smoking is continually stressed for the reasons discussed.

Oral antibiotics are routinely prescribed postoperatively. Antibiotic therapy is generally initiated after a culture has been performed. There is evidence that the underlying bone may be part of the inflammatory process, creating osteitis.[10] We prefer the combination of clindamycin and trimethoprim–sulfamethoxazole for 2 weeks. This antibiotic combination covers most groups of bacteria thought to be pathological in chronic rhinosinusitis. One must remember the differences in microbiology in chronic rhinosinusitis from that most commonly encountered in acute infections. *Staphylococcus aureus*, Gram-negative rods such as *Pseudomonas aeruginosa* and anaerobic organisms are prevalent in chronic rhinosinusitis. Clindamycin is prescribed at 150 mg orally three times daily and at this dose no patients have developed pseudomembranous colitis in our practice. Other appropriate choices may be amoxicillin–clavulanate, cephalosporins and quinolones. Patients are encouraged to supplement their diets with *Acidophilus*, either by tablet or live active culture in commercially available yoghurt.

Postoperative oral steroid medication is used fairly liberally in patients with nasal polyps or significant inflammation, but not in the absence of visible inflammatory changes. Dosage and duration of oral prednisone may vary based on the severity of inflammation and patient weight. A typical regimen for patients with nasal polyposis or extensive inflammation encountered intraoperatively consists of 0.2 mg/kg/day of prednisone daily for 1 month, it is then tapered to 0.1 mg/kg/day for 2 weeks, then 0.1 mg/kg/day every other day for 2 weeks. As the systemic corticosteroids are tapered off, topical therapy is initiated.

Topical therapies are of great benefit postoperatively and both sprays and irrigations have been shown to penetrate the sinuses more thoroughly after surgery.[11] Intranasal corticosteroids appear to have a number of benefits for the postoperative patient. Drug distribution is improved in the postoperative patient, and the subsequent anti-inflammatory effect is known to delay or prevent polyp recurrence.[12] A 5-year prospective, randomized, double-blind, placebo-controlled study demonstrated improved patient subjective scores and endoscopic scores, as well as a decreased need for the administration of oral steroids.[13] Intranasal steroids may also have a beneficial effect on mucosal innate immunity, and their use is associated with a decreased colonization by *S. aureus*, a common postoperative pathogen.[14] Culture-directed topical therapy with mupirocin has been effective for *S. aureus*, and gentamicin for *Pseudomonas*.[15]

Budesonide respules (Pulmicort 0.5 mg/2 mL) may be mixed into saline irrigations or applied directly twice daily for higher potency. Anecdotally, this is highly effective. Topical steroid drops may also be used to target the frontal recess specifically, if this is an area of concern. Mygind's head hanging position is favoured to direct steroid drops into the frontal recess. The patient is instructed to assume a supine position, and instil a few drops near the frontal recess on each side, and stay in a head-hanging position for approximately 15 minutes. The position is well tolerated, and a directed instillation for this time period provides mucosal contact to the appropriate area. If the patient cannot tolerate Mygind's position, consider Moffat's position (see Chapter 4 for details).

FOLLOW–UP AND DEBRIDEMENT

The role of postoperative debridement is a matter of controversy as we lack well-designed studies. There is expert consensus on the need for some degree of debridement and manipulation in the postoperative setting. Debridement of crusts, fibrinous debris, blood clot and bone chips is necessary to achieve a successful long-term result. Cleaning the operative cavity can decrease the likelihood of infection by the removal of debris that is a medium for bacteria and reduce mucus trapping. The serial removal of fibrinous debris decreases the scaffolding that allows synechiae to form or turbinates to adhere to adjacent tissue. During debridement, visible bone fragments should be removed to minimize the risk of scarring, osteitis and chronic inflammation. Excellent long-term results and low incidence of synechiae formation has been credited to meticulous postoperative debridement.[2,16] However, this can be uncomfortable for the patient, and may even create new epithelial injury. Within the first week, the removal of crusts was found to be associated with a 23 per cent incidence of new epithelial avulsion, a finding which is absent with crust debridement at 2 weeks postoperatively.[17] It should be noted that normal mucociliary clearance does

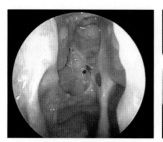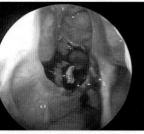

Figure 18.5 Paired images of sphenoid sinus ostia before and after debridement in the office. A J-curette and a mushroom punch were used to open the stenotic ostium.

not return for at least 6 weeks after surgery. Debridement supplements the use of saline washes until mucociliary clearance returns.

In the past, postoperative debridement was carried out daily during the first postoperative week.[18] Our current postoperative routine is based only on many years of experience. We currently remove middle meatal spacers and debride at 1 week, remove frontal sinus stents and debride at 2 weeks, and then examine and debride at 4 weeks. The degree and frequency of debridement are tailored to the procedure performed and to the individual patient. As described, biofilm formation has been documented on frontal sinus stents as early as 3 weeks, so removal should be performed prior to this time.[19]

At each visit, the nasal cavities are sprayed with topical ephedrine and 2 per cent tetracaine (Pontocaine) for decongestion and anaesthesia. Under endoscopic visualization, the middle meatus, sphenoid sinus and ethmoid cavities are cleaned with 7–10 French Frazier-style suction instruments. Otological instruments may be used in this setting. Fibrinous debris left at the sphenoid ostium can contribute to scarring and stenosis of its ostium (Fig. 18.5) and other sinuses can similarly be affected. If this occurs, a 3 mm curved olive-tip suction instrument is used with angled telescopes to clean the maxillary sinus, with particular attention to debriding any fibrinous tissue that can accumulate at the natural ostium. Attention is then turned superiorly with the same instruments, as well as additional specialized frontal punches, probes and through-cutters, to the frontal recess (Fig. 18.6). Confirmation of patency with the removal of debris from

the region of the frontal ostium and being able to pass small curved suction tips into the sinuses is ideal. In the clinic, surgical touch-ups can be performed as needed for the treatment of unfavourable scarring, to release synechiae, remove additional cell partitions or open stenotic ostia. Angled telescopes are necessary for full visualization of certain areas, such as the natural ostium of the maxillary sinus (Fig. 18.7). Small scar bands are easily managed in the office, and can prevent the recirculation phenomenon. Topical 4 per cent cocaine or injections of 1 per cent lidocaine may be used as needed for patient comfort (Fig. 18.8).

MANAGEMENT OF CONCURRENT DISEASE

Surgeons must never forget that surgery for chronic rhinosinusitis functions as a partial treatment for an ongoing medical disease process. The pathogenesis of inflammatory sinonasal disorders has a multifactorial aetiology. Each patient is unique in their presence of comorbid disease or risk factors, and each should be individually addressed. Smoking cessation, aggressive treatment of allergic disease and treatment of aspirin sensitivity is often helpful. A team approach with allergy and pulmonary consultation is recommended. Aspirin desensitization has been shown to decrease the frequency of sinus infections, polyp regrowth, use of systemic steroids, need for revision surgery and asthma-related hospitalizations, as well as improve the sense of smell in this subset of chronic rhinosinusitis patients.[20,21]

Culture-directed antibiotics or antifungals are indicated when pathological organisms are identified in the postoperative patient. Rarely, bacterial resistance to oral drug options may direct a patient towards a 6- or 8-week course of intravenous therapy. The indications for intravenous antibiotics in chronic rhinosinusitis patients are rare, and anti-inflammatory avenues of therapy should be exhausted first.[22] Our use of intravenous antibiotics has been restricted to cases in which infectious orbital or intracranial complications have been identified. We do not use intravenous antibiotic therapy for refractory chronic rhinosinusitis, with the belief that the outcome from this type of therapy does not offset its cost or side effects. Sterilization of the sinuses is an unrealistic goal. Instead, liberal irrigations and oral antibiotics are administered to

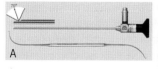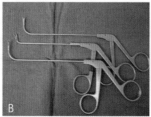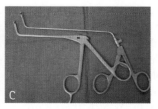

Figure 18.6 Advanced equipment is required for optimal results from endoscopic sinus surgery. (A) 45° and 70° endoscopes provide superior visualization in the frontal recess. (B, C) Angled through-cutting forceps and punches are necessary to perform complete debridement postoperatively.

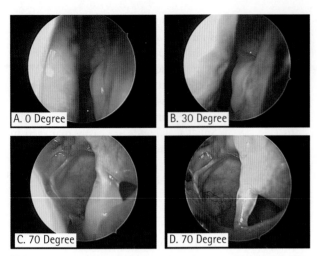

Figure 18.7 Endoscopic images in a postoperative patient with persistent postnasal drainage. (A, B) 0° and 30° endoscopes do not allow easy diagnosis. (C, D) 70° endoscopic view easily shows the recirculation phenomenon secondary to the natural ostium of the right maxillary sinus not meeting the surgically created ostium.

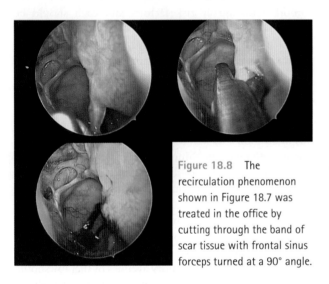

Figure 18.8 The recirculation phenomenon shown in Figure 18.7 was treated in the office by cutting through the band of scar tissue with frontal sinus forceps turned at a 90° angle.

decrease the bacterial load in expectation of the return of normal sinonasal flora.

CONCLUSION

Postoperative care for the sinus patient begins in the operating room and continues until symptoms resolve and endoscopic examination becomes normal. In some patients, this may last indefinitely. The goals for postoperative management include: the prevention of major and minor surgical complications, optimizing the surgical outcome and treating what is often a chronic disease to achieve a long-lasting result. As such, there is no set routine for postoperative care; rather the specifics of management should be tailored to the individual patient and the disease process. The mainstay of postoperative care includes perioperative and postoperative medical therapy, attention to debridement and the treatment of concurrent disease.

REFERENCES

1. Kennedy DW. Prognostic factors, outcomes and staging in ethmoid sinus surgery. *Laryngoscope* 1992; **102**: 1–18.
2. Senior BA, Kennedy DW, Tanabodee J *et al.* Long-term results of functional endoscopic sinus surgery. *Laryngoscope* 1998; **108**: 151–7.
3. Smith TL, Mendolia-Loffredo S, Loehrl TA *et al.* Predictive factors and outcomes in endoscopic sinus surgery for chronic rhinosinusitis. *Laryngoscope* 2005; **115**: 2199–205.
4. Mo JH, Han DH, Shin HW *et al.* No packing versus packing after endoscopic sinus surgery: pursuit of patients' comfort after surgery. *Am J Rhinol* 2008; **22**: 525–8.
5. Cruise AS, Amonoo-Kuofi K, Srouji I *et al.* A randomized trial of Rapid Rhino Riemann and Telfa nasal packs following endoscopic sinus surgery. *Clin Otolaryngol* 2006; **31**: 25–32.
6. Hockstein NG, Bales CB, Palmer JN. Transseptal suture to secure middle meatal spacers. *Ear Nose Throat J* 2006; **85**: 47–8.
7. Chandra RK, Conley DB, Kern RC. The effect of FloSeal on mucosal healing after endoscopic sinus surgery: a comparison with thrombin-soaked gelatin foam. *Am J Rhinol* 2003; **17**: 51–5.
8. Chandra RK, Conley DB, Haines GK 3rd *et al.* Long-term effects of FloSeal packing after endoscopic sinus surgery. *Am J Rhinol* 2005; **19**: 240–3.
9. Gross CW, Gross WE. Post-operative care for functional endoscopic sinus surgery. *Ear Nose Throat J* 1994; **73**: 476–9.
10. Kennedy DW, Senior BA, Gannon FH *et al.* Histology and histomorphometry of ethmoid bone in chronic rhinosinusitis. *Laryngoscope* 1998; **108**: 502–7.
11. Harvey RJ, Goddard JC, Wise SK *et al.* Effects of endoscopic sinus surgery and delivery device on cadaver sinus irrigation. *Otolaryngol Head Neck Surg* 2008; **139**: 137–42.
12. Stjärne P, Olsson P, Alenius M. Use of mometasone furoate to prevent polyp relapse after endoscopic sinus surgery. *Arch Otolaryngol Head Neck Surg* 2009; **135**: 296–302.
13. Rowe-Jones JM, Medcalf M, Durham SR *et al.* Functional endoscopic sinus surgery: 5 year follow up and results of a prospective, randomized, stratified, double-blind, placebo controlled study of postoperative fluticasone propionate aqueous nasal spray. *Rhinology* 2005; **43**: 2–10.
14. Desrosiers M, Abdolmohsen H, Frenkiel S *et al.* Intranasal corticosteroid use is associated with lower rates of bacterial recovery in chronic rhinosinusitis. *Otolaryngol Head Neck Surg* 2007; **136**: 605–9.

15. Ha KR, Psaltis AJ, Butcher AR *et al.* In vitro activity of mupirocin on clinical isolates of *Staphylococcus aureus* and its potential implications in chronic rhinosinusitis. *Laryngoscope* 2008; **118**: 535–40.

16. Bernstein JM, Lebowitz RA, Jacobs JB. Initial report on postoperative healing after endoscopic sinus surgery with the microdebrider. *Otolaryngol Head Neck Surg* 1998; **118**: 800–3.

17. Kuhn FA, Citardi MJ. Advances in postoperative care following functional endoscopic sinus surgery. *Otolaryngol Clin North Am* 1997; **30**: 479–90.

18. Lanza DC, Kennedy DW. Current concepts in the surgical management of chronic and recurrent acute sinusitis. *J Allergy Clin Immunol* 1992; **90**: 505–10.

19. Perloff JR, Palmer JN. Evidence of bacterial biofilms on frontal recess stents in patients with chronic rhinosinusitis. *Am J Rhinol* 2004; **18**: 377–80.

20. Rozsasi A, Polzehl D, Deutschle T *et al.* Long-term treatment with aspirin desensitization: a prospective clinical trial comparing 100 and 300 mg aspirin daily. *Allergy* 2008; **63**: 1228–34.

21. Stevenson DD, Hankammer MA, Mathison DA *et al.* Aspirin desensitization treatment of aspirin-sensitive patients with rhinosinusitis-asthma: long-term outcomes. *J Allergy Clin Immunol* 1996; **98**: 751–8.

22. Gross ND, McInnes RJ, Hwang PH. Outpatient intravenous antibiotics for chronic rhinosinusitis. *Laryngoscope* 2002; **112**: 1758–61.

19

Helping patients

NICHOLAS JONES

EXPECTATIONS

What do patients expect when they see a doctor? Some will have well-formed ideas whereas others will come with an open mind. It is worth finding out what the main motives for the visit are before examining the patient, and particularly before embarking on any recommendation about treatment. A sizeable proportion of patients come to seek reassurance that they do not have cancer or a life-threatening illness and that is all they want.

Patients might reasonably be expected to want a diagnosis, a prognosis, an explanation of their symptoms in the light of the disease process and a treatment plan. However, they may have a preconception that their disease is due to a process that differs from the medical diagnosis. This is often the case in patients with 'sinus headache', facial pain or catarrh as discussed in Chapter 2. It is worth taking time to discover what the patient's understanding of their disease process is so that their ideas about their symptoms and disease can be taken into consideration when explaining the medical construct of these processes.

Reassurance may be readily received with a clear explanation that outlines the cause of the patient's symptoms and addresses their concerns. However, in a small proportion of anxious individuals, the effect of firm reassurance after a thorough examination and explanation may fade. It is often counterproductive to ask these individuals to return as this may reinforce their concerns that the doctor may have some ongoing doubt. It may help to say to the patient that you will send them a copy of your letter to the referring doctor for them to read and take in their own time.

Patients often feel vulnerable when they come to see a specialist in secondary care.[1] It helps if you put the patient at ease as much as possible and be open, clear and supportive. Some patients come hoping for, if not expecting, a cure of their symptoms. Many find it difficult to accept that there is no cure, paradoxically particularly if they regard their diagnosis as 'minor', as the media often report advances in the management of what are perceived as more complex disease processes.

Several studies have found that over 75 per cent of patients have tried alternative therapy before seeking specialist advice. Many have surfed the internet for advice, but it is not easy for anyone without experience to decipher what is good or bad information. If patients attend with printed extracts it is worth studying these in front of the patient, time allowing, so that they can see that your advice is given having considered this information.

Anyone offering medical advice should not overplay the benefit of any treatment they propose. To be overenthusiastic or excessively optimistic runs the risk of the patient being both disappointed and disgruntled. That does not mean that all sense of hope for an improvement should be dashed but it is wise to qualify what the patient might realistically expect. This situation is not helped by claims that a treatment 'works' or has been shown to produce a 'statistically significant improvement' when in reality the studies on which these are based only show that the mean patient symptom score has reduced from 8 to 6 out of 10 in severity, in other words the patients still had a mean symptom score of 6 out of 10. Look at how many studies show high residual symptom scores or fail to improve some symptoms particularly in subgroups such as those with aspirin sensitivity and asthma.[2,3]

EXPLANATIONS

It is worth taking time to listen to the patient so that they feel that their viewpoint has been taken seriously. Listening is as important, if not more, as providing an explanation. Make an effort to let the patient know that you can appreciate their viewpoint however much it may differ from your own. Only then through a clear explanation might you be able to help them understand a different explanation for their symptoms.

It may be difficult to help a patient to accept that their symptoms are due to a variation in the normal spectrum of what is many people's experience. Surgery is sometimes thought by some to be the solution to their symptoms, particularly if a relative or a primary care doctor has encouraged this idea. Using analogies such as 'asthma of the nose' in chronic rhinosinusitis with idiopathic nasal polyposis and that surgery cannot cure these polyps any more than it can cure asthma can be helpful (Fig. 19.1).

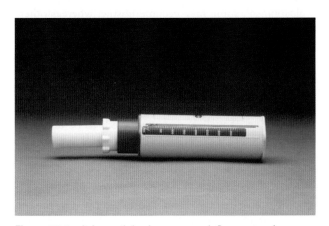

Figure 19.1   It is worth having some peak flow meters in a rhinology clinic given the frequent coexistence of upper and lower respiratory tract disease. Explaining to a patient with idiopathic nasal polyposis that it is like 'asthma of the nose' may help them to understand that surgery can no more be a cure for that than it can be for asthma.

Some symptoms are more readily improved, for example in patients who have idiopathic nasal polyps whose main complaint is nasal obstruction, whereas symptoms of headache or catarrh may not be helped.[4] If medical treatment is advocated then emphasize the need for compliance when this is important and mention the length of time they will be expected to take their medication (Fig. 19.2). Few patients like the prospect of a lifetime relying on regular medication so it may be helpful to suggest that every 6 months, or perhaps less, they have a holiday from their medication and see if their symptoms return. It is important to mention that if their symptoms return that they may need to be patient, as they were with their first course of treatment, as it may take a few weeks for the treatment to regain symptomatic benefit.

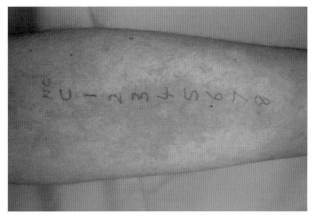

Figure 19.2   Skin prick tests show the patient that they have an intrinsic problem that will not be cured by surgery. The tests help explain to the patient with allergic rhinitis that it is their body's response and the reaction of the lining of their airway to inhaled allergens that is the problem and that treatment will be needed to reduce their reaction while their immune response reacts in this way.

CONSENT

In taking informed consent it is helpful to discuss what would happen without any treatment, what alternative treatment modalities exist (medical, different surgical procedures, alternative therapy) and their risks, the result of any personal audit or referring to the published complication rate, the likely outcome, what is involved, and what they might expect after treatment in both the short and long term.

It is worth discussing the symptoms that the patient may not have mentioned. For example the sense of smell may be reduced or have been lost in someone with idiopathic nasal polyps yet they may not mention this symptom. It may, or may not, return after surgery with concurrent medical treatment but the patient needs to be made aware of this. They may be grateful when their sense of smell returns after surgery only to be disappointed and possibly dissatisfied if it deteriorates after some time. Likewise, patients who are to have surgery for paranasal sinus disease and who have facial pain or headaches should be made aware that these symptoms may not be due to their sinuses and that they may need further medical treatment to deal with these symptoms if they fail to go, or return days, weeks or several months after their sinus surgery.

PREPARATION FOR SURGERY

If surgery is to be done then patients appreciate being given clear advice about the practical aspects of what they should do beforehand and afterwards in order to help them plan appropriately. For example, the need to stop medication or alternative treatments that may affect their anaesthetic or surgery, as well as what they should do about taking their regular proton pump inhibitor or antihypertensive medication on the morning of their surgery.

How much time they need to allow off work is important, as is what they might expect in terms of discomfort, nasal obstruction, secretions and how long their recovery period will be. The ability to travel or fly is of great importance to the patient, and when they can safely go on holiday. It is best to be cautious about the amount of time they will need off work as they can always return earlier if they recover quickly.

POSTOPERATIVE CARE

'Communication and interpersonal skills once again become of paramount importance.'[1]

'The technical act of an operation is seldom what gets surgeons into trouble. More likely sources of criticism are matters of judgement, working relationships with colleagues and most commonly communication.'[5]

It is very important to establish good postoperative pain control as the small subgroup that develops persistent neuropathic pain after surgery often gives a history of severe pain after surgery as though this has initiated some central firing of neuronal pathways.[6]

Advising the patient in the few minutes after a general anaesthetic provides immediate reassurance but many of the details are forgotten. Even if the patient nods in answer to any statement and answers appropriately at that time this information is rarely stored or retrieved by the patient. Although this early conversation can be very reassuring for the patient it is best done again several hours later to ensure that they have retained what has been said.

SOMATIZATION

Somatizing patients attribute their distressing symptoms to a physical illness that cannot be fully accounted for by organic disease. Often the distress caused by the symptoms is out of proportion when compared with that of someone with organic disease, and there may be symptoms of depression and anxiety. In prevalence studies approximately 25 per cent of patients attending an ENT surgeon have somatization. Typical symptoms include fullness in the head or ears, dizziness without vertigo, catarrh or a dry sore throat. There are often many recurrent symptoms that change in nature. It is common for these patients to seek many opinions. It is important to exclude any organic pathology that can present with these symptoms by doing a thorough examination and any relevant investigation. If the patient is thought be somatizing, it is important to then minimize the number of investigations, withdraw unnecessary treatment, address any psychological problems, and while fully acknowledging the patient's symptoms, they need unambiguous reassurance. If the patient's ability to function is impaired by their condition, it may be necessary to seek psychiatric help.

Some patients medicalize their symptoms and an explanation with clear reassurance may prevent a patient going down the path of unnecessary medical treatment or surgery.

PATIENTS' REACTIONS TO UNWANTED NEWS

It may be that a patient has come with a preconceived idea about the diagnosis or what can be achieved or that they are upset or anxious about a diagnosis. Patients react to these stressful situations in different ways. Some may be philosophical, some may become hostile, whereas others deny or do not appear to understand what has been said to them. Whatever their reaction, it is often worth allowing them time to express their anxieties and find out what they have been told means to them. Often a patient's concerns centre around the effect the diagnosis will have on their spouse or children, particularly if they are dependants. Any mention of malignancy often needs to be tempered with the news that no sudden catastrophic event is likely to happen in malignancy of the paranasal sinuses even if there is intracranial involvement. If a patient becomes abusive or aggressive it is unwise to repost with the same attitude. Repeating information with a nurse present and ideally one of the patient's relatives will often calm the situation.

PATIENTS VARY

People's symptomatic behaviour is most influenced by that of their mother and how she responded to illness. Family and ethnic culture can play a major role in patients' illness behaviour and the symptoms they describe. There are many factors that can influence illness behaviour such as the patient who is seeking legal redress after an injury or wrongdoing. They may dwell on their symptoms, if not exaggerate them, with the hope of monetary gain, but all too often this results in chronic symptoms. A slow resolution of the legal process is often associated with the patient's symptoms persisting. Someone who is keen to join friends on a holiday may well make a more rapid recovery as their plight is more readily forgotten. The sooner someone starts to function, the sooner they are likely to recover as they are doing their own rehabilitation and become less medicalized by the process.

PATIENTS' VIEWS ABOUT THE ASSESSMENT OF SURGEONS

> 'In general, as patients we really have very little insight into the processes and procedures that our surgeons go through ... the trust is so inherent in the patient–doctor relationship that in many ways, it is taken for granted by patients that doctors are appropriately and regularly assessed.'[1]

However, Rajé and Bentley[1] go on to cite desirable qualities that include patient communication and interpersonal skills, empathy, to listen to patients, to respect patients' autonomy, be trustworthy and to act in the interest of our patients.

SHORTFALLS IN DOCTOR–PATIENT COMMUNICATION

It is not good when the doctor–patient relationship breaks down. This is unusual but not rare and it is important to recognize when this has happened. Under these circumstances, offering the patient a referral to another surgeon is a good option. Copying patients into any correspondence is often useful in the spirit of trying to communicate with the patient and be open. The worst example that this author has witnessed was when a surgeon had a complication and he moved the patient to a side room and never went to talk to the patient or their relatives and left their care to the junior staff. The patient was very annoyed and unhappy about this attitude. Patients often understand that surgery is not an exact science. However, an explanation and an effort to address the patient's current concerns and situation helps a great deal.

If a complaint arises, it is best to explore this openly with the patient and tell them what has happened, an apology, what to expect, and what is being done to minimize any sequelae.

REFERENCES

1. Rajé F, Bentley L. How patients want their surgeons assessed. *ENT News* 2009; **18**: 44–6.
2. Smith TL, Mendolina-Loffredo S, Loehrl TA *et al.* Predictive factors and outcomes in endoscopic sinus surgery for chronic rhinosinusitis. *Laryngoscope* 2005; **115**: 2199–205.
3. Litvack JR, Mace J, Smith TL. Does olfactory function improve after endoscopic sinus surgery? *Otolaryngol Head Neck Surg* 2009; **140**: 312–19.
4. Litvack JR, Fong K, Mace J *et al.* Predictors of olfactory dysfunction in patients with chronic rhinosinuitis. *Laryngoscope* 2008; **118**: 2225–30.
5. Rowley D. The surgeon's job: how should we assess the trainee? *J R Soc Med* 2004; **97**: 363–5.
6. Khan O, Majumdar S, Jones NS. Facial pain after sinus surgery and facial trauma. *Clin Otolaryngol* 2002; **27**: 171–4.

20

Case studies

CASE STUDY 20.1: ANTERIOR CLINOID MUCOCOELE

Presented by Dharmbir S Sethi

A 50-year-old Chinese man with no past medical history presented to the emergency department with a 2-day history of pain in the left eye. The pain was of sudden onset and associated with chemosis of the affected eye. There was no associated headache, vomiting, fever or any nasal symptoms.

Physical examination revealed mild proptosis of the left eye and there was diplopia in all directions of gaze due to third, fourth and sixth cranial nerve palsy. Pupils were equal in size and responded well to light stimulus. Visual acuity and examination of the fundus were normal. The next day the patient developed severe periorbital pain, diminished light reflex and an abnormal optic disc.

Computed tomography (CT) showed a destructive soft tissue lesion, whose epicentre was at the clinoid process, creating pressure on the left optic nerve and mild protrusion into the left sphenoid sinus (Fig. 20.1.1). Magnetic resonance imaging (MRI) revealed a lobulated mass located between the optic nerve and carotid artery with elevated signal intensity on T1- and T2-weighted imaging, suggestive of mucocoele (Figs 20.1.2 and 20.1.3).

The patient subsequently underwent emergency endoscopic drainage of the mucocoele under image guidance. Wide bilateral sphenoidotomy was performed to gain wide access to the lesion. The left optico-carotid recess was blocked by a soft tissue mass that was covered by erythematous mucosa. The location of the lesion was confirmed with an intraoperative image-guided system (Fig. 20.1.4). The mucosa overlying the lesion was peeled

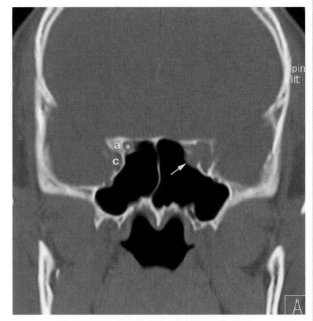

Figure 20.1.1 Coronal computed tomography (CT) scan of the patient showing an expansile lesion at the left anterior clinoid process. The arrow points to the mucosal bulge at the optico-carotid recess. Note the optic nerve (asterisk), carotid artery (c) and the anterior clinoid process (a) on the right side.

off and the capsule was exposed. A sharp number 11 blade was used to carefully incise the capsule. Thick mucoid secretions were encountered and drained. The mucocoele cavity opening was bounded superiorly by the optic nerve and inferiorly by the cavernous carotid artery (Fig. 20.1.5). The cavity was then inspected with a 30° endoscope and showed no connection to the intracranial cavity. The

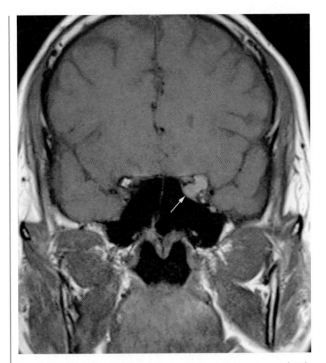

Figure 20.1.2   T1-weighted coronal magnetic resonance (MR) image with contrast showing the mucocoele at the anterior clinoid process (arrow).

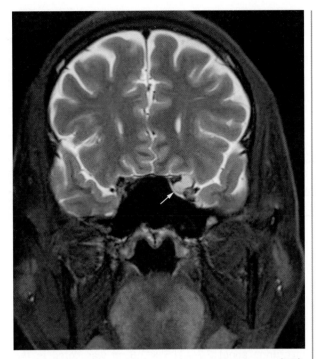

Figure 20.1.3   T2-weighted coronal magnetic resonance (MR) image showing the mucocoele at the anterior clinoid process (arrow).

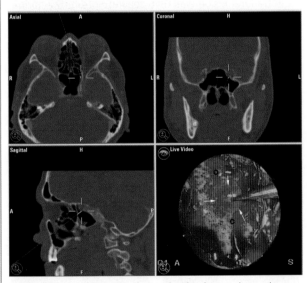

Figure 20.1.4   Intraoperative navigation image shows the probe on the mucosal surface of the mucocoele. The arrows show the mucosal boundaries of the mucocoele located between the optic nerve (o) and the carotid artery (c).

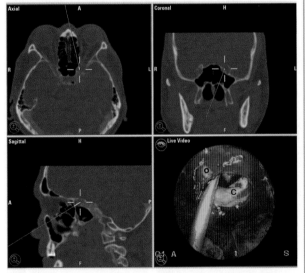

Figure 20.1.5   Intraoperative navigation image shows the probe in the cavity of the mucocoele. The mucocoele was drained by making an incision on the mucosal bulge between the optic nerve (o) and the carotid artery (c).

immediate postoperative course was uneventful. Both the orbital pain and diplopia reduced in the immediate postoperative period.

Mucocoeles of the anterior clinoid process are extremely rare and to our knowledge none has been reported in the otolaryngology literature.

CASE STUDY 20.2: AN UNUSUAL FINDING WITH BILATERAL ENCEPHALOCOELES

Presented by Dharmbir S Sethi

A 51-year-old man had been treated recently for meningitis in his home country. The patient was in coma for 5 days but recovered completely. He then presented at our institution for further management. He had undergone bilateral endoscopic sinus surgery 8 years earlier but was unable to provide details of the procedure and any postoperative events. The patient also reported intermittent episodes of clear rhinorrhoea during recent years. No investigation has been done to establish cerebrospinal fluid (CSF) leak diagnosis.

We undertook a nasal endoscopic examination, which showed large encephalocoeles bilaterally. A CT scan of the paranasal sinuses showed bilateral large skull base defects in the ethmoid roof with encephalocoeles (Fig. 20.2.1). An MRI evaluation confirmed the presence of the bilateral encephalocoeles. In addition, another lesion measuring about 2.5 × 1.5 × 1.6 cm was noted in the floor of the anterior cranial fossa extending to the lateral ventricle (Fig. 20.2.2). While the diagnosis of iatrogenic skull base defects with resultant encephalocoeles was clear, the radiological opinion on the intra-axial lesion was divided with the likelihood of this being an abscess. A neurosurgical opinion was obtained. In view of the intra-axial lesion, a craniotomy to approach the lesion and repair the skull base defects was advocated.

An external subfrontal approach was chosen for skull base exploration and repair. A bicoronal skin incision was made and a galeal flap created preserving the pericranium. A pericranial flap was then elevated separately exposing the frontal bone. A wide frontal sinusotomy was performed

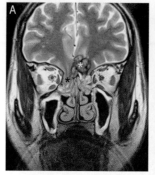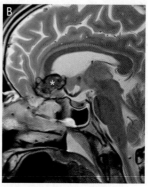

Figure 20.2.2   (A) T2-weighted sequence coronal magnetic resonance (MR) image showing the encephalocoele (black asterisk) and the intracranial lesion (white asterisk). The lesion shows areas of heterogeneous enhancement that is both hyperintense and hypointense. (B) T2-weighted sequence sagittal MR image showing the intracranial lesion (asterisk).

with suturing and division of the superior sagittal sinus. A dural window was then created and the frontal lobe was retracted. The bilateral skull base defect was identified and the herniating non-functioning brain tissue was resected. The intradural lesion was then separated from the normal brain tissue and resected. Inspection of the lesion core contents showed gauze fibres and extensive gliosis (Fig. 20.2.3). Skull base reconstruction was done using a free temporalis muscle–fascia graft inserted into the skull base defect and covered by vascularized pericranial flap. Postoperatively the patient was advised bed rest and intravenous antibiotic therapy was administered. No postoperative lumbar drain was used. The postoperative course was uneventful.

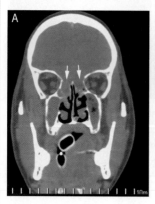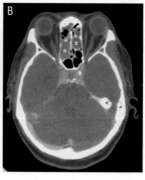

Figure 20.2.1   (A) Coronal computed tomography (CT) scan showing bilateral bony defects in the skull base (arrows). (B) Axial CT scan showing bilateral bony defects in the skull base (asterisks).

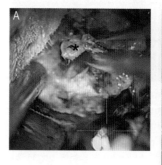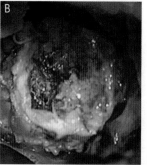

Figure 20.2.3   (A) Intraoperative view of the intracranial lesion incised open. Linen fibres are being removed from the encapsulated mass. (B) The mass lesion has been opened to reveal a retained piece of gauze, which has been removed.

CASE STUDY 20.3: ALLERGIC FUNGAL RHINOSINUSITIS AND POLYPOSIS

Presented by Nicholas Jones

A 46-year-old man from the Middle East presented with an 18-month history of marked bilateral nasal obstruction and a loss of sense of smell. He had discoloured nasal discharge that was sometimes yellow, sometimes green. He had sneezing bouts more than four times a day throughout the year. His primary care physician had prescribed two courses of broad-spectrum oral antibiotics (including against anaerobes) to no avail. He had a 5-year history of mild asthma but without any sensitivity to aspirin or non-steroidal anti-inflammatory drugs.

On inspection he had large bilateral pale, painless, mobile nasal polyps covered with light yellow mucopus. He had no diplopia, proptosis or epiphora. Skin prick tests showed him to be weakly positive to grass pollen and very positive to *Aspergillus*. A CT scan (Fig. 20.3.1) showed opacification of his paranasal sinuses with various densities within the sinuses along with some erosion of the anterior skull base and medial wall of the orbit.

A diagnosis of allergic aspergillosis was made. Although there was erosion of the skull base and medial wall of the orbit, this history and appearance was not indicative of chronic invasive aspergillosis as there was evidence of allergy to *Aspergillus* and the skin prick test was supported by specific IgE titres or raised titres of *Aspergillus precipitans* if there was any doubt. The erosion was due to tissue expansion and not invasion.

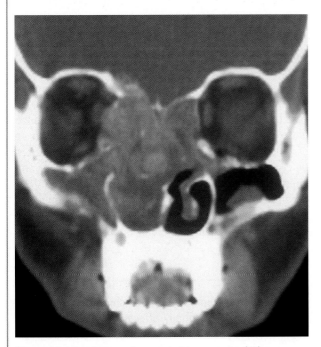

Figure 20.3.1 A coronal computed tomography (CT) scan showing opacification of the majority of the paranasal sinuses whose contents show varying densities. There is expansion into the orbit and anterior skull base with erosion of bone.

His liver function was tested and found to be normal before oral itraconazole was started 100 mg twice daily for 6 weeks prior to surgery. His liver function was tested every 4 weeks. (Although it is common for itraconazole to produce a small increase in liver function test levels, it should be stopped on the rare occasion when there is a moderate rise in liver function tests as occasionally it can induce a hepatitis. Itraconazole should be avoided if there is a history of liver disease or cardiac disease or if the patient is taking calcium channel blockers.)

In such patients, prednisolone (40 mg for an 80 kg man, 30 mg for a 60 kg woman) is also prescribed for 5 days prior to the surgery, to be taken with breakfast. This further reduces any oedema and inflammation of the nasal lining of the nose and makes surgery less bloody. At surgery the appearance almost resembles an 'auto fronto-sphenoethmoidectomy' as itraconazole usually eradicates most of the infection and the oral steroids will have reduced much of the oedema in the lining of the nose. Within the sinuses there may be some residual green-brown debris, which is removed when the partitions that divide the sinuses are removed wherever this is possible. The secretions are sent for fungal and bacterial culture and the polyps for histological examination, mentioning the possibility of a fungal infection. Little surgery is required other than to remove the lamellae separating the sinuses. After the fronto-sphenoethmoidectomy has been completed the cavity is lined with oxidized cellulose for haemostasis and to enhance the chance of the patient being discharged the same day. Patients in our unit are discharged on the same day as the surgery as long as there is a carer with them, they have a telephone and transport, and there are no medical contraindications. Postoperatively, patients are advised to douche their nose at least three times a day and they are prescribed betamethasone nose drops, two drops to each nostril in the 'nostril up position'. We have found that a 6-week postoperative course of itraconazole with liver function tests done every 4 weeks reduces the recurrence rate. Patients should be warned that allergic aspergillosis often recurs. They should also be reminded of the importance of compliance in taking postoperative topical nasal steroids in order to reduce the recurrence rate.

The present patient has remained disease-free for more than 8 years.

Recommended reading

1. Bent JP, Kuhn FA. The diagnosis of allergic fungal sinusitis. *Otolaryngol Head Neck Surg* 1994; **111**: 580–8.
2. Daudia A, Jones NS. Advances in the management of aspergillus of the paranasal sinuses. *J Laryngol Otol* 2008; **122**: 331–5.
3. DeShazo RD, O'Brien M, Chapin K *et al.* Criteria for diagnosis of sinus mycetoma. *J Allergy Clin Immunol* 1997; **99**: 475–85.

4. DeShazo RD, Swain RE. Diagnostic criteria for allergic fungal sinusitis. *J Allergy Clin Immunol* 1995; **96**: 24–35.
5. Kuhn FA, Javer AR. Allergic fungal rhinosinusitis. Perioperative management, prevention of recurrence, and role of steroids and antifungal agents. *Otolaryngol Clin North Am* 2000; **33**: 419–32.

CASE STUDY 20.4: FACIAL PAIN AND DIPLOPIA

Presented by Nicholas Jones

A 35-year-old woman presented with progressive left-sided facial pain in the distribution of the maxillary nerve. She had ophthalmoplegia looking medially with her left eye (Figs 20.4.1 and 20.4.2) but no diplopia reading or looking in other directions. She had not been feeling well for the last few weeks and felt as though she had a prolonged upper respiratory tract infection. She was referred to a neurologist who arranged for CT and MRI. These were presented at an interdisciplinary skull base meeting. The MR image showed some minimal changes of the meninges on the left around the cavernous sinus and near the foramen rotundum. The CT scan was reported as showing that there had been a middle meatal sinusotomy (Fig. 20.4.3). The neurologists were uncertain of the cause.

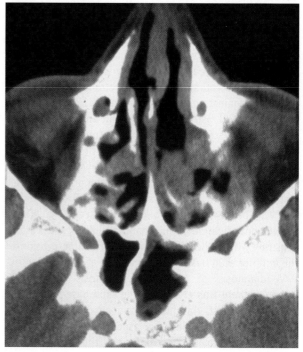

Figure 20.4.3   An axial computed tomography (CT) scan of the sinuses showing bony erosion of the medial wall of the left maxillary sinus. The patient had not had any surgery.

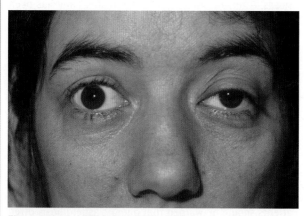

Figure 20.4.1   Mild ptosis of the left eye.

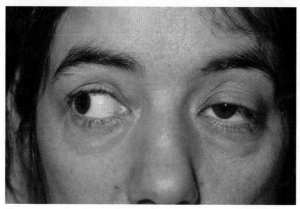

Figure 20.4.2   Ophthalmoplegia of the left eye looking medially.

On further enquiry it was noted that the patient had not had any sinus surgery. Examination of her nose revealed an inflamed lining covered by slimy mucus (Fig. 20.4.4). The full blood picture was normal, C-reactive protein was raised and c-antineutrophil cytoplasmic antibody titre (c-ANCA) was also normal. A nasal biopsy was done under local anaesthesia and a diagnosis of Wegener's granulomatosis was made. She was immediately started on cyclophosphamide and high doses of prednisolone and improved. Her renal function was preserved. Her c-ANCA became positive 3 weeks later. She required maintenance treatment for 4 years, having one relapse during this period, and has remained well for the past 10 years.

Comments

Wegener's granulomatosis is a chronic multisystem vasculitis that preferentially affects the respiratory tract and kidneys but can occur in any organ system. Diagnosis is usually based on clinical features, typical pathological features and the presence of circulating cytoplasmic autoantibodies to neutrophil cytoplasmic antigens (c-ANCA). The classic triad of pathological features is:[1]

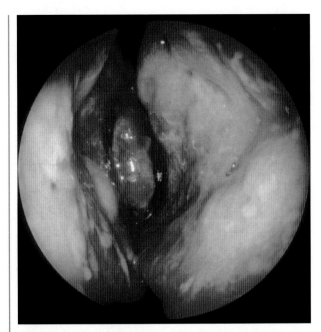

Figure 20.4.4   Endonasal view of the right nasal airway showing an inflamed lining with stagnant mucoid material indicating that the cilia were not functioning.

- vasculitis of small arteries and veins
- giant cells
- epithelioid cell granulomas.

It is unusual for all these features to be seen in every biopsy in Wegener's granulomatosis even when there is florid involvement of the nose. Nasal biopsy shows classic (all three) features in only 10 per cent of patients. A negative biopsy is by no way indicative that the disease is not present.

Serum c-ANCA is said to have a 92 per cent sensitivity and 96 per cent specificity for the disease.[2] c-ANCA is a useful test at presentation for diagnosis, but again a negative result does not rule out the disease.

Without treatment Wagener's granulomatosis is a progressive disease that ultimately leads to organ failure and can be fatal. Relapse correlates poorly with c-ANCA level and there is limited evidence as to how relapse is best predicted. Pulmonary and renal disease is seen at presentation in about a third of patients. The most important factors in making a diagnosis are the clinical features and/or a positive c-ANCA and/or a biopsy of affected tissue, whether renal, nasal mucosa, sclera or skin. Occasionally patients can present with a negative c-ANCA and nasal biopsy but become c-ANCA positive later as in the present patient, so where there is clinical suspicion it is worth repeating these.

Low relapse rates are achieved with prompt and rigorous initial immunosuppression even in limited disease. This produces less progression to multisystem disease and hence a lower mortality rate. The higher mortality seen in some series may be the result of less rigorous immunosuppression resulting in an increased incidence of renal disease.[3,4]

References

1. Rasmussen N, Petersen H, Andersen V. Histopathological findings in biopsies from patients with Wegener's granulomatosis. *APMIS Suppl* 1990; **19**: 15–16.
2. Bajema IM, Hagen EC, van der Woude FJ *et al*. Wegener's granulomatosis: a meta-analysis of 349 case reports. *J Lab Clin Med* 1997; **129**: 17–22.
3. Takwoingi YM, Dempster JH. Wegener's granulomatosis: an analysis of 33 patients seen over a 10 year period. *Clin Otolaryngol* 2003; **28**: 187–94.
4. Sproson E, Lanyon P, Al-Deiri *et al*. Lessons learnt in the management of Wegener's granulomatosis: Long-term follow-up of 60 patients. *Rhinology* 2007; **45**: 63–7.

CASE STUDY 20.5: FRONTAL SINUS OSTEOMA

Presented by Nicholas Jones

A 70-year-old retired soldier presented to his general physician with a year-long history of what he described as sinusitis. A CT scan was ordered and this showed an osteoma of the frontal sinuses (Fig. 20.5.1). He was referred to an otolaryngologist who elected to remove the osteoma via an external approach using coronal incision and an osteoplastic flap. During the procedure the surgeon inadvertently traversed the posterior wall of the frontal sinus entering the sagittal venous sinus, causing massive bleeding. This was stopped with a combination of oxidized cellulose and bone wax and the osteoma

was removed. The patient had a persistent CSF leak postoperatively, which was confirmed by being positive on immunofixation of β2 transferrin. He then underwent another external procedure by this author to close the dural defect and stop the CSF leak, which was successful.

The patient's original symptoms of 'sinusitis' continued. This was not a surprise as a detailed history before the second procedure had revealed that the patient's main symptoms were of pressure across the forehead without any exacerbating or relieving factors. He had never had any other nasal symptoms (blockage, purulent secretions – just clear CSF, or an altered sense of smell). The patient had been made aware before he had his second procedure that these symptoms might not be helped by surgery as they had the characteristics of tension-type headache.

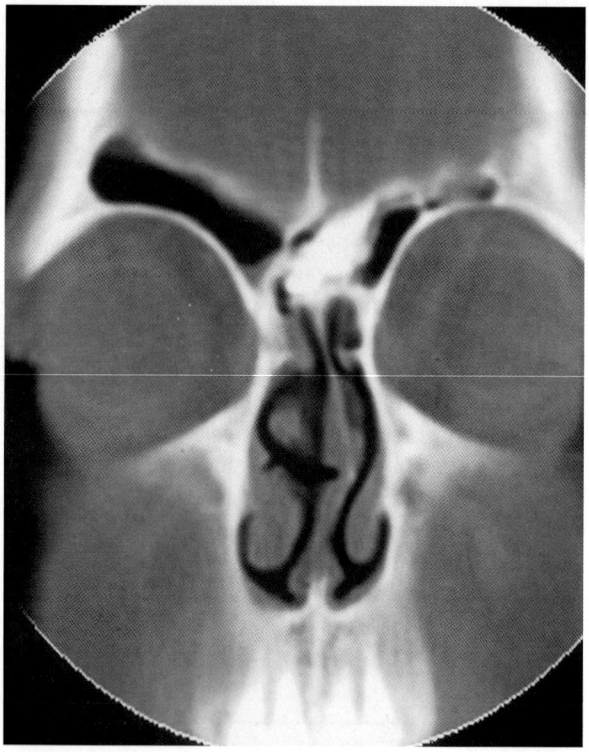

Figure 20.5.1   A coronal computed tomography (CT) scan of the left frontal sinus and a supraseptal cell. Note the sinuses are aerated and there are no mucosal changes.

Comments

Paranasal sinus osteomas are usually found as an incidental finding which occurs in approximately 1 in every 300 individuals. They rarely cause any symptoms unless they produce a cosmetic deformity; occasionally they can impair drainage of the frontal sinus and be associated with genuine sinusitis or a mucocoele. If there is genuine sinusitis, there are nasal symptoms of purulent discharge, obstruction, sometimes hyposmia and an increase in discomfort when there is an upper respiratory tract infection or an exacerbation of the infection when the drainage of the sinus is almost completely or completely blocked. There will usually be visible endoscopic changes.

The present patient was warned before their second procedure that the surgery might not help his symptoms of frontal discomfort and that he might need medical treatment if his symptoms persisted after closure of the CSF leak (note his osteoma had already been removed). About a third of patients with tension-type headache or midfacial segment pain have a reprieve from their symptoms should they inadvertently have surgery, but any reprieve is usually short lived. It appears that surgical trauma can temporarily reset the firing of neurones more centrally, probably in the caudal nucleus of the trigeminal nerve. However, such patients' symptoms almost always return as they did in the present patient.

Case study continued

A diagnosis of tension-type headache was made and the patient responded to low-dose amitriptyline (10 mg) after 6 weeks. His symptoms required the dose to be increased to 20 mg for them to be completely controlled and this was continued for a further 6 months. Following this, amitriptyline was stopped. His symptoms did not return and he has been pain-free for several years.

Further comments

The motto of this case study is: osteomas rarely cause facial pain. Most facial pain without any nasal symptoms is not due to sinusitis. Many patients incorrectly label themselves as having sinusitis. Osteomas are found incidentally when people are having scans for other reasons – beware of symptoms that are attributed to them! The problem occurs when a CT scan is done for symptoms such as headache or facial pain and an osteoma is found. It is easy to attribute the pain to the osteoma but it is not the cause.

CASE STUDY 20.6: PENETRATING INJURY OF THE ANTERIOR SKULL BASE

Presented by Nicholas Jones

A 30-year-old schizophrenic man attempted to commit suicide by inserting a ballpoint pen up each nostril and then ramming his head on a tabletop to force these up his nose and into his brain. Having found that this did not kill him he managed to pull out one pen. On pulling out the other, the pen broke half way leaving one part impacted in the man's brain (Fig. 20.6.1). He had clear rhinorrhoea from the side from which he had removed the pen and a clean punched-out hole in the roof of the nose in the area of the cribriform plate could be seen at rigid endoscopy. He was conscious when he was admitted and was assessed by the on-call psychiatric team.

Following rigid nasal endoscopy and a CT scan, an MR angiogram was done to check the proximity of the pen to any major vessel before an attempt was made to remove it. The concern was that the pen might tamponade a punctured vessel. The pen was found to be near an intracerebral vessel but not to have damaged it (Fig. 20.6.2). The pen was removed although it was firmly wedged in and through the anterior skull base. The plastic of the pen had already cracked and fragmented and it was removed in pieces and then put together to try to ensure that no fragment had been left *in situ*. The defect in the skull base was then

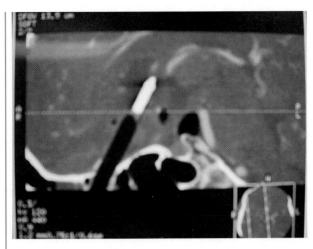

Figure 20.6.1   A sagittal computed tomography (CT) scan showing the end of a ball point pen that had penetrated the anterior cranial fossa.

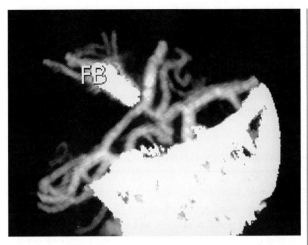

Figure 20.6.2   A magnetic resonance angiogram showing the proximity of the ball point pen (FB) to an intracranial vessel, although the vessel was not damaged.

defined endoscopically and its mucosal edges freshened. The defect was repaired with bone from a radical inferior turbinectomy, its mucosa having been dissected off it. The bone was wedged in the two defects on either side and the mucosa from the turbinate was placed over the bone grafts on each side. No attempt

was made to underlay the free mucosal graft. Oxidized cellulose was placed over the mucosa to support it. The patient was recovered 30° head up for 24 hours and given a 10-day prophylactic course of co-amoxiclav. He made an uneventful recovery and his schizophrenia has since been under better control.

CASE STUDY 20.7: PERIORBITAL INFECTION

Presented by Nicholas Jones

A 10-year-old boy presented after an upper respiratory tract infection with a left periorbital swelling (Fig. 20.7.1) and discomfort. He also could not open his eye and had moderate proptosis. One doctor commented that they thought that most of the swelling looked to be in the upper eyelid.

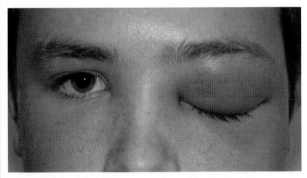

Figure 20.7.1   Left periorbital swelling consistent with periorbital cellulitis, and also consistent with periorbital abscess.

The key question that needed to be answered was whether he had a collection of subperiosteal pus in the

posterior compartment of his eye that threatened his vision. It was so painful that it was not possible to lift his eyelid and test his vision, in part because of his protective blepharospasm, which prevented this from being done. An ophthalmologist was also unable to check either his vision or the afferent reflexes of that eye.

Comments

Symptoms and signs at presentation often make it difficult to distinguish pre-septal from post-septal infection and this can result in inappropriate investigation and management, for example the overuse of CT or failure to recognize a periorbital abscess. To prevent the mismanagement of such cases and the development of such complications, interdisciplinary guidelines of how to manage such cases have been published.[1] These provide guidance on the criteria for admission of such patients and emphasize the importance of joint care between ENT, paediatrics and ophthalmology, the appropriate investigations to be performed (including which patients warrant CT), recommended antibiotic therapy and when there is a need for surgical intervention (see below).

The rise in retro-orbital pressure is akin to that which occurs in retro-orbital haemorrhage although the latter is of a more acute onset. Because the increase in pressure in the posterior compartment is less abrupt with a periorbital abscess, twice daily monitoring of visual acuity, colour vision and eye movement is thought to be sufficient, as there are no reports of an irreversible loss of vision that has occurred in a shorter period that has not been reversed by decompression. A paper by Slavin et al.[2] exemplifies cases of irreversible visual loss over a period, without regular monitoring, of 1 day or more.

Case study continued

Because it was not possible to test this boy's vision or his afferent pupil reflex an urgent CT scan was done. This showed a periorbital abscess and the boy was transferred to the operating theatre where this was drained via an external approach. He made an uneventful recovery and a scar was barely, if at all, discernible 1 year later.

Guidelines for the management of periorbital cellulitis/abscess[1]

Indications for admission:

- majority of patients with periorbital swelling
- proptosis
- diplopia or ophthalmoplegia
- reduced visual acuity
- reduced light reflexes or abnormal swinging light test
- for those in whom a full eye examination is not possible
- toxic or systemically unwell patients
- central nervous signs or symptoms.

Indications for CT scanning:

- central signs
- inability to accurately assess vision
- gross proptosis, ophthalmoplegia, deteriorating visual acuity or colour vision, bilateral oedema
- no improvement or deterioration at 24 hours
- swinging pyrexia not resolving within 36 hours.

Treatment plan:

- intravenous access, blood for full blood count, urea and electrolytes, blood culture
- cefuroxime (100 mg/kg/day in three doses) and metronidazole (7.5 mg/kg three times daily, maximum 400 mg)
- nasal ephedrine 0.5 per cent nose drops three times daily in a head back, nostril up position

- adequate analgesia
- arrange ophthalmic, ENT and paediatric opinions.

Twice-daily assessment of colour vision, acuity, eye movement and pupil reflexes is performed. If gross proptosis, ophthalmoplegia or concern, hourly assessment is indicated.

Controversy

That this boy had an external approach and not an endoscopic approach in a text that describes many of the advances that have occurred in endoscopic sinus surgery may seem surprising. It is *possible* to drain most periorbital abscesses endoscopically, unless there is a large lateral component that occasionally occurs. This was not the case in this boy. The reason that an external approach was favoured is that in an acutely infected situation the mucosa bleeds a lot and this can make visibility difficult. The other problem is that a moderate amount of the lamina papyracea has to be removed in order to ensure adequate drainage of the abscess. This has the potential for the orbital contents to prolapse medially, even though it is imperative to maintain the periorbital tissue, otherwise orbital fat will flow into the area. The combination of bleeding, poor visibility, the periorbital tissue coming medially where the lamina papyracea was, are all a recipe for narrowing the frontal recess. Episodes of periorbital infection are usually 'one-off' for the individual and are not associated with recurrent acute infection or chronic infective sinusitis except in rare cases of immunodeficiency. Maintaining the integrity of the frontal recess is therefore important. For this reason an external approach is often best. The incision should be in the upper third of the side of the nose and it should be broken (e.g. the shape of the silhouette of a seagull) in order to minimize any chance of the scar webbing. The scar is often slightly red for 9 months but after that it gradually fades so that it can barely be seen, except by the observant rhinologist!

References

1. Howe L, Jones NS. Guidelines for the management of periorbital cellulitis/abscess. *Clin Otolaryngol* 2004; **29**: 725–8.
2. Slavin M, Glaser JS. Acute severe irreversible visual loss with sphenoethmoiditis –'posterior' orbital cellulitis. *Arch Ophthalmol* 1987; **105**: 345–8.

CASE STUDY 20.8: UNRESPONSIVE BILATERAL PURULENT RHINOSINUSITIS

Presented by Nicholas Jones

A 33-year-old mother presented to her primary care physician with an unusual history. This comprised bilateral nasal obstruction, hyposmia and a persistent mucky nasal discharge all day long that had been present for several weeks. (It is relatively unusual for someone to have a mucky nasal discharge that means the patient can blow discoloured mucus into a tissue all day long. It is not uncommon for someone to report a mucky collection of mucus in the morning that is often due to mucus stagnating in the postnasal area in a snorer or mouth breather. The latter does *not* indicate that the patient has an infective rhinosinusitis but may just have mucus stagnating in their naso- or oropharynx while they are snoring overnight that has become discoloured by the commensals that are present.) The patient failed to respond to a 2-week course of a broad spectrum antibiotic and metronidazole (the prevalence of anaerobes in chronic infective rhinosinusitis is high and this is often the right choice of antibiotic spectrum in chronic bacterial rhinosinusitis).

Endoscopy revealed bilateral purulent nasal secretions (see Fig. 20.8.1).

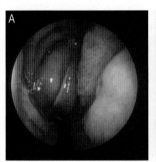 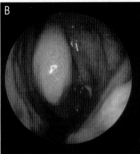

Figure 20.8.1   Endoscopic view showing a purulent nasal discharge: (A) left nasal airway. (B) right nasal airway.

Comment

Persistent or recurrent ear or sinus infections, not responding to antibiotics as would usually happen, or which are associated with unusual or opportunistic infections, should alert the doctor to a possible underlying immunodeficiency.[1]

The majority of patients with a primary immunodeficiency will have a history of recurrent ENT infections.[2] Although primary immunodeficiency is uncommon it needs to be considered in all patients with recurrent infections. An audit showed that a large proportion of UK patients with antibody deficiency had been seen in ENT outpatients without the underlying diagnosis being made.[3] The same report found that the average delay from onset of recognizable symptoms of antibody deficiency to diagnosis was 6.26 years. Early diagnosis of these syndromes is imperative to treat them to prevent irreversible organ damage. This includes the following issues.

- These patients need appropriate antibiotics in maximum dosages for at least 14 days.
- Counselling of patients is necessary, both in explaining current symptoms and in planning future management. Genetic counselling is also required for certain immunodeficiency diagnoses.
- Immunoglobulin replacement therapy should be available for antibody deficiency.
- There is an increased incidence of malignancy and autoimmune diseases in patients with immunodeficiency diseases.

It is important to remember that primary immune deficiencies, especially antibody deficiencies, can present at any age. The incidence of common variable immunodeficiency has two peaks, one in the first 5 years of life and the second in the second decade, but it should still be considered in the elderly.

Antibody deficiencies are the commonest primary immunodeficiency, and are also the most likely to present with recurrent ENT infections.[4] Primary defects of cell-mediated immunity, neutrophil function or complement activity are relatively rare, and although ENT infections may occur in these diseases, they are more likely to present with features outside the upper respiratory tract.

Investigation of patients with recurrent otorhinolaryngological infection

Specific recommendations have been made regarding the investigations that can be used to help exclude immunodeficiency as a contributing factor in the patient with recurrent otolaryngological infections.

First-line investigations:

- microbial samples for cultures
- full blood count, with differential white cell count
- immunoglobulins: IgG, IgA, IgM
- vaccine-specific IgG: tetanus, *Haemophilus influenzae* type b (Hib), pneumococcus
- urea and electrolytes, liver function tests, fasting plasma glucose
- human immunodeficiency virus (HIV) test.

Second-line investigations:

- nitroblue-tetrazolium reduction (NBT) test
- IgG subclasses
- functional complement assays
- tests of cell-mediated immunity.

Who should be investigated?

Ten warning signs for suspecting primary immunodeficiency have been suggested and ENT infections feature prominently among these (from the Jeffry Modell Foundation)[5]:

- eight or more new ear infections within 1 year
- two or more serious sinus infections within 1 year
- two or more months on antibiotics with little effect
- two or more pneumonias within 1 year
- failure of an infant to gain weight or grow normally
- recurrent deep skin or organ abscesses
- persistent thrush in the mouth or elsewhere on skin after age 1
- need for intravenous antibiotics to clear infections
- two or more deep-seated infections
- a family history of primary immunodeficiency.

A history should specifically enquire about recurrent lower respiratory or urinary tract infections, recurrent candidal infections, infections with unusual organisms, chronic diarrhoea, or (in infants) failure to thrive. Risk factors for HIV infection and a drug history including the use of steroids and second-line antirheumatic drugs should be sought. A detailed family history should be elicited, as many of the primary immunodeficiency disorders are hereditary (e.g. X-linked agammaglobulinaemia) or familial (e.g. common variable immune deficiency).

First-line investigations

CULTURE

It is important to obtain samples for bacterial, fungal and viral cultures, both to identify unusual organisms and to guide treatment according to sensitivities. Recurrent infections with common organisms can suggest immunodeficiency; for instance recurrent pneumococcal infections can result from specific defects in antibody production against polysaccharide antigens. Invasive *Aspergillus* infection may suggest a neutrophil or T cell defect.

FULL BLOOD COUNT, WITH DIFFERENTIAL WHITE CELL COUNT

It is essential that the differential white cell count is examined closely looking for the following features that can predispose to infection. Neutropenia is not uncommon and if persistent may contribute to infection. The lymphocyte count is normal in many immunodeficiencies, but can be reduced in HIV infection and certain rare primary syndromes, such as severe combined immune deficiency. Thrombocytopenia may be associated with immunodeficiency, and eosinophilia may suggest atopy or a vasculitis as a contributing factor to recurrent infection. It is important that the 'normal values' used as reference ranges are age-specific for the patient; remember that the normal lymphocyte count in an infant should be almost double that of an adult.

IMMUNOGLOBULIN LEVELS

Reduced immunoglobulin levels (IgG, IgA or IgM) characterize the majority of primary antibody deficiencies. Selective IgA deficiency is surprisingly common, occurring in approximately 1 in 500 Caucasians.[6,7] Patients with common variable immunodeficiency will usually have low levels of IgG and IgA, and often have recurrent pyogenic upper respiratory tract infections related to *Pneumococcus*, *Streptococcus* and *Haemophilus*.[8,9]

Increased immunoglobulin levels do not exclude immunodeficiency as increased IgG levels are frequently seen with HIV infection and in neutrophil defects such as chronic granulomatous disease.

IgG VACCINE RESPONSES (SPECIFIC IgG)

The generation of antibodies to specific antigens demonstrates an intact humoral immune system. Antibodies to commonly available vaccines such as Hib, pneumococcus and tetanus toxoid are measured. If specific antibody levels are low, the patient should be vaccinated and blood taken for specific IgG in 3–4 weeks. An adequate response to all three vaccines excludes a significant humoral immunodeficiency. An abnormal response needs to be discussed with an immunologist. No live vaccine (e.g. measles, rubella, mumps, Sabin polio) should be given when immunodeficiency is suspected.

HIV TEST – THINK OF IT!

Before embarking on other investigations for immune deficiency, the possibility of HIV infection should be critically evaluated. The decision to test for HIV in a patient with recurrent otorhinological infections should be prompted by a history of risk factors for HIV or infections with fungi such as *Candida* or *Aspergillus* or the herpes viruses. If such factors are present then all blood samples and biological materials should be labelled as high risk to avoid potential hazards to those handling these samples. Infections with unusual organisms such as *Pneumocystis* or *Toxoplasma* are virtually pathognomonic of a T lymphocyte defect. Remember that counselling and informed consent are required before taking blood for HIV testing.

Second-line immune function tests

If the above do not reveal a cause for the recurrent infections and the history is suggestive of immune deficiency then further investigations are required. It is advisable to involve an immunologist at this stage.

NBT TEST

This test detects chronic granulomatous disease, and in this condition the most common pathogen is *Staphylococcus aureus*, although *Aspergillus*, *Pseudomonas*, *Serratia* and *Klebsiella* infections are frequently seen.

IMMUNOGLOBULIN G SUBCLASSES

Assays for vaccine-specific IgG have largely superseded IgG subclass measurements. Transient IgG2 deficiency is common in childhood. Isolated IgG4 deficiency has not been found to be important. Patients with a clinically important IgG subclass deficiency will usually show defects in responses to immunization with pneumococcal or Hib vaccine. Essentially measurement of IgG subclasses is only useful if the total IgG is low. If total IgG is normal, an IgG subclass deficiency is unlikely to be important.

Patients with isolated IgG subclass deficiency are usually immunocompetent. An inadequate response to vaccination may be detected whether IgG subclasses are normal or abnormal. IgG subclass assay is therefore no longer considered to be an important test in defining antibody deficiency.

COMPLEMENT DEFICIENCIES

Deficiencies of various complement factors can cause recurrent infections with encapsulated organisms, typically meningococcus. These syndromes are rare and an assay for these factors is a low yield investigation. Should one be indicated on the basis of a positive family history or typical infections, functional assays that test all components in the classical and alternative pathways are required (e.g. CH50 and AP50).

TESTS OF CELL-MEDIATED IMMUNITY

In general, patients with primary defects of cell-mediated immunity (mostly severe combined immune deficiency or SCID) present with more severe infections than patients with antibody deficiencies only, and these individuals rarely survive beyond childhood without treatment. However, such defects are compatible with many months of apparently good health, and a clinical suspicion of SCID is regarded as a paediatric emergency. Affected infants typically present within the first few months of life with frequent episodes of diarrhoea, pneumonia, otitis media, sepsis and cutaneous infections. Persistent infection with organisms such as *Candida albicans*, *Pneumocystis carinii*, varicella, measles, cytomegalovirus and Epstein–Barr virus are common. Failure to thrive and a persistent rash are other important presenting features.

There are numerous tests for different aspects of cell-mediated immunity, both *in vitro* and *in vivo*. These include lymphocyte subset analysis, lymphocyte stimulation with antigens and mitogens, and delayed hypersensitivity skin tests. As disorders of cell-mediated immunity are relatively uncommon and the tests complex, urgent referral to an immunologist is recommended if this is suspected.

Non-immunological tests

CILIARY MOTILITY/STRUCTURE STUDIES

Primary ciliary dysmotility syndromes commonly have otorhinolaryngological infection as a prominent part of their history at diagnosis. Co-existent bronchiectasis, infertility in men and situs inversus are suggestive. The simple saccharin test is a useful screening test, but false-positive results may occur in the presence of infection.[10] Phase-contrast microscopy of a nasal brushing or electron microscopic examination of a nasal biopsy are more accurate.

SWEAT SODIUM CONCENTRATION

Cystic fibrosis is a possible but unlikely cause of isolated recurrent upper respiratory tract infections. A child with chronic sinusitis associated with intranasal polyposis should have cystic fibrosis excluded, as mild forms of the disease can occur. Sweat sodium concentration remains the standard investigation, but genetic testing for some alleles of cystic fibrosis is now available.

SERUM BIOCHEMISTRY

Diabetes, malnutrition, hepatic and renal failure, lymphoproliferative disorders, and therapy with certain drugs (e.g. steroids) or radiotherapy are relatively common causes of impaired immune function. Most of these will be evident from the history, but the addition of a basic biochemical profile is appropriate. Urea and electrolytes, liver function tests and fasting blood sugar levels are sufficient.

Clinical case continued

The patient had a normal white cell count. Mixed organisms including *Pneumococcus* were repeatedly cultured from pus coming out of the middle meatus. Titres for *Haemophilus*, pneumococcus and tetanus were unrecordable. Vaccination for *Haemophilus influenzae* type b (Hib), pneumococcus and tetanus toxoid produced no increase in antibody levels after 1 month. The patient was referred to an immunologist where further investigations revealed a severe immunodeficiency with a range of IgG subclasses thought to be secondary to a change in the antiepileptic medication that the patient had been prescribed. The patient remains well on immunoglobulin replacement therapy and they have not required surgery.

References

1. International Union of Immunological Societies. Primary immunodeficiency diseases. Report of an IUIS Scientific Committee. *Clin Exp Immunol* 1999; **118** Suppl 1: 1–28.

2. Polmar SH. The role of the immunologist in sinus disease. *J Allergy Clin Immunol* 1992; **90**: 511–14; discussion 514–15.
3. Spickett GP, Chapel HM. *Report on the audit of patients with primary antibody deficiency in the United Kingdom 1993–1996*. Newcastle upon Tyne Hospitals NHS Trust, 1998.
4. Buckley RH. Primary immunodeficiency diseases. In: Paul WE, ed. *Fundamental immunology*. Philadelphia: Lippincott-Raven, 1999.
5. Jeffry Modell Foundation (www.info4pi.org).
6. Schaffer FM, Monteiro RC, Volanakis JE *et al*. IgA deficiency. *Immunodefic Rev* 1991; **3**: 15–44.
7. Buckley RH. Clinical and immunologic features of selective IgA deficiency. *Birth Defects Orig Artic Ser* 1975; **11**: 134–42.
8. Primary immunodeficiency diseases. Report of a WHO scientific group. *Clin Exp Immunol* 1997; **109** Suppl 1: 1–28.
9. Cunningham-Rundles C. Clinical and immunologic analyses of 103 patients with common variable immunodeficiency. *J Clin Immunol* 1989; **9**: 22–33.
10. Lale AM, Mason JD, Jones NS. Mucociliary transport and its assessment: a review. *Clin Otolaryngol* 1998; **23**: 388–96.

CASE STUDY 20.9: *DE NOVO* FACIAL PAIN AFTER SURGERY

Presented by Nicholas Jones

A 53-year-old accountant had persistent right-sided purulent rhinosinusitis that failed to respond to repeated 2-week courses of antibiotics that covered a wide range of aerobic organisms including *Pneumococcus*, *Haemophilus*, staphylococci as well as anaerobes. His main symptoms were of nasal obstruction and a persistent purulent discharge throughout the day and he had no pain – it is common not to have pain in chronic infective sinusitis unless there is an acute exacerbation.[1] Pus aspirated from the middle meatus cultured mixed organisms which were sensitive to the antibiotics that had been prescribed. A screen of his immunity showed a normal white cell count and antibody titres to *Pneumococcus*, *Haemophilus* and tetanus. He had right endoscopic sinus surgery to open up his maxillary and ethmoid sinuses.

Five days after surgery he reattended with severe right-sided pain that affected the lateral side of his nose and periorbital area. At endoscopy he was noted to have bone exposed that was not covered with mucosa and it was not granulating (Fig. 20.9.1). He was apyrexial. He described his pain as being a very severe dull ache with a throbbing quality and he scored it 10 out of 10 for severity. His pain was not controlled with a combination of paracetamol, ibuprofen and codeine phosphate. He required moderate doses of morphine to partially control his pain. His pain failed to abate. Over the next few days his pain developed a gnawing and burning quality.

Comment

In cases of facial pain secondary to sinusitis, endoscopic sinus surgery has been shown to alleviate facial pain in approximately 75 per cent of cases.[2] However, patients with paranasal sinus disease can have incidental facial pain from other causes and it helps to raise this possibility

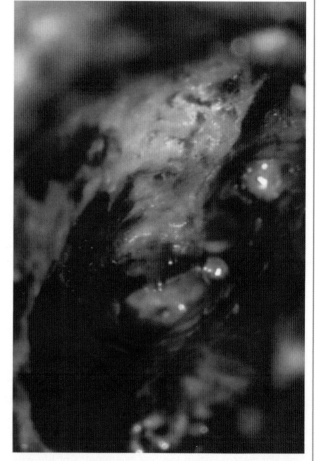

Figure 20.9.1 Endoscopic view of the right lateral nasal wall showing exposed white bone. These findings are in keeping with osteitis and this is analogous to the osteitis that occurs in a dry socket occurring after a difficult dental extraction.

preoperatively and counsel the patient that this may be the case.[3–6]

In a cohort of 136 patients who had endoscopic sinus surgery (ESS) done by the author, one patient with nasal polyposis and aspirin sensitivity went on to develop *de novo* pain after a thorough fronto-sphenoethmoidectomy in spite of no postoperative evidence of endoscopic disease and with patent ostia.[3] Little attention has been focused on postsurgical and post-traumatic facial pain. Indeed, there is no mention of traumatic or postsurgical pain in the current classification systems[7,8] although post-traumatic headache is recognized. Acquadro *et al.*[2] noted that in those patients with preoperative pain who underwent endoscopic sinus surgery, 7 per cent developed a new type of pain, and 2 per cent reported a worsening of their facial pain but none developed *de novo* pain if they had had no preoperative pain. Indeed to date, there have been few reported cases of facial pain following ESS in previously pain-free patients. This fact is particularly surprising given that open sinus surgery, in particular the Caldwell–Luc procedures, have long been known to cause *de novo* facial pain. One study noted this complication in 46 per cent of all patients who had undergone a Caldwell–Luc procedure,[9] including some patients who had no prior facial pain.

Trauma causes pain that is mediated by myelinated Aδ and unmyelinated C fibres. Prolonged stimulation of these can activate *N*-methyl-D-aspartate (NMDA) and cause central sensitization. An alteration in central processing can then lead to an alteration in pain thresholds producing hyperalgesia or even lead to spontaneous firing of neurones and may produce reverberating circuits. It is also possible that antidromic flow in C fibres can cause the release of substance P or that efferent sympathetic flow can release noradrenaline (norepinephrine); both these mechanisms have the potential to sensitize peripheral receptors.[10] Trauma can be an initiating factor in this process by either altering the fibres within the trigeminal nucleus or by altering its somatosensory input, thereby altering nociceptive fibres to or within the caudal nucleus of the trigeminal nerve. Altering the neuroplasticity of the nerves to and within the trigeminal nucleus can result in neuropathic pain. A peripheral injury or inflammation may induce neuroplastic changes in the trigeminal brainstem sensory nuclear complex and produce central sensitization.[11] An alteration in nerve function through neuroplasticity either peripherally or centrally may have contributed to pain in these patients.

The main treatment in most patients with post-traumatic facial pain without paranasal sinus disease is with neurological pharmacological agents. Gabapentin is a second-generation anticonvulsant that does not affect sodium channels of γ-aminobutyric acid (GABA) receptors and is the first-line treatment of choice closely followed by pregabalin. Amitriptyline has been shown to be effective in relieving traumatic neuralgia[12] in doses of 75 mg or more, and even in lower doses it works synergistically with gabapentin. Duloxetine may help if there is a moderate degree of patient anxiety. Problems with sleeping and depression also need to be addressed.

Local anaesthetic nerve blocks can break a cycle of persistent pain. Lidocaine patches may also provide some relief. Opioids are effective but need to be prescribed with caution because the patient may develop dependence. Transcutaneous electrical stimulation and acupuncture have also been advocated by some pain control physicians. The management of patients with pain unresponsive to medical treatment should involve pain coping strategies that involve a pain management team and psychologist.

In patients whose pain is initiated by trauma or surgery, the pain is likely to be neuropathic in origin, whether by a peripheral and/or central mechanism, and these patients often have a deep gnawing, burning unpleasant quality to their pain[3]. Less commonly patients complain of dysaesthesia, paroxysms of pain, shooting, staging or electric shocks.[13] The cardinal symptoms are spontaneous pain and an abnormal response to non-painful or painful stimuli.

Case study continued

A diagnosis of a local osteitis and neuropathic pain was made. The patient was started on gabapentin, which was built up to 600 mg three times a day. After 6 weeks it became possible to withdraw the morphine. The patient remained on gabapentin for 8 months before it was reduced and his pain has not recurred. (Note it is not necessary to have an osteitis to get neuropathic pain.)

References

1. Clifton N, Jones NS. The prevalence of facial pain in 108 consecutive patients with paranasal mucopurulent discharge at endoscopy. *J Laryngol Otol* 2007; **121**: 345–8.
2. Acquadro MA, Salman SD, Joseph MP. Analysis of pain and endoscopic sinus surgery for sinusitis. *Ann Otol Rhinol Laryngol* 1997; **106**: 305–9.
3. Khan OA, Majumdar S, Jones NS. Facial pain following sinonasal surgery or facial trauma. *Clin Otolaryngol* 2002; **27**: 171–4.
4. Tarabichi M. Characteristics of sinus-related pain. *Otolaryngol Head Neck Surg* 2000; **122**: 84–7.
5. Salman SD. Questions awaiting answers. *Curr Opin Otolaryngol Head Neck Surg* 1999; **7**: 1.
6. Ruoff GE. When sinus headache isn't sinus headache. *Headache Quarterly* 1997; **8**: 22–31.
7. Merskey H, Bogduk N, eds. *International Association for the Study of Pain. Classification of chronic pain.* Seattle: IAPS Press, 1994:59–95.
8. Headache Classification Committee of the International Headache Society. Classification and diagnostic criteria for headache disorders, cranial neuralgias and facial pain. *Cephalgia* 1988; **8** Suppl 7: 1–93.
9. Low WK. Complications of Caldwell-Luc operation and how to avoid them. *Aust NZ J Surg* 1995; **65**: 582–5.
10. Romer HC. Medical management of facial pain. *Hosp Med* 2001; **62**: 607–10.

11. Sessle BJ. Acute and chronic craniofacial pain: brainstem mechanisms of nocioceptive transmission and neuroplasticity, and other clinical correlates. *Crit Rev Oral Biol Med* 2000; **11**: 57–91.

12. Solberg WK, Graff-Radford SB. Orodental considerations of facial pain. *Semin Neurol* 1988; **8**: 318–23.

13. Freynhagen R, Bennett MI. Diagnosis and management of neuropathic pain. *BMJ* 2009; **339**: 391–5.

Index

Illustrations (figures and tables) are comprehensively referred to from the text. Therefore, significant material in them have only been given a page reference in the absence of their concommitant mention in the text referring to those illustrations.